Clinical Methods
A Key to Diagnosis in Paediatrics

Clinical Methods
A Key to Diagnosis in Paediatrics

Dilip Mukherjee
MD (Paed), DCH, PhD, FIAP, FAMS
Professor of Paediatrics
Ex-Dean, Vivekananda Institute of Medical Sciences
Ramakrishna Mission Seva Pratishthan
Kolkata-700 026, India

Indraneel Banerjee
MD (Paed), MRCPCh (UK)
Consultant Paediatric Endocrinologist
Department of Paediatric Endocrinology
Royal Manchester Children's Hospital (UK)

TM

JAYPEE BROTHERS MEDICAL PUBLISHERS (P) LTD

New Delhi • Ahmedabad • Bengaluru • Chennai
Hyderabad • Kochi • Kolkata • Lucknow • Mumbai • Nagpur

Published by

Jitendar P Vij
Jaypee Brothers Medical Publishers (P) Ltd
B-3, EMCA House, 23/23B Ansari Road, Daryaganj
New Delhi 110 002, India
Phones: +91-11-23272143, +91-11-23272703, +91-11-23282021, +91-11-23245672, Rel: +91-11-32558559
Fax: +91-11-23276490, +91-11-23245683 e-mail: jaypee@jaypeebrothers.com
Visit our website: www.jaypeebrothers.com

Branches

- 2/B, Akruti Society, Jodhpur Gam Road Satellite
  Ahmedabad 380 015 Phones: +91-79-26926233, Rel: +91-79-32988717, Fax: +91-79-26927094
  e-mail: ahmedabad@jaypeebrothers.com
- 202 Batavia Chambers, 8 Kumara Krupa Road, Kumara Park East
  Bengaluru 560 001 Phones: +91-80-22285971, +91-80-22382956, +91-80-22372664, Rel: +91-80-32714073
  Fax: +91-80-22281761 e-mail: bangalore@jaypeebrothers.com
- 282 IIIrd Floor, Khaleel Shirazi Estate, Fountain Plaza, Pantheon Road
  Chennai 600 008 Phones: +91-44-28193265, +91-44-28194897, Rel: +91-44-32972089
  Fax: +91-44-28193231 e-mail: chennai@jaypeebrothers.com
- 4-2-1067/1-3, 1st Floor, Balaji Building, Ramkote Cross Road
  Hyderabad 500 095 Phones: +91-40-66610020, +91-40-24758498, Rel:+91-40-32940929
  Fax:+91-40-24758499, e-mail: hyderabad@jaypeebrothers.com
- No. 41/3098, B & B1, Kuruvi Building, St. Vincent Road
  Kochi 682 018, Kerala Phone: +91-484-4036109, +91-484-2395739, +91-484-2395740
  e-mail: kochi@jaypeebrothers.com
- 1-A Indian Mirror Street, Wellington Square
  Kolkata 700 013 Phones: +91-33-22651926, +91-33-22276404, +91-33-22276415, Rel: +91-33-32901926
  Fax: +91-33-22656075, e-mail: kolkata@jaypeebrothers.com
- Lekhraj Market III, B-2, Sector-4, Faizabad Road, Indira Nagar
  Lucknow 226 016 Phones: +91-522-3040553, +91-522-3040554 e-mail: lucknow@jaypeebrothers.com
- 106 Amit Industrial Estate, 61 Dr SS Rao Road, Near MGM Hospital, Parel
  Mumbai 400012 Phones: +91-22-24124863, +91-22-24104532, Rel: +91-22-32926896
  Fax: +91-22-24160828, e-mail: mumbai@jaypeebrothers.com
- "KAMALPUSHPA" 38, Reshimbag, Opp. Mohota Science College, Umred Road
  Nagpur 440 009 (MS) Phone: Rel: +91-712-3245220, Fax: +91-712-2704275 e-mail: nagpur@jaypeebrothers.com

Clinical Methods—A Key to Diagnosis in Paediatrics

First Edition: **2008,** Reprint: 2024
ISBN 81-8448-193-4

Typeset at JPBMP typesetting unit
Printed in India

This book is dedicated to all who are involved in the care of the children and specially the residents and the postgraduate students in paediatrics

Foreword

Standard textbooks serve as reference material but are no substitutes for books that deal with practical aspects of clinical paediatrics. There are few books that focus on clinical approach to childhood diseases but this book titled *"Clinical Methods – A Key to Diagnosis in Paediatrics"* is unique in many ways.

Opening chapter emphasizes systematic approach to detailed history taking that nearly offers clue to probable diagnosis. Importance of each point in the history is analysed with probable interpretations. Physical examination follows in the next chapter that is aimed at sharpening clinical skills. Subsequent chapters deal with individual systems. Appropriate stress on anatomy is a special feature in the chapter on Neurology. Endocrinological and metabolic system is a welcome addition that universally lacks in most of the publications. Special mention must be made for inclusion of child behaviour and psychology that is often neglected though extremely relevant. Each chapter includes many tables that provide useful information.

Another unique feature of this book is the Appendices that include growth charts, body surface area chart, ECGs and radiological images. This adds significantly to the academic value of the book. The book also includes many clinical photographs that offer visual impressions of various conditions.

This book is authored by two experienced paediatricians — Dr. Dilip Mukherjee and Dr. Indraneel Banerjee who have very thoughtfully presented their ideas on clinical methods.

Never before such a complete book was published on clinical methods and I strongly recommend it to all the students and practitioners alike.

YK Amdekar MD, DCH
Former Professor of Paediatrics
Grant Medical College and J.J. Group of Hospitals
Mumbai
President of Indian Academy of Paediatrics 1995
Consultant Paediatrician Jaslok Hospital and Breach Candy Hospital
Mumbai

Preface

Clinical Paediatrics is a very challenging and interesting subject. Clinical medicine in adults has been more or less standardised but in children there are wide variations across ages and individuals which make it more complex. Further, we faced everyday with new knowledge of disease states and better understanding of pathology. We therefore need to constantly refine our clinical methods to account for this recent acquisition of information.

Our humble endeavour in this regard has been chiefly aimed at the postgraduate students and all those involved in the care of the child. It shall be our greatest reward if this book can be of any service to them.

A word of caution–clinical paediatrics is an eminently practical subject. The many cases you see, the variety you come across, the better will be your insight to diagnose and treat. However quality can never be compromised for quantity. Examine each case thoroughly, searching for all possibilities with an observant eye and trained ear. Do not take things for granted – your meticulous approach will be handsomely rewarded. This book is not meant to be armchair reading, rather it is for practice, discussion, comparison and criticism.

It is important to follow-up a case and see through the natural progression. Examine the same case periodically for differences of symptoms and sign, no matter how subtle. Do not be disheartened if your provisional diagnosis does not always tally with the actual diagnosis made after performing investigations. Remember to make a clinical diagnosis as would be expected of a clinician. In most cases the clinical diagnosis would fit in with the real diagnosis, but not always. In such situations be satisfied that your approach and rationality are justified in the formulation of a working diagnosis.

Develop a sense of regard for the child or newborn baby. Never take a patient as a mere name or a diagnosis. Cultivate a rapport with the patient and the guardian and you will positively find your history taking and examinations less bumpy and more satisfying. Happy reading!

Dilip Mukherjee
Indraneel Banerjee

Acknowledgements

We express our great sense of gratitude to Dr Prachi, Clinical Psychologist and Stress Counsellor, UN Department of Safety and Security (UNDSS), New Delhi for kindly contributing as guest author for chapter on Psychological Assessment of Children. We are really indebted to her for her contribution which as added a new dimension to this book. We are grateful to Prof YK Amdekar, Ex-Prof of JJ Hospital, Mumbai and renowned consultant paediatrician and a versatile genius in the field of paediatrics for kindly agreeing to write the foreword for this book. We express our gratitude to him for his generosity.

We are also grateful to Prof AK Dutta the Director Professor of the Department of Paediatrics of Lady Hardinge Medical College, New Delhi for kindly going through the manuscript and encouraging us very much.

Dr Debjani Das and Dr Sutapa Halder the postgraduate students of the department of paediatrics of Ramakrishna Mission Seva Pratisthan, Vivekananda Institute of Medical Sciences have kindly drawn all the sketches for this book. Dr Anindya Saha, Dr Arpan Agarwal and Dr Suparna Guha (MD, Paed) of our department who has taken all the photographs for this book. Dr Surajit Santra has taken the arduous trouble to incorporate and edit the photos and the sketches in the CD for the book. Dr Taraknath Ghosh, MD (Paed) and Ex-registrar of our department, and Dr Soumitra Masani our PGT have gone through the entire book and did the primary editing job for us. We are grateful to all of them and also to other residents and the senior colleagues of our department for their suggestions and comments.

We are really grateful to Parimal Kar for doing the composing and typing of this manuscript.

We are also grateful to M/s. Jaypee Brothers Medical Publishers (P) Ltd for their cooperation and help to publish this book.

Contents

1 History

INTRODUCTION

Obtaining a good history is an art and gets better with practice. A sound history is vital to diagnosis as this is the structure on which to build upon. A problem history is most often from parents and not directly from the child. This entails a degree of bias which should not be ignored but rather weighed for its true worth. Communication is most essential in this process. The doctor-parent or doctor-patient relationship is not one way, rather it is a two-way process involving two people studying each other. The doctor must put the informant at ease and encourage him or her to talk freely.

History is not just limited to questions and answers. It helps to start a conversation by greeting the patient, addressing him or her by name, identifying a common town of origin or a mutual interest in pets. All this while, watch the parent's and patient's gestural language. The eyes and hands may tell you more than what is actually said.

Concentration is very important in a conversation. Your undivided attention must be devoted to hearing the complaint; otherwise the response from the patient's end will be incomplete. Gentleness is all-important, more so in a physical examination. The patient should be reassured and not frightened or put off.

Behavioural problems often make it more difficult for the interviewer. It helps to strike up a communication directly with the patient, be it verbal or non-verbal. Establishing a rapport with the distressed child relieves much anxiety relating to the disease.

The doctor, in an interview with the child and parents, must have a well balanced attitude. It would be unwise to allow your feelings to surface into confrontation. Barriers of language, culture or manners may tend to put you on the wrong track, and in such situations evaluation and re-evaluation of what has been said and what has been missed, is essential.

Let the informant unfold the story in his own words. Only when he or she has done so should he or she be asked to expand on what appears to be the more important aspects of the story. Specific leading questions should only be asked after you have reached the heart of the problem and have framed in your own mind a possible diagnosis and a differential diagnosis list.

It is important that you practice this art over and over again so as not to miss the salient points of interest. Time is important and often at a premium. In an unstructured setting, for example, in a busy emergency, you have to get all the details in a few minutes. This takes a lot of practice and practice builds on premonition. The following headings are relevant in history (Table 1.1):

Table 1.1: History taking
Name, age, sex and address
Presenting complaint
History of present illness
History of prior illnesses/past illness
Family history
Social history
Past medical/surgical treatment history
Antenatal and birth history
Postnatal history
Dietary history
Immunization history

PRESENTING COMPLAINT

Try to define the main complaint and its duration. The presenting complaint is simply the problem that makes the patient seek medical help. This is usually confined to one or two key points. Multiple presenting complaints themselves represent the problem rather than the diagnosis. The timing and duration of symptomatic events is important since the chronology provides clues to the underlying pathology. Sometime the duration of actual presenting complaints is bypassed and the onset taken at the point of trivial complaints. This error has to be corrected as you go on taking the history.

THE HISTORY OF THE PRESENT ILLNESS

Ask the informant to give you a detailed account of the illness from the beginning. A history may not always start with a chief complaint, and may start with other relatively minor complaints. Ideally you should allow the narrator to continue without any interruption, but for people who are either quite reticent or too talkative and deviating from the symptoms, you will need to gently encourage them to stay on track.

Symptom Analysis

Each symptom has to be analysed thoroughly and qualified suitably. As an example, an illness starting with pain should be described as:

- Timing and duration: When did the pain start? Does it come and go? How long does it last on average?
- Character: What the pain feels like stabbing, burning, pricking, dull aching, colicky
- Severity: Whether it interferes with daily activities or keeps the child awake at night
- Radiation: Whether it stays at one place or spreads along the distribution of a nerve
- Referral: Whether the pain at a site originates at a different site
- Shifting: Whether the pain shifts from the original site to a new location
- Aggravating factor: What brings it on and what worsens it?
- Relieving factor: What makes it better?

Likewise, symptoms of fever can be described as:

- Duration of illness
- Height of temperature
- Type of fever (remittent, intermittent, continued - Chap 2, page 28)
- Character (i.e., quotidian) — associated with chills or rigor
- Associated convulsions
- Associated malaise, headache
- Descriptions of related symptoms.

Similar analysis of the other illness complaints will help us draw a pen picture of the child's problems. Relating one symptom to the other will then help you towards a differential diagnosis. The pattern of evolution of the complaints tells you of the natural history of a disease. Find out if the illness began insidously and gradually worsen or was it intermittent? Was the onset acute, then slowly getting better, but not fully disappeared? Is there a relation to a previously diagnosed illness? Of the symptoms presented, which ones are more relevant than others? Are there pieces of information that appear out of place? Do you need to revisit those issues and work out the connection, if at all? A good history is like an intricate network – it is your job to set this up so that you can make sense of it all.

An outline of the questions related to individual systems is given below:

General

Weight

- Is it increasing, decreasing or stationary?
- If the child has lost weight recently – has the child been unwell? Has he or she strenuously exercised to lose weight?
- Is there a family history of obesity, type 2 diabetes mellitus or early cardiovascular morbidity?

Sleep

- Has the sleeping pattern changed?
- Is there difficulty in getting to sleep or unsual early waking?
- Does the child snare at night?
- Is the patient sleepy and tired during the day?
- Have the parents noticed any convulsions during sleep?
- Any odd behaviour during sleep?
- If the child is of an age of bladder continence, does he or she have nocturnal enuresis?

Energy

- Is it loss of energy or boredom?
- Is it part of a general malaise?
- Is there unusual fatiguability?
- What time of the day is there lethargy?
- Can the child play with his/her friends?
- Is the child so tired that he/she does not want to be with his/her friends?

The Gastrointestinal System (Table 1.2)

Gastrointestinal symptoms can be of upper or lower tracts. The following questions should help you get to the bottom of the problem.

Table 1.2: GI system
• Pain • Appetite • Vomiting • Water brash • Heart burn • Dysphagia • Diarrhoea • Constipation

Pain

- What site is the pain?
- Judge the severity
- Is it localized or diffuse? Is it persistent or intermittent?
- Does it radiate in any particular direction?
- For how long has the patient had it?
- Are there intervals of freedom? If so, for how long?
- What is its relation to meals (if any)?
- Does it wake the patient at night? Does the child wake up in the night screaming with pain?
- What things aggravate it? What affords relief (food, anatacid, vomiting)?
- Does any particular posture relieve the pain?
- Is it relieved by defaecation or by the passage of flatus?
- Is there underlying anxiety or tension suggesting a functional non-organic aetiology?
- What medication does the child have for the pain?

Appetite

- Is it increased or reduced?
- Does the child dislike certain foods?
- Does the child eat good size portions at mealtimes?

Vomiting

- How serious a problem is this?
- Does the child throw up after milk feeds (gastro-oesophageal reflux)?
- Is abdominal pain relieved by vomiting (gastritis)?
- Is there vomiting in the morning (raised intracranial pressure)?
- What does the child throw up?
- Check if the vomitus is bilious (intestinal obstruction)
- Does it ever contain fresh blood (mucosal tear)?
- Does it ever look like coffee grounds (gastric mucosal haemorrhage)?
- Is the child having regular intermittent vomiting episodes as in intermittent malrotation?
- Is the child passing urine? Large fluid loss may result in dehydration
- Is the child on any medication that is emetogenic, for example opioids?
- Is this is gastroenteritis, or is there a more serious underlying illness like diabetic ketoacidosis, pyelonephritis or metabolic disorder?

Water Brash

- Does the patient ever experience excessive secretion of saliva into the mouth, with regurgitation of mouthfuls of clear, tasteless fluid?

Heartburn

- Does the patient suffer from pain behind the sternum?
- Does it come on especially when lying down?

Dysphagia

- Record the child's words—what does he/she mean by difficulty of swallowing?
- Where does the food appear to stick?
- Is it worse with liquids or with solids?
- Is swallowing painful?
- Is there underlying anxiety that itself could be responsible for difficulty of swallowing?

Diarrhoea

- What is the duration of diarrhoea?
- How frequent and at what times are the motions during the day?
- What is their relation to meals?
- Does the child have loose motions after eating certain types of food?
- Has the child eaten unusual food in the recent past?
- Is there a possibility of food poisoning?
- What colour are the motions?
- Has the patient ever passed any blood or mucus with stool (dysentery, inflammatory bowel disease)?
- Are they unformed, porridge-like, frothy, or watery (chronic diarrhoea, malabsorption)?
- Do they float in the lavatory pan or are they difficult to flush away (malabsorption)?
- Is the diarrhoea painless?
- Is there colicky abdominal pain, suggestive of colitis?
- Does the patient use laxatives?
- How is the child's appetite?
- Is the child gaining weight appropriately?

Constipation

- How often does the child "go" to the toilet?
- Get the parents or child to describe the motions—small, dry, hard and pellety, elongated but hard or tubular and formed
- Is this a long standing problem (habit constipation, megacolon)?
- Does the child avoid the toilet because it is painful to defaecate?
- Does the child consume reasonable amounts of fruit, vegetables and greens?
- Can this be explained by change in circumstances, medicines, etc.?
- Is the child constantly wearing nappies and will not pass motions if taken off (habit)?
- Is there soiling of clothes suggestive of overflow incontinence of stools secondary to constipation?
- Did the child open his or her bowels in the first day of life (Hirschprung disease)
- Is the child taking medication to relieve constipation? If so, what dose?
- Is there any colicky pain? Is the pain aggravated when using laxatives like senna?
- Is there blood in the stools (anal fissure)?

Liver and Gallbladder

Jaundice

- Has the child noticed any yellow discolouration of conjunctivae or skin, or high coloured urine?
- Are the motions pale or dark?
- Does the skin itch?
- Any bruises or unusual skin marks?
- Have there been any other cases of jaundice among family or friends?
- Any foreign travel?
- Was any injection given in the last 3 or 4 months?

Pain

- Where is it?
- Has the patient ever had attacks of very severe pain, coming on suddenly and lasting for a few hours?

- If so, did the pain radiate and in what direction?
- Was there any jaundice after the pain subsided?
- Did the pain radiate to the tip of the shoulder or the middle of the back?

The Cardiovascular System

If the symptoms point to disease of the circulatory system, enquire about the following:

Dyspnoea

- When does this come on? Is it present at rest or only on exertion?
- What degree of exertion is necessary to produce it?
- Judge the severity of dyspnoea. Does it impede routine daily activity?
- Are there attacks of breathlessness at night (paroxysmal nocturnal dyspnoea)?
- Does the patient have to sleep sitting up (orthopnoea)?
- Does the child have palpitations and how long do they last?
- Does the heart give an occasional thump now and then?
- Is the pulse rate increased on occasion and is it regular or irregular?

Cough

- Enquire about cough, sputum and haemoptysis, as detailed in the section on the respiratory system

Oedema

- Do the heels or ankles swell?
- Does the face also swell up?

Other Symptoms

- Are there cramp-like pains in the calves when walking relieved by rest? Or
- Is there undue coldness, redness or blueness of the extremities?
- Is there a past history of rheumatic fever or chorea?

Haemopoietic System

If the clinical features suggest a blood disorder, enquire about the following:

- Tiredness, lethargy, feeling miserable (anaemia)
- Infections involving the mouth, skin, lungs, urinary tract and perianal area (bone marrow aplasia)
- Blood loss from gums, nose, bruising, rectum as well as malaena (black stools) and menstrual irregularity (bleeding disorder)
- Is bleeding or bruising out of proportion to degree of trauma (bleeding or clotting diathesis)?
- Does the child appear to be pale?
- Are there red skin spots (purpura, petechiae) and changes in skin colour?
- Is bleeding or skin rash associated with pallor?
- What about diet–ask for consumption of meat and green vegetables
- If the child is drinking far too much milk there may be iron deficiency anaemia
- Does the child go about barefoot–hook-worms can cause enough blood loss to cause significant anaemia
- Any excessive bleeding after dental extraction or tonsillectomy
- Has the child ingested drugs known to cause bone marrow aplasia or haemolytic anaemia?
- Is there a family history of blood disorders (haemolytic disease)?
- Has the child noticed any glandular enlargements (lymphoma, leukaemia)?

The Respiratory System

Parents will often tell you that their child has been coughing for some time or been rather wheezy. Asthma is a common problem, so explore atopy and allergy. Do think about tuberculosis as a possible diagnosis, even though this may not be very obvious. You should also ask for possible exposure to animal, mineral or vegetable dusts to search for an explanation for chronic cough.

Cough

- What is the duration of the cough?
- Did the cough start recently or is it present for weeks or even months?
- Is it chronic persistent (tuberculosis, bronchiectasis) or chronic episodic (asthma)?
- Is it dry or productive?
- In the child less than a year, is the cough "fruity" (bronchiolitis)?
- If this a baby, does the cough sound like a "whoop" (pertussis)?
- Enquire if the child had surgery (tetralogy of Fallot repair) – viral upper respiratory tract infections can trigger a "TOF" cough
- At what time of the day or night is it worst?
- Has the child used inhalers (relievers like salbutamol) and do they help?
- Are there family members who smoke around the child?
- Does the child have eczema or family history of atopy, suggesting a predisposition to asthma?
- Is it worsened by any particular conditions, such as cold or dust?
- Is it painful or not?
- Is the child taking medication (like captopril) that may aggravate the cough?
- Are there associated symptoms to worry about pulmonary tuberculosis?
- Are there family members with a chronic coughing illness suggesting tuberculosis?
- Is there a functional element in the history (habit cough)?

Sputum

- How much? (in children more than 6 years of age).
- When is expectoration maximal?
- What is the consistency, colour, and odour?
- Is it purulent (bacterial infection)?
- Is it ever blood-stained, and if so whether with streaks or clots (tuberculosis, bronchiectasis, trauma, pulmonary sequestration, haemosiderosis)?
- Does the child do chest physiotherapy to help produce sputum (bronchiectasis)?

Breathing

- Is there increased work of breathing?
- Is the child unusually tachpnoeic?
- Does dyspnoea occur at rest, or after varying degrees of exertion?
- Describe the level of activity that brings out dyspnoea
- Does the child snare at night?
- Does he or she fall asleep easily during the day, suggesting obstructive sleep apnoea?

Wheeze

- Is it wheeze or stridor?
- Is it constant or intermittent?
- Is the child a "happy wheezer" (viral wheeze)?
- Does anything provoke it?
- Does the child become wheezy with viral upper respiratory infections?
- Is it worse at any particular time of day or night?
- What relieves it?
- Is there a history suggestive of foreign body inhalation?
- What is the dose of inhaled reliever medication?
- What about the technique of inhaler use?
- Is the child growing well (severe asthma)?
- Is the child missing a lot of school days? (severity of asthma)?
- Can the child play a full game (assess functional ability)?

Chest Pain

- Where is it – all over the chest or central and retrosternal?
- Is the pain unilateral (pleural effusion)?

- Is it aggravated by deep breathing or coughing?
- Describe the pain character – sharp, stabbing (pleuritic) or dull, aching (haematoma, trauma, neuralgia).
- Is it associated with an increase in cough, sputum or dyspnoea (pneumonia)?
- Is the onset sudden and sharp and accompanied by significant dyspnoea (spontaneous pneumothorax)?

The Urinary System

Pain on micturition, haematuria, oliguria and oedema are pointers in the direction of a renal or urology problem. Probe further if you feel that the waterworks are at fault.

- Is there less urine (oliguria)?
- Is the child passing urine too frequently (polyuria—diabetes mellitus, insipidus)?
- Is the child drinking large amounts of fluids (polydipsia)?
- Will the child drink water instead of juice (compulsive juice drinking)?
- Does the child wake up often through the night for a wee (polyuria)?
- Is the child at an age of continence?
- Is there nocturnal enuresis? If so, how many nights a week?
- Is there day time incontinence and accidents when the child is awake (bladder detrusor weakness)?
- What methods have the parents tried to make the child continent?
- Explore the child's social circumstances
- What is the colour of the urine?
- Is there blood in urine?
- If there blood in urine, at what stage of the micturition is it (upper renal tract – constant, lower tract—end of micturition)?
- Is micturition painful? Does the child have a burning or stinging sensation (cystitis)?
- Any pain shooting down to the groin or genitalia (calculi)?
- Is the child passing less urine (oliguria)?
- Is there a record of fluid intake-output? Have the nappies been weighed to estimate urine output?
- Is the child losing fluid elsewhere (e.g. diarrhoea, vomiting)?
- Is urine output disproportionate to the oral intake?
- Is there a history of diarrhoea preceding oliguria (haemolytic uraemic syndrome)?
- Does the face or ankles swell (nephrotic syndrome, renal failure)?
- What medications is the child on?
- Is the child on long term steroids?
- Are the side effects from medication (Cushingoid appearance, infections from steroid use)?
- Is the child on dialysis? If so, what type?
- Has the child had a renal transplant?
- What immunosuppressives is the child using?
- Is the child on antihypertensives?
- If so is hypertension well controlled?
- Has the child been admitted to intensive care with headaches, blurring of vision, drowsiness or fits (hypertensive encephalopathy)?
- Is the child gaining weight and growing well (poor growth and inadequate weight gain in renal failure)?

Skin Diseases

Itch

- Has the child got an itchy skin problem (eczema, contact dermatitis, scabies)?
- Whereabouts is the itch (between fingers in scabies, flexures in eczema)?
- Does the child have jaundice (obstructive jaundice)?
- Enquire carefully into the patient's hygiene – clothing, cleanliness etc (scabies)
- Is there any exposure to chemical substances or other irritants? Ask about recent drug therapy.

- Is there a history of asthma, hay fever or any other allergic disorder (atopic dermatitis)?
- Is there contact with animals, insects, or plants (contact dermatitis)?
- Does the child have dry skin (eczema)?
- What topical medications have been used?
- Is there a family history of skin disease, asthma, hay fever, urticaria (atopy)?

Rash

- Where is the rash?
- What colour is the rash (red—measles, enterovirus, meningococcal infections)?
- Is the rash vesicular (chicken pox, folliculitis, burns)?
- Is the rash associated with joint swelling (Henoch-Schonlein purpura, juvenile idiopathic arthritis, vasculitis, inflammatory bowel disease)?
- Is the rash brought on by specific food ingestion (cow's milk protein intolerance)?

Pigmentation

- Are there patches of skin depigmentation (vitiligo, psoriasis, pityriasis)?
- Is there generalised pigmentation of the skin with associated mucosal pigmentation (Addison disease)?
- Are there leathery, dark patches over the neck and axillae (acanthosis nigricans)?

Hair

- Is there loss of hair (alopecia)?
- Is the child on cytotoxic chemotherapy (alopecia)?
- Is the child on sodium valproate (hypertrichosis)?
- Is there excess hair in a girl (hypertrichosis or hirutism)? What is the distribution (forearm, arm, legs—hypertrichosis; moustache, sideburns, chest—androgenic)
- Is there irregularity of periods associated with excess hair (polycystic ovarian syndrome)?

Neurology

Headaches, convulsions, limb weakness, altered consciousness should alert you to investigate the child's neurology.

Headache

- How often does the child have headaches?
- How long do they last?
- Is it one side only (migraine)?
- Are the headaches relieved by sleep (migraine)?
- Do the headaches occur in the evening after coming back from school (tiredness)?
- What exactly does the child mean by the term "headache" (headache an attention seeking device in preschool children)?
- Do headaches occur early in the morning and improve by the end of the day (space occupying lesions)?
- Any associated visual perceptions (acute – migraine, chronic—craniopharyngioma, optic nerve glioma)?
- Any family history of headaches with or without visual disturbances (migraine)?
- Is there loss of balance (cerebellar astrocytoma)?
- Does the child have an intracranial shunt? If so when it was last revised?
- Was there weakness of the limbs at any stage (migraine, stroke, vasculitis, tumours)?
- What medication does the child take to relieve the headaches?

Convulsion

- Is it a convulsion—get a first hand account (jerking of limbs, incontinence, biting of tongue, eyes rolling back—suggest tonic clonic seizures)
- Any post ictal symptoms (headaches, paralysis)?
- Was the child standing when it happened (syncope)?
- Was the episode brought about by exercise (hypertrophic cardiomyopathy)?

- Is there a family history of sudden death (hypertrophic cardiomyopathy)?
- Does the child have episodes where he or she appears vacant and inattentive (behavioural, absence seizures)?
- Does the child show abnormal behaviour (complex partial seizures)?
- Is it a morning seizure with numbness of the face, drooling and garbled vocalization (Rolandic seizure)?
- Was the convulsion triggered off by flashing lights (photosensitive epilepsy) or accompanied by lauging bouts (gelastic seizure)?
- Is there warning or aura (focal seizures)?
- Was there loss of consciousness (generalized epilepsy) or not (partial epilepsy)?
- What is the treatment history?
- Assess the compliance with anticonvulsants.

Dizziness

- Is dizziness induced by moving the head in a particular way or assuming a particular posture (positional vertigo)?
- Did it follow an injury or a presumed viral infection (inner ear abnormality)?
- Is there a history of long standing aminoglycoside use (inner ear toxicity)?
- Does the child appear unusually anxious (panic attack)?
- Was the episode following intake of medication (hypotension following antihypertensive ingestion)?
- Did dizziness precede headaches (migraine)?

Weakness

- Is the weakness transient? (atypical hemiplegic migraine)
- Is the weakness present from birth (spinal muscular atrophy, cerebral palsy, congenital myopathies)?
- Was the onset of weakness acute (vasculitis, injury, infections) or chronic (tumours, degenerative disease)?
- Is the weakness generalized (malnutrition, chronic illness) or localized (nerve or muscle lesions)?
- Is there weakness in the lower limbs with sphincter incontinence (transverse myelitis)?
- Any paraesthesia (Guillain-Barre syndrome)?
- Any history of trauma to back or surgical intervention (spinal injury)?
- Was the child treated for tuberculosis (spinal tuberculosis)?
- Is weakness associated with headaches or dizziness (brain tumour, vasculitis)?
- Any associated mouth ulcers and skin rash? (Behcet syndrome).

Locomotor System

Symptoms related to this system are covered elsewhere. However, you may find to it important to ask a few pertinent questions.

- How far can the child walk (functional ability)?
- Can the child run without hindrance (excludes major abnormalities)?
- Is there swelling of one or more joints (juvenile idiopathic arthritis, vasculitis)?
- Is joint swelling accompanied by high temperatures (osteomyelitis, vasculitis, juvenile idiopathic arthritis)?
- Was joint swelling preceded by gastroenteritis (reactive arthritis)?
- Is the child's walking distance getting progressively short (Duchenne dystrophy)?
- Does the child receive physiotherapy?
- Is there use of pain relieving medication?
- Does the child use orthopaedic devices (ankle foot orthoses for Charcot Marie Tooth disease, special boots for talipes equinovarus)?
- Was there any surgery to limit the child's movement?

HISTORY OF PRIOR ILLNESS/PAST ILLNESS

Search for any past illness and whether it bears a relation to the present illness. A history of fever and sore throat is relevant in the context of acute glomerulonephritis. Children with immune deficiency often have recurrent hospital admissions. Children with inadequate weight gain may have had chronic illnesses in the past. Diseases like juvenile idiopathic arthritis or chronic renal failure can lead to growth failure. Prior steroid use may be the cause of later problems of obesity. Always consider the child's current problems in the context of previous episodes of illness and treatment. Do not, however, assume that the present and past problems are associated all the time. The child may have different pathologies at different points in time.

SOCIAL HISTORY

No history will be complete without a thorough evaluation of the child's social and economic background. Many diseases are borne out of the child's circumstances. Malnutrition occurs in children of families of meagre income. Obesity occurs relatively commonly where the family income has received a boost. Diseases may be spread by poor quality of housing and sanitation. Hookworm infestation, giardiasis, scabies are typical examples.

It is important to estimate the living condition of the family. Ask about the number of family members, the number of rooms, water supply and waste disposal facilities. It helps to understand the family's economic structure. This is often a delicate matter and not all families will be keen to discuss their financial status. If you manage to extricate this information you may compare this against a socio-economic scale such as that given in Table 1.3. You should remember this table holds little relevance in real life as burgeoning costs and inflation have rendered it obsolete. You could devise a scale along similar lines depending upon the economic prosperity and average income of people of your region.

Table 1.3: Socio-economic class as per BJ Prasad

Class	*Per capita income in Rs per month*
I	1536 and above
II	770-1535
III	360-769
IV	150-359
V	Less than 150

FAMILY HISTORY

Note the patient's position in the family and the ages of siblings if any. Also record the state of health, important illnesses and cause of death of immediate relatives. Draw a family tree going back three generations. Ask about consanguinity as this is important for autosomal recessive conditions. Document diseases in each family member—a detailed description will help you understand if the child is likely to be a carrier or case of an autosomal recessive condition. Often the child is the index case and diagnosis in other family members may be made after the diagnosis in the child. In a child with Langer mesomelia, check the heights of the parents, uncles and aunts as they may have undiagnosed Leri-Weill dyschondrosteosis (haploinsufficiency of SHOX). Very often a child will have died in the family from an unknown disease. It may be relevant to know the circumstances leading to death. For example, a child may have died of thalassaemia major and secondary infections prior to actual diagnosis. This indicates that the parents are carriers and hence exclusion of thalassaemia in the other children is important.

Enquire about associated diseases in other family members – coeliac disease in a child with type 1 diabetes mellitus, tumours in multiple endocrine neoplasia and stillbirths in congenital adrenal hyperplasia. Further, enquire about close relations with persons outside the family. It may be important to know of a next door neighbour with tuberculosis who may have infected the child.

Treatment History

Document medical or surgical treatment, if any. Record details of medicines—their dose, duration, complications and efficacy. Previous surgical intervention is important to know in the context of a child with possible intestinal obstruction. Chemotherapy and craniospinal radiation can damage the hypothalamus and pituitary gland resulting in hypopituitarism. Sodium valproate for epilepsy can lead to weight gain in puberty. Carbamazepine can give rise to Stevens-Johnson syndrome acutely. Long term steroids in nephrotic syndrome lead to obesity and stunting of height. Previous treatment for urinary tract infection is important in the child with chronic renal failure.

ANTENATAL, BIRTH AND POSTNATAL HISTORY

Data on any untoward event in pregnancy (rubella) may be important as a causation of disease in the infant (congenital rubella). Equally important is the history of drugs taken which may adversely affect the fetus (fetal hydantoin, fetal alchol syndromes). Record if the antenatal scan was normal. What was the growth of the fetus in utero? Was the baby born premature? Was there any perinatal asphyxia? Document the treatment if the child was in the neonatal unit. Intraventricular haemorrhage may have a bearing in a child with dystonic cerebral palsy. Extrahepatic portal vein thrombosis may be due to umbilical venous catheterization in the newborn period. A child with metabolic syndrome may have been born small for gestational age.

IMMUNIZATION HISTORY

Note whether the child received oral polio, BCG, triple antigen and measles as per the immunisation programme. Ask the mother whether a BCG left a scar or not. A BCG vaccine without a scar is best taken as having had no conversion. Also enquire about the other vaccines namely hepatitis B, rabies, MMR. Ask for any serious side effects after the first triple antigen dose.

Developmental History

Gather information from the parents on the child's play, speech and social interactions. You should be able to assess the age at which the child functions in gross motor, fine motor, personal-social and speech-language areas. You can calculate the Development Quotient (DQ) as ratio of developmental age for chronological age. A DQ of less than 70 is taken as developmental delay. You can quantify the child's developmental age with the aid of an inventory (a screening test like the Denver Development Screening Test or a comprehensive Griffith Development Assessment) but in the bedside situation it helps to be aware of the common milestones as given below.

You should remember that there is considerable variation in individuals and that you should allow for social and cultural situations. A child with limb weakness will perform below par in gross motor skills. A child with recurrent otitis media may lag behind in speech and language areas. Children with chronic illnesses may falsely appear to have global developmental delay.

MILESTONES OF DEVELOPMENT

Neonatal Period (1st 4 weeks)

Prone : Lies in flexed attitude, turns head from side to side, head sags on ventral suspension.
Supine : Generally flexed and a little stiff.
Visual : May fixate face or light in line of vision, 'Doll's eye' movement of eyes on turning head.
Reflex : Moro response active, stepping and placing reflexes, grasp reflex active
Social : Visual preference for human face.

4 Weeks

Prone : Legs more extended, holds chin up momentary, lifts head from plane of body on ventral suspension.
Supine : Tonic neck posture predominates, head lags on pull to sit position.

Visual : Watches person, follows moving object.

Social : Body movements in cadence with voice of other in social contact, beginning to smile.

8 Weeks

Prone : Raises head slightly further, head sustained in line of body on ventral suspension.

Supine : Tonic neck posture predominates, head lags on pull to sit.

Visual : Follows moving objects.

Social : Smiles on social contact, listens to voice and coos.

12 Weeks

Prone : Lifts head and chest arms extended, head above plane of body on ventral suspension.

Supine : Tonic neck posture predominates, reaches towards and misses objects, waves at toy, shows hand regard.

Sitting : Head lag partially compensated on pull to sit, early head control with bobbing motions, back rounded, leans forward.

Reflex : Moro disappears, makes defensive movements or selective withdrawal reactions.

Social : Sustained social contact, listens to music, says "aah, ngah." (hatching socially).

16 Weeks

Prone : Lifts head and chest, head in approximately vertical axis, legs extended.

Supine : Symmetric posture predominates, hands in midline, reaches and grasps objects and brings them to mouth.

Sitting : No head lag on pull to sit, head steady, enjoys sitting with full trunk support.

Standing : When held erect, pushes with feet

Adaptive : Sees pellet, but makes no move to it

Social : Laughs aloud, may show displeasure if social contact is broken, excited at sight of food.

28 Weeks

Prone : Rolls over, pivots.

Supine : Rolls over (Back to stomach - 6 mon), squirming movements.

Sitting : Sits briefly with support of pelvis, leans forward on hands, back rounded.

Standing : May support most of weight, bounces actively.

Adaptive : Reaches out for and grasps large object (voluntary grasp at 20 wk), grasps using radial palm, rakes at pellet, transfers object from hand to hand, bangs cubes on table.

Language: Polysyllabic vowel sounds formed (Da, Ma, Ba, Ka).

Social : Prefers mother, babbly, enjoys mirror, responds to changes in emotional content of social contact.

40 Weeks

Sitting : Sits up alone and indefinitely without support, back straight.

Standing : Pulls to standing position, 'cruises' or walks holding to furniture.

Motor : Crawls (creeps—44 wk)

Adaptive : Grasps objects with thumb and forefinger, pokes at things with forefinger, picks up pellet with assisted pincer movement, uncovers hidden toy, atttempts to retrieve dropped object (object constancy), releases object grasped by other person, clicks 2 cubes in imitation.

Language: Repetitive consonant sounds (mama, dada).

Social : Responds to sound of name, plays peek-a-boo ('tuki') or pat-a-cake ('tai-tai'), waves bye - bye ('ta-ta').

52 Weeks (1 year)

Motor : Walks with one hand held (48 wk), rises independently, takes seveal steps.
Adaptive : Picks up pellet with unassisted pincer movement of forefinger and thumb, releases object to other person on request or gesture, may kiss on request, rings a bell.
Language: A few words besides 'mama, dada.'
Social : Plays simple ball game, makes postural adjustment to dressing.

15 months

Motor : Walks alone, crawls up stairs.
Adaptive : Makes tower of 3 cubes, makes a line with crayon, inserts pellet in bottle.
Language: Jargon, follows simple commands, may name a familiar object (ball), looks with interest at coloured pictures.
Social : Indicates some desires or needs by pointing, hugs parents.

18 months

Motor : Runs stiffly, sits on small chair, walks up stairs with one hand held, explores drawers and waste baskets, manages spoon without rotating near mouth, turns 2-3 pages of book at a time.
Adaptive : Makes a tower of 4 cubes, imitates scribbling, imitates vertical stroke, dumps pellet from bottle.
Language: Ten words (average), names pictures (4), identifies one or more parts of body, identifies 3 parts on doll.
Social : Feeds self, a seeks help when in trouble, may complain when wet, or soiled, kisses parents with pucker, alternates between clinging and resistance.

24 months

Motor : Runs well (walks backward - 21 mon), walks up and down stairs, one step at a time, opens door, climbs on furniture, jumps.
Adaptive : Tower of 7 cubes, circular scribbling, imitates horizontal stroke, folds paper once imitatively, parallel play but not playing with other children.
Language: Puts 3 words together (subject, verb object), vocabulary of 100 words or more.
Social : Helps undress, listens to story with pictures, dry at night if lifted out late in the evening.

30 months

Motor : Goes upstairs alternating feet, jumps on both feet.
Adaptive : Tower of 9 cubes, makes vertical and horizontal strokes, but generally will not join them to make a cross, imitates circular stroke, forming closed figure.
Language: Refers to self by pronoun "I," knows name.
Social : Helps put things away, pretends in play.

36 months

Motor : Rides tricycle, stands momentarily on one foot.
Adaptive : Tower of 10 cubes, imitates construction of "bridge" of 3 cubes, copies circle, imitates cross.
Language: Knows age, sex, counts 3 objects correctly, repeats 3 numbers or a sentence of 6 syllables.
Social : Parallel play with other children, unbuttons clothing, puts on shoes, washes, handedness established.

48 months

Motor : Hops on one foot, throws ball overhand, uses scissors to cut out pictures, climbs well.

Adaptive : Copies bridge from model, imitates construction of "gate" of 5 cubes, copies cross and square, draws a man with 2-4 parts besides head, names longer of 2 lines.

Language: Counts 4 coins, tells story.

Social : Goes to toilet alone plays with several children.

60 months

Motor : Walks easily on narrow line, runs lightly on toes, skips on alternate feet.

Adaptive : Draws triangle form copy, names heavier of 2 weights.

Language: Names 4 colours, repeats sentence of 10 syllables, counts 10 coins correctly, fully, nine-letter vision chart at 6 meters and near-vision testing card (Stycar), delights at reciting, gives full birthday, home address.

Social : Dresses and underesses, asks questions about meaning of words, domestic role play, chooses own friends, enjoys jokes and riddles.

SCHOOL PERFORMANCE

School is often the window to judge a child's overall health. Check if he or she finds it difficult with numbers and concepts (Turner syndrome). Is there a problem with inattention, hyperactivity or impulsiveness (attention deficit disorder)? Has there been a recent steady decline in school work (autoimmune hypothyroidism)? Is the child missing school frequently (chronic illness)? Is the child isolated and avoiding contact with other children (autism spectrum)?

Dietary History

A proper dietary history is important to assess the nutritional state. Record the child's average daily intake of food in terms of calories and grammes of protein. A rigorous dietary assessment is crucial to evaluating the extent of malnutrition. In infants, note the the duration of breast feeding, weaning foods and weight gain.

A list of commonly used food items and their calories and proteins are given in Table 1.4.

Table 1.4: Calorie and protein value of commonly used foods

	Kcal	*Protein*
1 Medium chapati (25g)	85	3
1 Medium katori Rice (25g)	86	2
1 Slice bread (25g)	60	2
1 Medium katora bread (25g)	86	6
1 Medium sized egg	60	6
1 Piece fish	60	9
2 Pieces Meat	60	10
Cow's milk (250 ml)	165	8
Curd (100 gm)	60	3
Leafy vegetable (100 gm)		
1/3 cup (cooked)	28	3
1/2 cup cooked potato (100 gm)	100	2
1 Medium sized apple (100 gm)	60	-
1 Medium sized orange (100 gm)	48	-
1 Medium sized Banana (100 gm)	120	-
Oil and ghee 2 tsp	90	-
Sugar (25 gm) 5 tsp	100	-
Jaggery (15 gm) 1 small cup	96	-

Plan of Diagnosis (Table 1.5)

A careful history will help you piece together a credible story. There will be positive pointers as well as important negative attributes that will you build a multi-layered pen picture. A good history will be multidimensional and allow you to choose the thread to follow further with your examination.

Table 1.5: Plan of diagnosis

History	-	Suggest something
General survey	-	Suggest specific system for clinical diagnosis
Specific system	-	Points toward clinical diagnosis
Investigation	-	Probable diagnosis
Successful specific treatment/ Surgery/Autopsy	-	Final diagnosis

2 GENERAL SURVEY

The general survey is essential to form an opinion about the child before proceeding to the systemic examination. You should pick up clues as you go along. Think of the examination as a jigsaw puzzle and how you can fit the pieces. The more meticulous you are the better. However, not all pieces of information will make sense at the same time. It may be that you will come back to a sign or a lesion and understand its meaning in retrospect.

Observe the child's appearance and activity and note how the child adjusts to his or her environment. Simple observation can give you vital clues, so it is important that you **observe the child at play or in the way he walks or interacts.** Like the interview, establish a rapport with the child and do appear non-threatening in your approach. Record height, weight and head circumference as detailed in the section on anthropometry.

Note the apparent age of the child and whether it tallies with the stated age. A 'nutritional dwarf' will pass off as a normal for a lower age – anthropometry should resolve this. Is the child cooperative, alert, playful, retracted or anxious?

It is useful to have **a system by which you can assess systematically** in order - anaemia, cyanosis, jaundice, oedema, clubbing and the tell tale signs of any disease. One-way would be to start with examination of the hands and to proceed upwards. In the hands you could note the presence of pallor, asymmetry, muscle weakness, liver, palms, clubbing, pulse, perfusion and blood pressure. Whilst you are going from a distal to proximal aspect you will have noted any scars, wasting, venous prominences, lymph nodes and spider naevi. At the neck, note lymph node enlargements, jugular venous engorgement, carotid pulsation and the thyroid gland. Look at the mouth for the health of teeth, gums, pallor, cyanosis, jaundice, granulomas, mucositis and general hygiene. The face is a vast source of information. There will be clues for anaemia, syndromes, facies, and a whole lot more. These will be dealt with in greater detail through the text.

Whilst examining a child, always keep an eye out for anything noteworthy. It may be a ventriculoperitoneal shunt, a pleural drain or a central venous catheter. These adjuncts are crucial that you do not miss them, for they will add up to the final diagnosis. As you perform a general survey, you should think through the positive points in your examination. At the end of your survey, chalk out a plan of the system which is likely to be affected. This may not be all that clear, so be prepared to examine a number of systems, often in a certain order.

Look for the following points in general survey:

PALLOR

Look for pallor with the **child facing sunlight** and not in a room lit by artificial light. Look at the lower palpebral conjunctiva, tip and dorsum of tongue, oral mucosa, creases of the palm and sole and the skin in general.

Table 2.1: Causes of pallor
• The "unwell" child
• Anaemia
• Shock states
• Nephrotic syndrome
• Congestive cardiac failure

It may sometimes be difficult to differentiate anaemia from other causes of pallor (Table 2.1). Pallor is also difficult to assess in the presence of icterus. Pallor due to anaemia may be graded roughly in clinical terms as mild, moderate, and severe:

- Mild—slightly less than normal
- Moderate—conjunctival capillaries appear prominent on a pale base
- Severe—capillaries appear as pale as those in the conjunctive; pallor evident in the palmar creases.

Icterus

Like pallor, **look for jaundice in daylight**. The sites are the sclera, palate, under surface of tongue, palms and soles. A lemon yellow tint indicates haemolytic anaemia; dark yellow or orange tint suggests obstructive jaundice (also look for scratch marks and shiny nails). In the neonate, discolouration of the face (= 5 mg/dl), trunk (= 10 mg/dl), knee onwards (15 mg/dl) and soles (20 mg/dl) gives a rough estimate (not to be relied on) of the degree of juandice.

Cyanosis

This is the bluish discolouration of the skin and mucous membrane due to the presence of reduced haemoglobin in the blood. Clinically cyanosis is present when the oxygen saturation is bellow 85 percent. Normal saturations are greater than 93 percent—a child who is cyanosed is at serious risk of hypoxia.

Types

a. *Central cyanosis (due to excessive oxygen desaturation of the arterial blood):* This is examined in all warm mucosal surfaces (and also peripheral sites). The common causes (Table 2.2) are:

Table 2.2: Central cyanosis—causes
Lung Causes
• Respiratory failure
• Pneumothorax
• Severe pneumonia
• Lobar collapse
Heart causes:
• Fallot's Tetralogy
• Persistent fetal circulation
• Transposition of great arteries
• Eisenmenger's syndrome
Abnormal Haemoglobins:
• Abnormal haemoglobins such as sulphalemoglobinaemia and methaemoglobinaemia also give rise to central cyanosis

b. *Peripheral cyanosis:* This occurs in the presence of normal arterial oxygen saturation (Table 2.3) and is due to pronounced oxygen desaturation of the venocapillary and capillary beds. Peripheral cyanois occurs in the tip of nose and nails, lips and ear lobules.

Table 2.3: Peripheral cyanosis
• Fever and rigor
• Cold exposure
• Shock
• Local vasomotor disturbance

In newborns, cyanosis of the acral parts (acrocyanosis) is common and is a variety of peripheral cyanosis. A number of neonates have "perioral cyanosis," due to prominent superficial venous plexuses in that region.

c. *Differential cyanosis:* It is as follows

- Hands blue, feet pink–Coarctation of aorta with transposition of great arteries
- Hands pink, feet blue–Patent ductus arteriosus with reversal of shunt due to pulmonary hypertension.

Pigmentation

Look for abnormal pigmentation on the face, back, spinal prominences, buccal mucosa, gums and on the palmar creases (Table 2.4).

Table 2.4: Pigmentation
• *Hyperpigmentation*
– Ethnic
– Mongolian spot
– Kwashiorkor
– Cafe-au-lait spots
– Polyposis coli
– Addison's disease
– Kala-azar
• *Hypopigmentation*
– Albinism
– Protein energy malnutrition
– Phenylketonuria
– Pityriasis versicolor
– Pityriasis alba

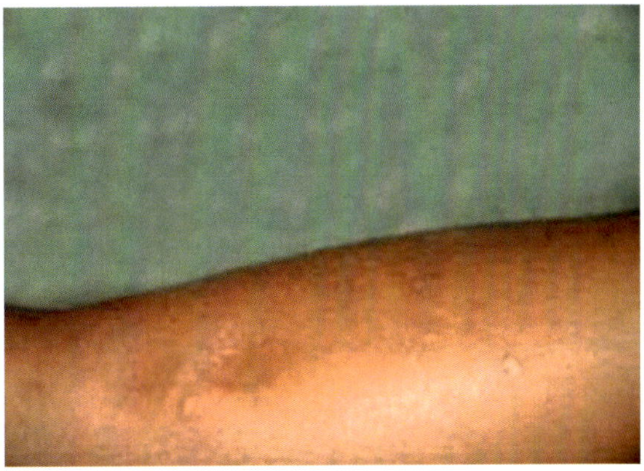

Fig. 2.1: Pitting oedema

Oedema

An excess of fluid in the subcutaneous tissue causing swelling of the tissues is known as oedema. The best place to examine for this is over the medial malleolus of the tibia. In the supine child, it may be more useful to examine over the sacral alae. Press over the area firmly with the ball of thumb for 20-30 seconds and allow a depression to form (if there is a swelling). Wait for the same duration of time and allow for the dimple to disappear. Palpate and make sure that the dimple persists (Fig. 2.1). Oedema due to fluid accumulation pits on pressure and the skin returns to its previous state when time is allowed. Oedema due to lymphatic obstruction does not pit on pressure (Table 2.5).

Table 2.5: Types of oedema
a. Generalized (Due to changes of hydrostatic pressure, osmolality or renal malfunction)
– Nephrotic syndrome
– Congestive cardiac failure
– Kwashiorkor
– Fulminant hepatic failure
– Cirrhosis
b. Localized (Due to local changes in capillary permeability)
– Angioneurotic oedema
– Urticaria
– Cellulitis

Clubbing (Figs 2.2A and B)

This physical sign is characterized by swelling of the terminal phalanges of the fingers and toes. The tissues at the base of the nail are thickened and the angle between the nail base and the adjacent skin of the finger is obliterated. The nail loses its longitudinal ridges and becomes convex from above downwards as well as from side to side. In extreme cases, the terminal segment of the finger becomes bulbous like a drumstick.

You can assess clubbing by different ways as follows:

i. Keep the nail bed at the level of the eye and look for the angle at the nail bed. Clubbing is present if this angle is lost. Once clubbing is established, you can test fluctuation. Stabilize the child's finger distally with your thumbs and steady the proximal phalangeal joint with the middle fingers. Test for fluctuation using your index fingers. Then test for subperiosteal thickening (hypertrophic pulmonary osteoarthropathy) by palpating the bones of the wrist and ankle.

ii. In normal nails, when both thumbnails are placed in apposition, there is a diamond shaped gap, which is obliterated in clubbing (Schamroth's window test) (Figs 2.2A and B).

iii. The comparison of the depth of the index finger at the base of the nail with its depth at the distal interphalangeal joint is a good method to recognize digital clubbing. The depth at the base of the nail is normally smaller. A depth at the nail base equal to that at the distal interphalangeal joint is

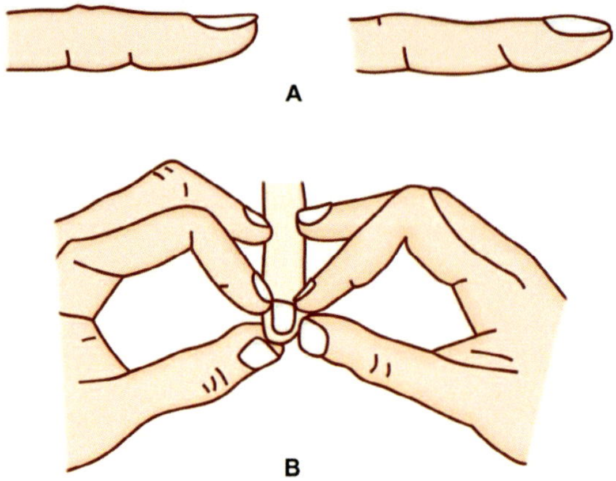

Figs 2.2A and B: Clubbing

said to be 2.5 standard deviations above normal.

Hypervascularity and opening of anastamotic channels in the nail bed occurs due to anoxic (Fallot's tetralogy), toxic (infective endocarditis) influences, alteration of local prostaglandin metabolism, growth factors and other unknown mechanisms. Clubbing is a slow process and is unlikely to be an acute event. You can use this information to judge if the process has been going on for some time. **Some clinicians grade clubbing but this is of little practical significance.** Say if clubbing is present or absent.

When commenting on clubbing, also make a note of cyanosis. You can home in on the diagnosis in a child who is cyanosed and also has clubbing. Familial clubbing is by far the commonest cause of clubbing in a well child. Compare with the hands of the parents in cases of confusion. Here are some other causes of clubbing that you may come across (Table 2.6).

Table 2.6: Causes of clubbing

- Cardiac
  - Cyanotic congenital heart disease
  - Infective endocarditis
- Pulmonary
  - Lung abscess
  - Bronchiectasis
  - Cystic fibrosis
  - Chronic lung disease
    - Empyema
    - Tuberculosis
  - Pleural mesothelioma
- Gastrointestinal
  - Coeliac disease
  - Inflammatory bowel disease
  - Polyposis coli
  - Chronic active hepatitis
- Others
  - Familial
  - Hodgkin lymphoma
  - Thyrotoxicosis

Decubitus

This is the posture of the patient in bed. This does not apply to infants and young children (who may be judged as to whether they are lying comfortably in the mother's lap or not).

Types

a. Of choice–comfortable in all positions.
b. Propped up–due to dyspnoea (congestive cardiac failure due to rheumatic valvular disease, pneumonia, bronchial asthma, huge ascites).
c. Trepopnoea–a child with pleural effusion and/or hydropneumothorax lies comfortably on the affected side (splints the hemithorax) and becomes dypnoeic if lies on the opposite side.
d. Curled up–biliary colic, meningitis.
e. Opisthotonus–kernicterus, tetanus, rabies, cerebral palsy.
f. Listless–encephalopathy.

Facies

This refers to the expression on the face of the child. Some diseases are thought to take on a typical facial appearance. It is more sensible to describe the appearance than label as a certain facies. For example, in a child with thalassaemia major, describe the (high cheekbones), maxillary protuberance and mild discolouration of the conjunctivae. It may also appear to be **insensitive to speak of a "Down's facies"** when you can convey the same information in your description of a rounded face, almond shaped eyes and protruding tongue. However, you should be familiar with some "typical" facies and their associations with syndromes or diseases. You should look out for the following possibilities:

i. Anxiety and apprehension may be due to pain, fear of the examiner or impending respiratory failure.
ii. A child with a vacant look who is not interacting with the environment may have severe learning difficulties and mental retardation.
iii. Down's syndrome–upward slant of eyes, prominent epicanthic fold, small nose, with depressed nasalbridge, wide palpebral fissures small oral cavity with fissured, protuberant tongue. In Down's syndrome the widest part is at the centre of the eye. This is in contrast to ethnic variants where the widest part is at the junction of middle and inner thirds (Fig. 2.3).
iv. "Hepatic facies"– shrunken eyes, hollowed out temporal fossa, pinched up nose, parched lips, muddy complexion and icteric tinge.
v. Thickened facial outlines (coarse features), wrinkling of eyebrows, thick tongue and a dull uninterested look suggest hypothyroidism or mucopolysaccharidosis.
vi. Moon face–steroid therapy, nephrotic syndrome, Cushing syndrome, pulmonary stenosis (Fig. 2.4).
vii. Facies of bilateral facial palsy (loss of facial expression) may occur with Guillain-Barre syndrome.
viii. Malar flush–high colour on the cheeks is said to be associated with mitral stenosis (an oestrogen effect, due to unmetabolized oestrogens in circulation)
ix. Risus sardonicus–raised eyebrows and drawn out angles of the mouth (tetanus).
x. Congenital cry facies–deviation of the angle of the mouth to one side due to an absent depressor anguli oris. A facial palsy needs to be excluded.
xi. Conotruncal facies–hypertelorism, narrow palpebral fissure, bloated eyelids, small mouth, deformed ear lobes. Examples are Fallot's tetralogy, transposition of great arteries and the chromosome 22-deletion syndromes (like di George syndrome).
xii. Haemolytic facies–pallor, prominent malar bones, depressed bridge of the nose, frontal bossing (Fig. 2.5).
xiii. Anhidrotic ectodermal dysplasia– frontal bossing, malar hypoplasia, recessing columella, lack of eyebrows, absent/conical teeth, wrinkled and hyperpigmentated periorbital skin.

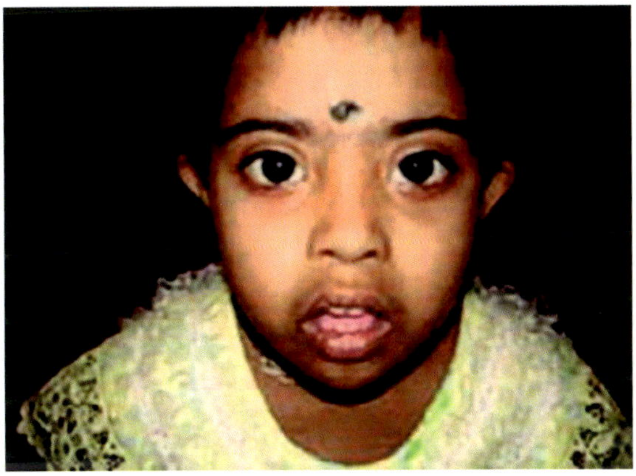

Fig. 2.3: Facies of Down syndrome

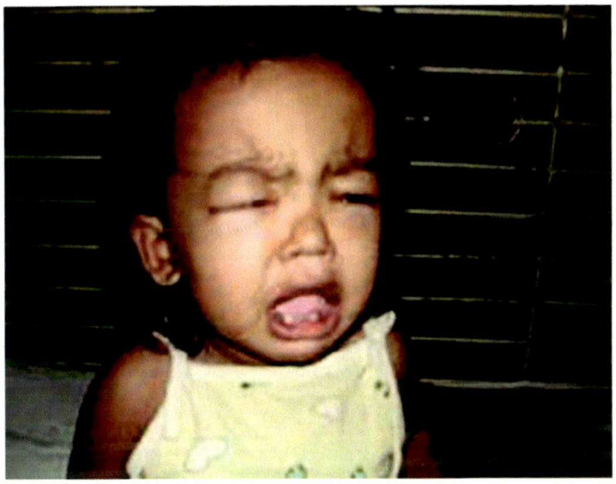

Fig. 2.4: Moon facies

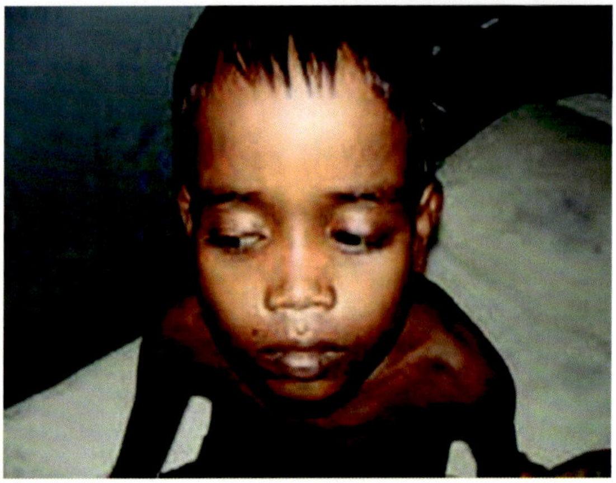

Fig. 2.5: Facies of haemolytic anaemia

xiv. Williams' syndrome–broad upper lip, small mandible, prominent maxilla, upturned nose and a "cocktail party chatter."

xv. Noonan's syndrome–triangular face, posteriorly rotated ears, ptosis, downslanting palpebral fissures, deep grooved philtrum.

xvi. Russell-Silver syndrome – triangular face, pseudohydrocephalic appearance, downturned corners of the mouth, lateral asymmetry.

Cry

Babies normally cry and this is not always a distress signal. With practise you will be able to differentiate the cry of a well baby from that of the sick newborn. The neonate with an infection has an irritable cry and may be difficult to console. He or she will not generally be pacified by measures like feeding. Irritable cry also occurs in other causes of cerebral irritation and painful conditions of the skeletal system (osteomyelitis, arthritis, periostitis).

A high-pitched shrill cry is heard in conditions of raised intracranial tension (like meningitis) and tetanus. Hoarse cry is a feature of hypothyroidism, laryngotracheobronchitis or left recurrent laryngeal nerve paralysis. A weak cry is heard in neuromuscular paralysis of the respiratory muscles as in diaphragmatic palsy. A cry is sometimes accompanied by stridor as in acute laryngotracheobronchitis.

Infants often hold their breath at the height of crying. They may go blue or white in what is described as a breath holding spell. A child with Tetralogy of Fallot (without repair) may end up with a cyanotic spell when crying.

Pulse

Pulse is the lateral expansion of the arterial wall imparted by the column of blood due to ventricular systole. Clinically there are different areas to feel for a pulse (Table 2.7) (Figs 2.6 and 2.6a). They are:

1. Radial pulse: Keep the child's forearm in slight pronation and wrist in mild flexion. Feel with the tips of 3 fingers of your hand, compressing the vessel against the bone of the radius.
2. Brachial pulse: It is felt just medial to the tendon of the biceps brachii in the lower part of the arm.
3. Carotid pulse: The carotid may be gently compressed against the transverse process of the cervical vertebrae. For quick localisation (as in a cardiac arrest), palpate the thyroid cartilage (the most prominent point in the neck) and slide the fingers down to the groove in front of the sternocleidomastoid. Care should be taken not to palpate both carotids simultaneously (danger of critically reducing cerebral arterial supply). It is good practice to palpate the carotid whilst listening to the heart. A carotid thrill with a murmur in the right second intercostal space is almost always an aortic stenosis.
4. Femoral pulse: The femoral arteries lie midway between the antero-superior iliac

Table 2.7: Pulses to check
1. Radial
2. Brachial
3. Carotid
4. Femoral
5. Popliteal
6. Post-tibial
7. Dorsalis pedis

spine and pubic tubercle. They are easily palpated against the underlying femur. Newborn femoral arteries should be routinely checked for coarctation of the aorta.

5. Popliteal pulse: They are not routinely checked and are difficult to detect. They are examined with the patient's knees flexed at an angle of 120 degrees. The fingertips of both hands are placed in the popliteal fossa, with the thumbs restng on the child's patellae.
6. Posterior tibial pulse: This is detected 1 cm behind the medial malleolus of the tibia.
7. Dorsal pedis pulse: You can feel this over the dorsum of the foot by compressing over the tarsal bones.

Once a pulse has been localized, make observations about the following (Table 2.8).

Table 2.8: Peripheral pulse

Presence or absence (palpability)

- Rate
- Rhythm
- Volume
- Tension
- Equality
- Delay
- Character

Palpability

When you feel for a pulse, be sure that you are not feeling the pulsation in the tips of your own fingers. Absence of a femoral pulse may signify coarctation of the aorta. Hypoplastic left heart syndromes may present with left outflow tract obstruction and absence of a femoral pulse. A child in shock may have a pulse that is difficult to palpate. In such a situation palpate a bigger vessel like the carotid artery. Absent femorals can also be iatrogenic - umbilical artery catheters can lead to ileal/femoral artery spasm or thrombosis.

Rate

Use one of the radial pulses to assess the rate. For the character and volume, we should examine the carotid artery, which is the closest pulse to the ascending aorta (the true arterial waveform may be modified as one moves to the periphery). The pulse rate is counted in beats per minute. Ensure that the child is relaxed (so as to eliminate tachycardia due to nervousness) and note the pulse for a full minute. In emergency situations, one minute is a luxury. A pragmatic way is to count beat for six seconds and multiply the figure by ten to arrive at the pulse rate in beats per minute.

Normal pulse rates for various ages are given in Table 2.9.

Table 2.9: Normal pulse rate

Age	*Pulse rate/min*
Newborn	100 - 170
<1 yr	80 - 160
2 yrs	80 - 130
4 yrs	80 - 120
6 yrs	75 - 100
8-10 yrs	70 - 90
Adolescent	55 - 90

Tachycardia is an unusually fast pulse rate when the rate exceeds the normal limits for age. Tachycardia is usually sinus tachycardia, as with anxiety or fever. Bradycardia is when there is unusual slowing of the heart rate. These can occur with heart blocks and conduction defects. There is some usage of a term called relative tachycardia. In this case the pulse rate rises by more than 10 beats per minute per degree rise of temperature (°C) e.g., in rheumatic carditis, thyrotoxicosis.

Rhythm

The pulse rhythm is either regular or irregular. If it is irregular, try to assess if it is completely irregular (the so called "irregularly irregular" pulse) or is there any pattern to the regularity. Commonly an entirely normal rhythm is occassionally interrupted by some slight irregularity. This occurs with atrial ectopics that may be conducted to the ventricles or premature ventricular beats (extrasystoles). The pulse of atrial fibrillation is completely irregular. Sinus arrythmia (heart rate increases with inspiration and decreases with expiration) is a normally occurring rhythm disturbance with no underlying heart condition.

Volume

The volume of a pulse gives an idea of the pulse pressure. Pulse pressure in turn depends on the stroke volume and compliance of the vessel wall. Low volume pulse is associated with shock, cardiomyopathy and significant aortic stenosis. High volume pulse occurs typically with fever or high output states like anaemia and thyrotoxicosis.

Tension

Feel the 'tension' of a pulse by rolling the artery and gauging the elasticity of its walls. However this is a very subjective test and has been largely replaced by the use of the sphygmomanometer. Blood pressure recording is a more reliable measurement of tension.

Equality

Compare both radial pulses for equality. Suspect a coarctation if a pulse is absent on one side. Some types of anastamoses (for a primary coarctation) leave an absent pulse. It is also common to find an absent pulse in a Blalock-Taussig shunt (not a modified shunt) on that side.

Delay

Compare the femorals with the radials to ascertain any radio-femoral delay. There should normally be no delay (in fact the femoral pulse arrives faster than the radial) unless there is any obstruction like a coarctation.

Character

Occasionally, a pulse is assigned a special character. To understand the character, let us first see what the normal arterial pulse looks like on a diagram.

Abnormalities of different parts of the waveform occur with different conditions (Table 2.10). They are:

Table 2.10: Abnormal pulses
1. Slow rising pulse
2. Hyperkinetic pulse
3. Bisferiens pulse
4. Dicrotic pulse
5. Pulsus alternans
6. Pulsus bigeminus
7. Pulsus paradoxus
8. Collapsing pulse

i. Slow rising pulse: There is slow upstroke with a delayed peak. The pulse in aortic stenosis is classically 'parvus et tardus' - a low volume and a prolonged systolic peak (Fig. 2.6b).
ii. Hyperkinetic pulse: There is a quick rise with good amplitude and is associated with an increased stroke volume (congenital heart block, anxiety, anaemia, fever, patent ductus arteriosus, aortic regurgitation) (Fig. 2.6c).
iii. Bisferiens pulse: There are 2 systolic peaks, as occurs in aortic regurgitation, with or without aortic stenosis. The first systolic peak is called the 'percussion wave.' A brief decline in pressure (mid-systolic increase of obstruction) is followed by a smaller, slow rising positive pulse wave (tidal wave). The latter is produced by continued ventricular ejection and reflected waves from the periphery (Fig. 2.6d).
iv. Dicrotic pulse: This is due to 2 palpable waves, one in systole, and another in diastole and occurs in those with low stroke volume, some adolescents, cardiac tamponade, severe heart failure and hypovolaemic shock (Fig. 2.6e).
v. Pulsus alternans: Alternating strong and weak pulse occurs in left ventricular failure. Unlike dicrotic pulse, each beat is

separate with no quantitative difference in systole and diastole (Fig. 2.6f).

vi. Pulsus bigeminus: Regular alteration of pressure pulse amplitude caused by premature ventricular contraction that follows each regular beat. The larger wave is followed by a small premature contraction and then by a pause. It usually occurs with digoxin toxicity or ischaemic states of the myocardium as in hypoxia.

vii. Pulsus paradoxus: It is an alteration of the decrease in systolic arterial pressure accompanying the reduced amplitude of the pulse that normally occurs during inspiration (pulsus normalis exaggeratus). Thus, a pulse is paradoxic if there is quickening during inspiration and slowing down in expiration. Some causes giving rise to a paradoxic pulse are:

- Rapidly developing pericardial effusion, cardiac tamponade
- Chronic constrictive pericarditis
- Restrictive cardiomyopathy
- Bronchial asthma
- Severe cardiac failure
- Superior mediastinal syndrome.

The mechanism of a paradoxic pulse is as follows. Normally, during inspiration, the right atrium is at a lower pressure and this sucks in blood from the vena cavae. At the same time the pulmonary veins dilate leading to a marginal decrease of left atrial volume. This in turn leads to lesser left ventricular filling. Thus, with inspiration there is a relative volume overload on the right compared with the left. As space is at a premium, bulging of the right side compresses the left side of the heart and decreases the left ventricular output even further. As cardiac output drops, blood pressure falls and there is a compensatory rise of pulse rate. The reverse takes place in expiration. In states of constrictive pericarditis or cardiac tamponade, the

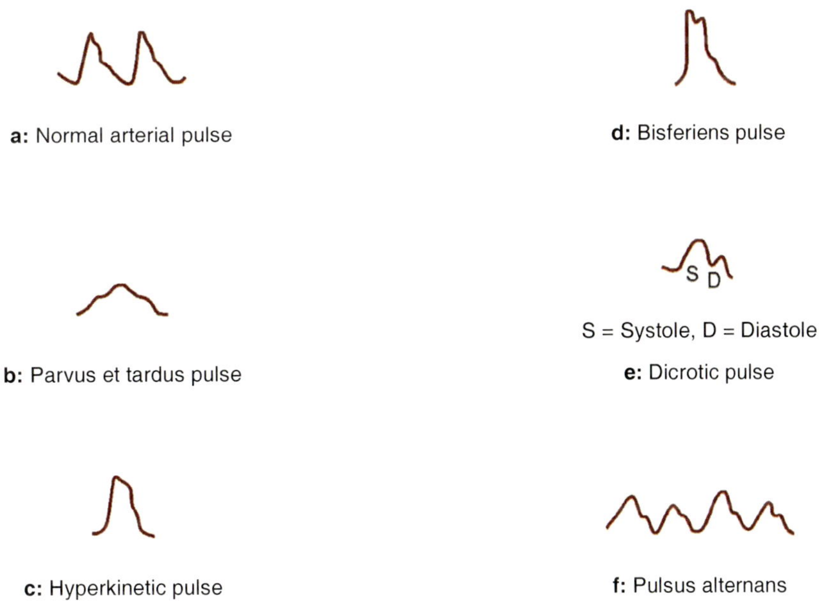

Fig. 2.6: Arterial pulse tracing

right ventricle further compresses the left ventricle, as the thickened pericardial sac allows no room to expand. In states of bronchial asthma, bronchiolitis, the negative intrathoraic pressure allows greater right atrial return and less of left atrial filling. Also hyperinflation stretches the pericardium resulting in a rise of intra-pericardial pressure.

Pulsus paradoxus can be effectively demonstrated using a sphygmomanometer. Ask the child (who has to cooperate) to breathe normally without exaggeration. Push up the mercury and then allow it fall. The first Korotkoff sound will be heard intermittently (varying with respiration). Note the first point and allow the mercury to fall until the first Korotkoff sound is heard continously. This will appear to be a "doubling" of the previous sounds heard. Note the pressure at this point. The difference between the two points noted is known as the pulsus paradoxus. A 10-20 mm Hg change is equivocal but a value of more than 20 mm Hg is suspicious of a significant aetiology.

viii. Collapsing (water-hammer) pulse: A collapsing pulse is characterized by a rapid upstroke and descent of the pulse wave. A water-hammer is a Victorian toy in the shape of a club. It contains half water and half vacuum. On inverting the toy, a sudden thud is felt on the palm due to the falling column of water. A similar feeling is obtained with a water-hammer pulse. Hold the child's wrist and feel the radial pulse with your palm at the finger bases. Then lift the hand upwards quickly. In the normal individual, the pulse appears feebler. In the high volume collapsing pulse, the pulse is felt to slow initially followed by an increased intensity.

Collapsing pulses can be of high volume or low volume. Highvolume collapsing pulse is caused by aortic regurgitation, patent ductus arteriosus, arterio-venous fistula and other conditions where there is a run-off of blood from one vessel to the other. Mitral regurgitation and ventricular septal defect can sometime give rise to low volume collapsing pulse.

The underlying mechanism of a high volume collapsing pulse is as follows. An increased stroke volume leads to the abrupt upstroke in the pulse wave. The collapsing character is a result of two factors: a diastolic run-off into the left ventricle, and a rapid run-off to the periphery because of low systemic vascular resistance.

In mitral regurgitation there is rapid run-off of blood into the left atrium. Similarly, blood flows into the right ventricle in a ventricular septal defect. In both instances there is rapid run-off without an increase in stroke volume. This leads to a low volume collapsing pulse.

PERFUSION

Capillary refill is a useful means of assessing skin perfusion. Press lightly for five seconds with the ball of the thumb in a central site, for example over the manubrium sterni. The area of the skin should blanch with pressure. Count how long it takes for the colour to return. The central capillary refill time should be less than two seconds. It may be prolonged if the child is underperfused from dehydration, septicaemia or cardiogenic shock. You may check capillary refill in the nailbeds, but do this only when you are certain that the child's circulation is intact and that the hands and feet are warm.

At the time that you check the child's capillary refill time, it is also useful to examine for the state of hydration. Check the skin turgor, mucous membranes and anterior fontanelle to estimate the state of hydration. Enquire if the child has passed urine–this gives you clues to the state of renal perfusion. Do also note if the child is alert and well orientated–a pointer for cerebral perfusion.

BLOOD PRESSURE

The blood pressure is recorded by a sphygmomanometer. An occlusion cuff is tied around the uper arm (right, by convention) and pressure in the manometer is increased. As the pressure is slowly reduced, Korot koff sounds are heard with the stethoscope over the brachial artery. The first sounds that occur (phase I) indicate the peak systolic pressure. The second and third phases are due to turbulent flow of blood through a partially occuluded vessel. The fourth phase occurs when the sounds become muffled and the fifth is when they disappear. The fifth phase corresponds more accurately to true diastolic pressure. These are following:

There should be some specifications that you should ensure.

i. Patient should be sitting or lying at ease.
ii. The manometer is placed so as to be at the same level as the cuff on the arm and the observer's eye.
iii. The cuff should be applied closely to the right upper arm, with the lower border not less than 2.5 cm from the cubital fossa.
iv. Cuff size should be correct for the arm. A narrow cuff will spuriously raise the blood pressure. A variety of sizes are available. The inflatable bag should be long enough to encircle the full circumference of the upper arm and should be of a width roughly equal to two-third of the arm length. For general use, cuffs are made as neonatal, infant, child and adult sizes.

You can use one of the many techniques of blood pressure measurement.

i. Palpatory method: Palpate the arterial pulse while the mercury in the manometer is allowed to fall. Note the point where there is a return of pulsation. This gives you the systolic blood pressure.
ii. Ausculatory method: Palpate the radial artery and inflate the cuff to a pressure of 30 mm Hg above the level at which the pulse can no longer be felt. Place the stethoscope lightly over the brachial artery and lower the pressure slowly. Listen carefully for the first sound, which indicates the systolic pressure. As you continue to lower the pressure, the sounds suddenly become faint and then disappear (diastolic pressure). The blood pressure should ideally be measured in the resting (static) and ambulatory phases. Record should also be kept of the blood pressure in the lower limb. This is useful in cases of suspected coarctation of the aorta. Tie the cuff over the thigh and auscultate the popliteal artery. Normally lower limb pressure is higher by 10-30 mm Hg in both systolic and diastolic pressures. This is due to the relatively smaller cuff size (trying to occlude the greater muscle bulk of the thigh). In coarcation, the recorded pressure is low and in aortic regurgitation it is higher by 40 mm Hg (Hill sign).
iii. Flush method: Squeeze the palm of the limb with the cuff tied on the same arm. Inflate the cuff while the pressure on the palm is maintained. The palm should look pale when you have the cuff inflated. Now reduce the pressure in the cuff slowly while observing for the first flush. The reading on the manometer at this point is somewhere between systolic and diastolic. This test can also be done by holding up the arm and applying a tight bandage from the hand up to the cuff and inflating. The bandage is then removed to reveal a white limb. The pressure is slowly reduced to note the point of first flush.
iv. Doppler: Automated oscillometric methods like "Dinamap" are a more convenient way of measuring blood pressure than the flush method. This is especially useful in neonates, where any of the above methods are unreliable (in the absence of an arterial catheter). This also comes in handy in continuous recording of blood pressure in an intensive care setting.
v. Invasive arterial recording: An arterial catheter is introduced and the arterial trace

recorded. A pressure transducer can then read off the systolic and diastolic pressure from the pressure wave. They are invaluable in umbilical or peripheral lines in sick newborns or ill children who may often need inotrope support.

For a quick calculation, the median (50th percentile) systolic blood pressure for children older than 1 year may be approximated by the formula 90 mm Hg + (2 × age in years). The corresponding diastolic blood pressure is 55 mm Hg + (2 × age in years). The lower limit (5th percentile) of systolic blood pressure (below which the child could well be in decompensated shock) is 70 mm Hg + (2 × age in years) (Table 2.11).

A child is said to have significant hypertension if the blood pressure is at or above the 95th centile for age. Blood pressure is normally about 2-5 mm Hg higher for boys than girls. Here are some figures from children in western children to denote hypertension (Table 2.12).

You may have noticed other uses of the sphygmomanometer apart from pure measurement of blood pressure. They are:

i. To detect orthostatic hypotension (Chap. 6, page 130).

ii. To detect pulsus paradoxus (see page 24).

iii. Hess test for thrombocytopenia/capillary fragility: Draw a 2.5 cm circle on the forearm and inflate a blood pressure cuff to a pressure between systolic and diastolic for 5 minutes. Normally less than 5-10 petechiae should erupt.

Table 2.11: A guide to the normal blood pressure values

	mm Hg
Birth (12 hours, less than 1000 g)	50/25
Birth (12 hours, 3 kg)	60/30
Neonate (96 hrs)	65/45
1 year	75/50
4 years	85/60
8 years	95/65
10 years	100/70

Table 2.12: Criteria for hypertension in western children

Age	*Blood pressure (mm Hg) at 95th centile*
Newborn	systolic 96
7 days	systolic 104
Child < 2 years	112/74
3-5 years	116/76
6-9 years	122/78
10-12 years	126/82

Respiration

Examine a child's respiration in the following categories:

- Rate
- Rhythm
- Depth
- Type
- Work of breathing
- Adventitious sounds
- Saturation.

Rate

Count the rate for a minute when the child has been at rest for a few minutes or whilst sleeping. Note also for rhythm, depth, position of discomfort, dypnoea, adventitious sounds, and odour in breath. The normal respiratory rates in children are given in Table 2.13.

Table 2.13: Normal respiratory rate in children

Age	*Respiration per minute*
Newborn	40-60
1-6 months	30-40
6 month - 2 years	20-30
Adolescents	12-20

Rhythm

Normal newborns (especially preterms) exhibit alternate periods of progressively deeper respiration until a pause is reached. This is known as periodic breathing. Cheyne-Stoke respiration is similar in older children with left ventricular failure or cerebral oedema. Biot's breathing is characterised by periods of apnoea alternating with 4-5 breaths of normal depth, and is associated with raised intracranial tension.

Depth

Shallow breathing is observed with ventilatory failure (narcotic overdose, cervical cord lesions). Rapid, deep breathing is seen in cases of metabolic acidosis (salicylate poisoning, diabetic ketoacidosis).

Type of Respiration

In older children, this is abdomino-thoracic. In newborns, the respiration is almost entirely diaphragmatic, and thus predominantly abdominal. During inspiration, the compliant chest wall is sucked in (instead of expanding) giving rise to 'paradoxic' breathing.

Work of Breathing

You should assess the effort it takes the child to breathe. The child without a respiratory problem has quiet breathing. The child with a chest infection has tachypnoea and has a noticeable effort in his breathing. Look at his or her chest for recessions–subcostal, intercostal and suprasternal. Check if the alae naesi are flaring. A child with severe acute asthma will often find it difficult to speak.

Adventitious Sounds

Sounds audible to normal ears are due to pathology in the upper airway (sniffling as in nasal obstruction, snaring noise of soft palate weakness, rattling sound of loose mucous in the trachea). The noise of stridor is typically inspiratory but in severe cases may be both inspiratory and expiratory. The expiratory noise of wheezing may also be audible in a child with asthma.

Wheezing is expiratory because the smaller airways collapse (patent in inspiration) during expiration forcing air through them. Stridor is inspiratory because the compliant subglottic tissue collapses due to negative pressure as a result of the air travelling through the narrow glottis at a high speed. On the other hand the distal airways (by virtue of the negative pressure of the pleural lining) cannot collapse and continue to expand. During expiration air is pushed out of the lungs but no pressure gradient exists for the subglottic tissues.

Adventitious sounds are suggestive of pathology but their absence should not make you assume normality. A child with a severe asthma may not shift enough air to wheeze. Similarly, a child who is seriously ill with epiglottitis may not produce an audible stridor.

Oxygen Saturation

Pulse oximetry is being used increasingly as bedside observation equipment. It incorporates the principle of the oxygen dissociation curve. A red and infra-red rich light source is used across an area rich in capillaries, like the pulp of the finger or the ear lobule. The light is then analysed at the other end after it passes through the tissue. Depending on the state of the oxygenation of haemoglobin in that tissue, certain parts of the red-rich light gets absorbed. What comes out at the receiving end of the probe is analysed by a microprocessor into a waveform. The machine then reads out a percentage of oxygen saturation.

Normal saturations are more than 93 percent. Saturations less than this indicate a degree of hypoxia but are rarely clinically detectable. Herein comes in the use of the pulse oximeter. It is a useful tool in any child with tachypnoea and increased work of breathing. However, you must be aware that oximetry does not record the partial pressure of oxygen and is not a substitute for monitoring blood gases. Saturations can give false readings if there is a motion artefact (moving probe) or improper signal quality (as in poor pickup from cold surfaces).

Temperature (Table 2.14)

Normal body temperature is considered to be between 36.6°C (97.7°F) and 37.2°C (99.0°F).

Table 2.14: The temperature ranges at different conditions

	Centigrade	Fahrenheit
Normal	36.6-37.2	98-99
Subnormal	< 36.6	< 98
Hypothermia	< 35	95
Febrile	> 37.2	> 99
Hyperpyrexia	> 41.6	> 107

When measuring temperature you should ensure:

i. The thermometer must be accurate. Mercury thermometers are the standard but sometimes cumbersome. Ear sensors are quick and reliable, provided they have been calibrated. Skin probes are handy in situations that demand a continous skin temperature (as in a child with shock) but cannot always be relied upon.
ii. Mercury thermometers must be kept in the oral cavity or under the axilla for 2-3 minutes. Ear thermometers (which measure core temperature to a degree) automatically read off when the signal is complete.
iii. Rectal temperatures (bulbous tip compared to the long tip of the oral thermometer) are to be taken carefully as the glass may break. Rectal temperatures are a useful method of measuring core temperature but may not always be practical. Remember that axillary temperature is less than the rectal temperature by 1°C, which in turn is less than the oral temperature by 0.5°C.
iv. Before inserting the thermometer, wash it with an antiseptic or in cold water and see that the mercury is well shaken down. Wash it again before replacing in its case.

In fever, the 'thermostatic' mechanism controlling heat gain and loss is set at a level higher than normal. While temperature is rising to this new level, heat is conserved, the skin vessels are constricted so that the body feels cold and the patient may shiver violently (rigor). When the higher temperature has been reached, heat loss becomes apparent, the skin vessels dilate and the body feels warm.

An infant with a high body temperature may be febrile or overheated. A febrile infant has a high set point temperature and behaves as if cold. Some infants can feel warm from a warm environment. In this situation he/she then makes an effort to lose that extra-heat. The clinical difference of the two is given in Table 2.15.

Table 2.15: Clinical difference of overheated and febrile infant

Overheated infant	Febrile infant
High rectal temperature	High rectal temperature
Warm hands and feet	Cold hands and feet
Abdominal exceeds hand skin temperature by less than 2°C	Abdominal exceeds hand skin temperature by more than 3°C
Pink skin	Pale skin
Extended posture	Lethargic
Healthy appearance	Looks unwell

There are textbook descriptions of fever—continued, remittent and intermittent. However, in practice the descriptions are less typical. Antipyretics will alter temperatures, especially if used on a regular basis. You should be more keen on describing the spikes and duration of fever than worry about the pattern it fits. The classical fever patterns are:

a. Continued: Fever does not fluctuate more than 1°C (1.5°F) during 24 hours, and at no time touches normal.
b. Remittent: Daily fluctuations exceed 2°C and does not touch the base line.
c. Intermittent: Fever present for several hours daily with return to normal. Three patterns of intermittent fever exist (and in connection with malaria) which are:
   - Quotidian: Paroxysm occurs daily
   - Tertian: Paroxysm occurs on alternate days.
   - Quartan: Paroxysm occurs every two days.

Fever may also be described in other ways.

i. Hectic: Temperature characterized by a great swing with return to normal, as in septicaemia, empyema.

ii. Crisis/lysis: A temperature falling quickly within 6-12 hours is known as crisis (lobar pneumonia). Alternately the fever subsides gradually over several days by lysis in infections untreated by antibiotics and in bronchopneumonia.

iii. Pel-Ebstein temperature: Regular alteration of recurrent bouts of pyrexia with a period of apyrexia (lymphomas).

iv. Relapsing fever: Characterised by cyclic periods of fever and normal temperatures (Borrelia recurrentis).

Jugular Venous Pressure (JVP)

The internal jugular vein is in direct communication with the right atrium and reflects pressure changes within the heart. The external jugular vein is more readily visible but is a less reliable means of predicting pressure changes in the right atrium. There are venous valves in the external jugular vein that do not allow accurate transmission of the pressure in the atria in the heart. Further the external jugular system passes through more fascial planes than the internal system and is more likely to be affected by extrinsic compression from other structures in the neck and upper thorax. In theory, therefore, the internal jugular venous pressure is an accurate marker of atrial venous pressure. However, the relatively short neck of infants makes detection of venous pulse extremely difficult in smaller children.

The venous pulse has 3 positive waves a, c and v and 2 negative waves (descents) x and y. The mechanisms of the individual waves are discussed in Table 2.16.

To examine the jugular venous pressure, adopt the following procedure. Make an incline of 45° on the bed with the examiner's hand/back rest and allow the child to recline on it. The neck should be supported so that the neck muscles, especially the sternocleidomastoids are relaxed. In normal children, the top of the venous column does not exceed 2 cm vertically above the sternal angle with the patient reclining at 45°. The sternal angle is taken as the reference point because the centre of the right atrium is at a depth of 5 cm from it in any position of the body. This means in a healthy child reclining at an angle of 45°, the mean level will be invisible. When reclining at a 90° angle the venous level should not be visible beyond the clavicle normally (Figs 2.7A to C).

If there is venous engorgement at the level of the middle of the neck at 45° inclinaton, or at the root of the neck at 90°, jugular venous pressure is likely to be elevated. The venous pulse will normally be exaggerated (but not beyond the lower third of the neck) when firm and gentle pressure is applied below the right costal arch (hepato-jugular reflux).

Note the vertical height of the pulsation above the sternal angle. Venous pulse is often confused with an arterial pulse. In general, the characteristics of a venous pulse are given in Table 2.17. They should help you distinguish true venous from arterial pulsations.

Table 2.16: Mechanisms of individual waves of JVP

a	Due to atrial contraction
c	Coincides with the onset of ventricular systole and results from the movement of the tricuspid valve ring into the right atrium as the right ventricular pressure rises
x	Due to atrial relaxation and downward displacement of the tricuspid value towards the apex of the right ventricle in systole
v	Due to passive rise in pressure as venous return to the atrium continues during ventricular systole whilst the tricuspid value is closed
y	As the tricuspid valve opens, blood enters the right ventricle rapidly and thus there is lowering of right atrial pressure

Table 2.17: Characteristics of jugular venous pulse

i. Soft, undulating, sinous
ii. Better seen in soft diffuse light e.g., a torch beam held tangentially across the neck
iii. Upper level falls with inspiration
iv. Changes with posture
v. y-descent is seen as a dominant inward motion (whereas the arterial pulse has an outward motion)

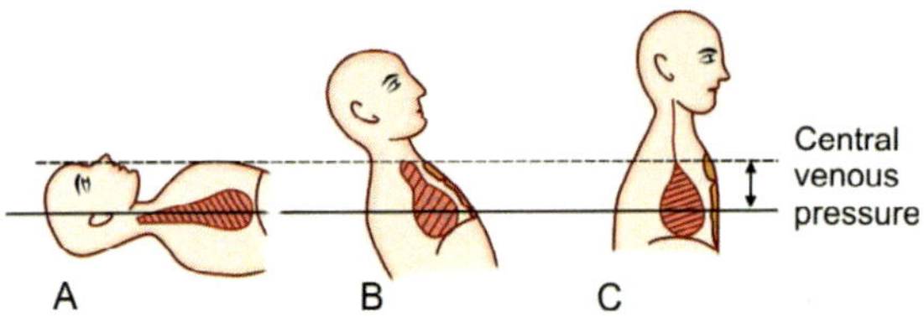

Figs 2.7A to C: (A) Jugular venous pressure in normal subject; (B) Reclining at 45°-point of transition between distended and collapsed vein; (C) Upright-upper part of vien collapsed and transition points obscured by sternum

The JVP can be elevated due a number of reasons. They are as follows:

i. Right heart failure
ii. Superior vena caval obstruction
iii. Pulmonary hypertension
iv. Tricuspid stenosis, atresia
v. Tricuspid regurgitation – A large c-v wave is formed by the regurgitation of blood into the right atrium during right ventricular systole. This wave is followed by a particularly prominent y descent.
vi. Complete heart block–Regular 'a' waves occur while carotid pulsation occurs at a slower independent rate. Occasionally atrial contraction occurs when the atrioventricular values are still closed, resulting in a 'canon wave.'
vii. Constrictive pericarditis (JVP raised, but not pulsatile).
viii. Cardiac tamponade (x descent only, no y descent).

Lymph Nodes

Examination of the lymph nodes is important in the context of infection and malignancy. Lymph nodes may be palpable due to minor abrasions or viral infections. A viral sore throat can give rise to large tonsillar nodes. A cut in the toes can track up to the inguinal nodes. To complete the picture, include a description of what you think are the possible causes of lymphadenopathy in the child. The palpable lymph node systems are given below:

i. *Cervical lymph nodes:* You can either examine from behind (with the neck slightly flexed) or from the front. The lymph node chains that you should palpate are: occipital and suboccipital, post auricular, anterior auricular, tonsillar, submandibular and submental groups, glands of the anterior and posterior triangles and lastly the supraclavicular group.
ii. *Axillary lymph nodes:* Raise the patient's arm and insert the examining hand high into the axilla. Lower the arm into a flexed position to rest across your examining arm. Palpate individually for anterior, posterior, medial, lateral and apical groups of lymph nodes. This is possible if only the child is not too ticklish.
iii. *Inguinal lymph glands:* These are found bilaterally along the groin creases. They are normally palpable (especially in children who go barefeet) and are likely to be of no significance on their own.
iv. *Other groups:* Epitrochlear (behind the medial condyle of the humerus), popliteal (back of the knee), retroperitoneal (deep palpation of the abdomen).

Lymph nodes are thought to be significant if the size of any of the lymph nodes (other than inguinal) is more than 1 cm in diameter. The corresponding size for the inguinal group is more than 1.5 cm. Lymphadenopathy can be localized or generalized. If two or more lymph node groups are enlarged, the term generalized lymphadenopathy is used. When you detect lymphadenopathy, look for the associated features:

1. Matted–Typically found in tuberculosis but may also be present in lymphoma, bacterial lymphadenitis and secondary deposits.
2. Mobility–Malignant nodes may be fixed to deeper structures. Any large adenopathy appears to immobile.

3. Tender, fluctuant, inflamed skin–These are the tell tale signs of lymphadenitis, with or without absess formation.
4. Draining areas–Commonly seborrhoea over scalp, poor oral hygiene, tonsillitis.

You should be wary of lymphadenopathy having a wider clinical significance. It is, therefore important to recognize the characteristics of lymph nodes when palpating them. Bear in mind the following diagnoses whenever you come across lymphadenopathy (Table 2.18).

You can consider lymphadenopathy to be either local or generalised. The causes for each of the categories are given in Table 2.19.

Thyroid

Inspect the neck for any general or local enlargement of the gland. The thyroid gland is normally sited just below the Adam's apple and should not be obviously visible in the healthy child. Sometimes it may be confused with fatty deposition in the same area. Not the thyroid as the child swallows—it should move up and down with swallowing. Palpate the gland if enlarged (minor degrees of enlargement are often better seen than felt). Comment on the following aspects of the thyroid gland:

a. Feel–solid, cystic, irregular.
b. Symmetry–enlarged on one side or smooth and symmetrical.
c. Pressure effects–difficulty of swallowing, hoarseness.
d. Abnormal site–ectopic thyroids are often lingual (look at the back of the tongue).
e. Associated features–exophthalmos, tachycardia, sweating, warmth (thyrotoxicosis), learning difficulties, lethargy, dry skin, delayed ankle reflex (hypothyroidism).

If you have hypo or hyperthyroidism as a possible diagnosis, do comment on the height and weight of the child. Hypothyroidism may lead to relative weight gain and poor growth. Hyperthyroidism can manifest itself as relative tall stature. Remember to check for medication before commenting on the state of the thyroid. Is the child taking thyroxine? Is he or she already on anti-thyroid medication like carbimazole?

Table 2.18: Important diagnoses associated with lymphadenopathy

- Leukaemia–generalised lymphadenopathy with pallor and bleeding
- Tuberculosis–"matted" nodes, failure to thrive and history of contact with TB
- Hodgkin lymphoma–isolated location, "rubbery" feel, fever, night sweats
- Kawasaki disease–marked cervical lymphadenopathy, fever, rash, mucositis, skin peeling

Table 2.19: Causes of localised and generalised lymphadenopathy

Causes of localised lymphadenopathy
- Local infection – throat, gums, hair follicles, wounds
- Lymphadenitis
- Atypical mycobacteria
- Hodgkin lymphoma
- Infectious mononucleosis

Causes of generalised lymphadenopathy
- Acute leukaemias
- Lymphomas
- Leishmaniasis
- Tuberculosis
- Autoimmune disorders
- HIV

Skin, Hair, Nails

Skin

Run your hand over the skin in general and look for dryness, pigmentation, scars, hydration and signs of nutritional deficiency. You need to define skin lesions according to the site, size, character and terminology. A useful description is given in Table 2.20.

In practice, it is not so easy to distinguish between petechiae and purpura. More often than not, a child with a bleeding disorder will have a combination of petechiae and purpura.

Hair

The pattern and distribution of hair is vital as an adjunct in coming to a diagnosis in many conditions. Look not only for scalp hair but also

Table 2.20: Skin lesions

Skin lesions	*Description*
Macule	Non-palpable area of altered colour
Papule	Palpable elevated area of skin < 0.5 cm
Plaque	Palpable discoid lesion > 2 cm
Nodule	Solid palpable lesion within the skin > 0.5 cm
Vesicle	Small fluid filled blister < 0.5 cm
Bulla	Large fluid filled blister > 0.5 cm
Pustule	Blister containing pus
Urticaria	Elevated lesion, reddish or white with red margin due to dermal oedema
Telangiectasia	Dilatation of superficial blood vessels, blanches on pressure
Petechiae	Subdermal bleed, size about 2 mm (pinhead)
Purpura	Subdermal bleed, size about 3 mm (larger than a pinhead)
Ecchymosis	Large extravasation of blood size >5 mm (bruise)

hair over the body and genitalia. You should be conversant with the Tanner staging of pubic and axillary hair in boys and girls. Hypertrichosis and hirsuitish are terms used to define excessive and abnormal hair growth, but they are not synonymous. Hirsutism is an androgen dependent male pattern of hair growth in females. The common sites of hirsutism are the moustache, sideburns, beard area and back (Table 2.21). Hypertrichosis is excessive hair growth in non-androgenic areas. Causes of hypertrichosis is given in Table 2.22.

Hypotrichosis is deficient hair growth, whereas hair loss (partial or complete) is called alopecia. Alopecia areata involves a patch of hair loss - if you look closely, you will find "exclamation mark" hairs in that part of the scalp. Tineasis, trichotillomania and idiopathic alopecia are generally cited as the reasons. Other causes of scanty hair (alopecia and hypotrichosis) are as follows (Table 2.23).

Nails

Nails are useful diagnostic markers in many chronic disorders. Look for clubbing, cyanosis, whitening, splinter haemorrhages and use the evidence to corroborate with your findings in other systems. It is often a good idea to use a magnifying glass to observe the nails. A handy clinical tool is the auroscope if you do not have a magnifying glass. You could describe nails as per Table 2.24.

Table 2.21: Causes of hirsutism

Gonadal
- Polycystic ovary syndrome
- Ovarian tumour

Adrenal
- Cushing syndrome
- Congenital adrenal hyperplasia
- Adrenal tumour

Drugs
- Minoxidil, Phenytoin
- Danazol, androgenic steroids, oral contraceptives
- Acetazolamide, penicillamine, phenothiazines

Congenital
- Trisomy 18
- Corelia de Lange syndrome
- Hurler syndrome
- Hypothyroidism

Table 2.22: Causes of hypertrichosis

Intrinsic factors
- Ethnic, familial traits

Extrinsic factors
- Local trauma
- Malnutrition
- Anorexia nervosa
- Phenytoin, corticosteroids, minoxidil, psoralen, penicillamine, streptomycin

Naevi
- Congenital pigmented naevi, hamartomas

Congenital disorders
- Mucopolysaaccharidoses
- Cornelia de Lange syndrome
- Lipodystrophy
- Hemihypertrophy
- Fetal hydantion and alcohol syndromes
- Trisomy 18
- Porphyrias

REGIONAL EXAMINATION

Head

Record the head circumference using standard methods outlined (see anthropometry). An

Table 2.23: Causes of alopecia

From birth/inherited
- Autosomal recessive anomaly, ectodermal dysplasia, Moynahan syndrome, aplasia cutis, epidermal naevus, progeria, hereditary hypotrichosis, keratosis pilaris, phenylketonuria, Menkes kinky hair syndrome, dyskeratosis congenita, Seckel dwarf, cartilage-hair hypoplasia, incontinentia pigmenti, Treacher-Collins syndrome

Endocrine
- Hypopituitarism, hypothyroidism, hypoparathyroidism, diabetes

Nutritional
- Protein energy malnutrition, iron and zinc deficiency, essential fatty acid deficiency, gluten-sensitive enteropathy

Toxic
- Cytotoxic chemotherapy, radiation therapy, heparin, hypervitaminosis A

Auto immune
- Alopecia areata, dermatomyositis

Traumatic
- Traction, trichotillomania

Cicatricial
- Lupus erythematosus, dermatomyositis, tinea, cicatricial pemphigoid, acne, leishmaniasis
- Trichodystrophies
- Trichorrhexis nodosa, pili torti, pili annulati

abnormally big head is called macrocephaly. Similarly, microcephaly is a head circumference that is small by 3 standard deviations from the expected normal for age and sex (use a head circumference growth chart). Common causes are described in Table 2.25.

There are many abnormal head shapes, not all of which are related to disease conditions (Fig. 2.8). The flat occiput of plagiocephaly, where the skull seems asymmetrical is a normal variant in infants. Plagiocephaly is commoner nowadays because of the advice given to mothers to lay their babies on the back (the "Back to Sleep" campaign to prevent cot death). Plagiocephaly, however, can also be related to craniosynostosis that needs surgical intervention. Palpate the sutures to see if they have fused prematurely in craniosynostosis. Overriding of the skull bones may lead you to believe that there is prominence of a suture. Check if the head circumference is small and if the anterior fontanelle is closed. If normal, it is unlikely to be a fusion problem. Look for clues that will point you in the right direction. The abnormality may be the result of a localised swelling like a cephalhaematoma, a dermoid or an abscess. Search for surgical scars and ventriculo-peritoneal shunts. Some abnormalities that should alert to you a serious problem are given in Table 2.26.

Table 2.24: Different types of nail and its causes

Small/absent–Ectodermal dysplasia, nail-patella syndrome, cartilage-hair hypoplasia, incontinentia pigmenti, trisomy 13, trisomy 18, Turner syndrome, fetal hydantoin and alcohol syndromes
Large–Hemihypertrophy, Rubenstein-Taybi syndrome, pachyonychia congenita
White nails–Trauma, pallor, cirrhosis, hypoalbuminaemia, tuberculosis, chronic arsenic poisoning, malignancies
Terry nails (white nail, with distal normal pink colour) – Hypoalbuminaemia of cirrhosis
Muehrcke lines (parallel white bands)–Hypoalbuminaemia
Lindsay nails (proximal part white, distal part pigmented) –normal variant, renal failure
Onycholysis (separation from nail bed)–Trauma, fungal infection, psoriasis, contact dermatitis, vincristine, bleomycin, chloramphenicol
Pitting–Psoriasis, alopecia areata, dermatitis, fungal infections
Beau lines (transverse grooves in nail plate)–Systemic disease (chronic illnesses), zinc deficiency (acrodermatitis enteropathica)
Pigmentation–Lichen planus, black and Asian children (melanonychia striata)
Green pigmentation–Pseudomonas infection of nail
Yellow nails–Icterus, carotinaemia, yellow nail syndrome
Azure half moons–Wilson's disease
Red half moons–Chronic renal failure
Splinter haemorrhages–Minor trauma, dermatomyositis, infective endocarditis, vasculitis, peptic ulcer disease, hypertension, chronic glomerulonephritis, cirrhosis, scurvy, neoplasms
Clubbing–See section on clubbing

Fontanelles

There are 6 fontanelles at birth, all of which may or may not be palpable. The most important ones are the anterior and posterior fontanelles. The fontanelles may be measured by joining the mid points of the 4 sides to form 2 diameters.

Table 2.25: Abnormal head circumferences

Microcephaly
- Primary
  - Autosomal recessive
  - Autosomal dominant
  - Trisomies
  - Cornelia de Lange syndrome
  - Smith Lemli Opitz syndrome
- Secondary
  - Intrauterine infections–CMV, Rubella, toxoplasmosis
  - Neuronal injury from meningitis, encephalitis, perinatal hypoxia
  - Malnutrition
  - Fetal alcohol syndrome

Macrocephaly
- Hydrocephalus, hydranencephaly
- Cranial thickening–Chronic anaemia, rickets, osteogenesis imperfecta
- Subdural effusion–Secondary to meningitis, non-accidental injury
- Metabolic–Mucopolysaccharidosis, Tay-Sachs, Alexander disease
- Sotos syndrome
- Neurofibromatosis

Table 2.26: Abnormal head shapes

- Dolicho/scaphocephaly–Head elongated in the anteroposterior diameter (children born prematurely)
- Prominent occiput (trisomy 18)
- Frontal bossing (thalassaemia, rickets, Hurler's syndrome, hydrocephlaus, malnutrition)
- Acrocephaly/oxycephaly/turricephaly – conical head (Apert's syndrome)
- Brachycephaly–Anteroposterior flattening (Down's syndrome)
- Trigonocephaly–Pointed metopic suture (craniosynostosis)
- Caput quadrantum–hot cross bun appearance (rickets)

The anterior fontanelle usually measures 2.5 cm × 2.5 cm at 3 months and closes by 9-18 months of age. The posterior fontanelle is small at birth (usually the size of a fingertip) and closes rapidly by 6 weeks of age.

It is best to examine the fontanelle when the baby is quiet and the head upright. You may find a bulge if he/she is crying and in the lying position. In such instances, change position and re-examine. You should always worry if the fontanelle feels tense and bulging in which case

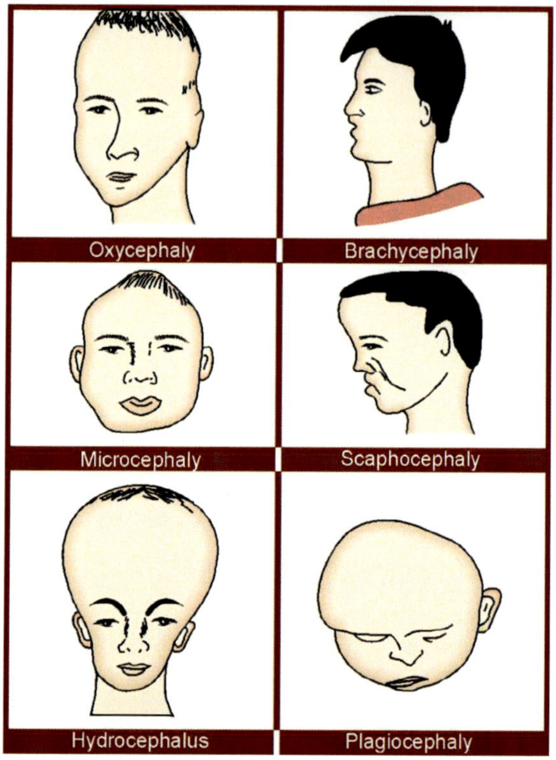

Fig. 2.8: Different types of abnormal head shapes: oxycephaly, brachycephaly, macrocephaly, scaphocephaly, hydrocephalus, plagiocephaly

meningitis needs to be considered. Some conditions give rise to a wide anterior fontanelle. Common causes are hydrocephalus, achondroplasia, prematurity, osteogenesis imperfecta, trisomies and vitamin D deficiency rickets.

Normally, a fontanelle is pulsatile because of transmitted pulsation of the CSF secretion from the choroid plexus. In raised intracranial tension, the normal pulsation is lost. The fontanelle then appears to be abnormally "full" and tense. Contrast the depressed fontanelle that you see in a child with significant dehydration.

Scalp

We discussed about the significance of hair in the chapter headed "skin, hair, nails." Here are a few additional features of scalp hair that you could comment in Table 2.27.

Table 2.27: Scalp hair

Colour

The colour of hair is genetically determined. Some conditions like phenylketonuria, albinism lead to uniformly hypopigmented hair. Children with kwashiorkor have alternating periods of relatively improved nutrition and this gives rise to an alternating pattern of hypopigmentation called the 'flag sign.' Partial hypopigmentation of the hair may also be found in Wardenberg, syndrome, Chediak-Higashi syndrome and pili anulati.

Texture

Fine thin hair is a feature of homocytinuria and Weaver's syndrome. Dry coarse hair is found in hypothyroidism and fetal alcohol syndrome.

Curled hair

This hair is an Afro-Caribbean characteristic, but twisted hair along its long axis (pili torti) along with fragility is found in Menkes syndrome.

Beaded appearance

This may be due to constriction at regular intervals (monilethrix) and nodular swellings along the shaft (trichorrhexis nodosa). More commonly look for lice and nits if the hair appears beaded.

Aberrant pattern

The normal pattern is characterized by a parietal whorl, located anterior to the position of the posterior fontanelle, from which the hair stream progresses outward covering the extent of scalp hair. Usually a single whorl is present to the left of the midline. Abnormal patterns are:

1. Absent parietal whorl or location more central or posterior (microcephaly)
2. Low hairline, often related to a short or webbed neck (Turner syndrome, Klippel-Feil anomaly)
3. Excess projection of hair into cheek (Treacher-Collins syndrome)

Run your hand through the child's hair and look under the hair for any scalp abnormalities. You may pick up scars from neurosurgical procedures that lie neatly hidden under locks of hair. You may also palpate the tube coming out of a ventriculoperitoneal (VP) shunt. Here are some abnormalities which you may come across in your examination (Table 2.28).

Table 2.28: Scalp abnormalities

a. Caput succedaneum–Diffuse, boggy, soft swelling of the scalp that disappears by the end of the first or second day
b. Scalp abscess, pyoderma
c. Seborrheic dermatitis (cradle cap)–Adherent scales and crusts that are large, moist, greasy and dirty yellow
d. Mastocytosis–Small brown to scales, crusting and petechial lesions
e. Distension of the scalp veins associated with raised intracranial tension
f. Scalp defects as in focal dermal hypoplasia, incontinentia pigmenti, Wolf-Hirschhorn syndrome
g. Subcutaneous nodules over occipital areas - rheumatic fever or rheumatoid arthritis
h. Cutis verticis gyrata–Characterized by 10-12 (1-2 cm thick) anteroposterior or transverse gyrate folds, often accompanied by mental retardation

Forehead

You may want to describe the forehead when commenting of the face of the child. This is particularly important when you are dealing with dysmorphic syndromes. Look carefully at the size and shape of the forehead and comment on the frontal hairline. Vertical height of the forehead is increased in hydrocephalus, Crouzon's disease and Apert's syndrome. A pointed forehead is seen in trigonocephaly and midline brain defects. Low frontal hairline is common in Hurler's syndrome, de Lange's syndrome and is often a feature in children with severe learning difficulties.

In a child with a large forehead and suspected hydrocephalus you could percuss for a "crackpot" sign (MacEwan's sign), which feels like a crumbling eggshell under your fingers. The sign is positive when sutures are separated due to raised intracranial tension. It is physiologically present during infancy as long as the anterior fontanelle is open.

Translucency is a test for subdural effusion, hydrocephalus, hydranencephaly and porencephaly. Use a flashlight, preferably with rubber foam encircling the end, and place it snugly over the frontal and occipital areas in a dark room. Look for a rim of translucency extending beyond 2.5 cm in frontal area and over 1 cm in the occipital region.

Intracranial bruit may be auscultated over the scalp. It may be present in 10 percent of normal children, some conditions of raised intracranial tension and artriovenous malformations. If you see a child with cardiovascular features of high output failure but no obvious lesion, it is good practice to put the stethoscope over the scalp. An A-V malformation involving the vein of Galen is a noteworthy example.

Neck

Children normally have relatively shorter necks compared to adults. A neck length (occipital protruberance to the C7 vertebral spine) of less than 1/13 of the occiput-heel length is defined as a short neck in children. Shortness of the neck in clinical practice is, however, a subjective term. The neck may appear short in webbing due to Turner syndrome. Short neck occurs in children with vertebral anomalies, platybasia and Klippel-Feil deformity. Other causes include chondrodystrophic congenital calicification, hypothyroidism, Sprengel deformity, Goldenhar, Hurler and Morquio syndromes.

The neck is a midline structure, but appears to be positioned to one side in a child with tortiocollis. To differentiate between tilting and tortiollis have the child lie on his back and examine from the head end of the table. In torticollis, the occiput is tilted to one side and the chin tilted to the other. In head tilting both the occiput and chin are tilted to the same side. Sternomastoid tumours commonly present with torticollis. In opisthotonus (tetanus, dystonic cerebral palsy) the occiput is tilted markedly backward. Neuromuscular disorders with altered curvature of the spine may also affect the appearance of the neck. In Caries spine, the child holds his neck stiff and walks carefully avoiding jarring movements.

Look out for any abnormality that catches your eye. There may be lymph node enlargement, thyroid swelling, thyroglossal cyst, branchial cyst or fistula. Branchial fistulas are located in the lower part of the neck and thyroglossal fistula situated higher up in the upper third of the neck. Observe if the carotids are 'dancing' and if there is a thrill or a venous hum. If there is a swelling, ascertain if it arises from a lymph node, muscle, bone or the skin.

Eyes

The eyes are a storehouse of information and you should reserve considerable time and effort in the eye examination. Whilst talking to or observing the child you may have picked up some features like squints, epicanthic folds or abnormal pigmentation. Make a mental note of these findings and correlate them when you test the eyes more formally.

It may be easier to **have a system** whereby you test all aspects of the eye in sequential fashion. A system is handy for practical purposes as it will enable you to cover most aspects the examination. With practice you should do this quickly and accurately. Before commencing your systematic examination you should make sure that the child can see well, otherwise it is meaningless to give him/her a command. To do this, use a Snellen chart to test visual acuity in children older than seven years (and possibly adapted to a local vernacular). In the absence of a formal chart, roughly test for visual acuity by asking the child to count the number of rails (at a distance) or the number of fingers (near vision). Also satisfy yourself that the child has some sense of colours. The Ishihara chart is not standardized for children less than 11 years, so it is not helpful in those younger. Use common primary colours on dresses, books, etc and ask the child "what colour is this?" This question presumes that the child's development is appropiate to understand the command.

Look carefully at the eyes and note if they are normally spaced out. Are they too far apart or are they too close to each other? Is there any obvious squint (manifest squint)? Is there any abnormality of the palpable fissure, eyelid, conjunctivae, cornea or iris? Do the eyes move equally in all directions? Is one eye completely static in movement in all directions (glass eye)?

Comment on all visible structures in each eye and say if they are normal. Next use a pen torch and use it from a distance. The light should fall equally (almost) on the pupils of both eyes. This is known as corneal reflection. If the spot of light appears wide of the centre, a squint is likely. Do the cover-uncover test if there is any suspicion. Bring the light to one eye (whilst you put the ulnar aspect of your hand over the nose to prevent light getting into the other eye) and observe for direct and consensual light reflexes. Repeat the same with the other eye. Move back and ask the child to follow the light source. You are now testing for extra-ocular muscle movement. Let the child know what you are about to do and encourage him/he to say if he/she sees double (diplopia) at any point. Define (with your pen torch) movements in vertical, horizontal, temporal and nasal directions in the shape of an "H" or an "X." Observe for nystagmus and corroborate with symptoms of diplopia. You should also be able to watch for signs of lid lag or ptosis.

You could now test for field of vision. Sit in front of the child (at one metre distance) with one eye closed. Use the child's own hand (or the parent's) to cover his/her corresponding eye (opposite to you). Keep the head still and encourage fixing his/her eye on your nose. Do the same for yourself. Wiggle your finger and bring it from outside inwards and compare against your own field of vision. Make a game of this to see if the child can see better than you can. Test in different directions and for each eye separately. Lastly use the ophthalmoscope to see the fundi of both eyes (see chapter on neurology). You should have by now assessed the 2nd, 3rd, 4th and 6th cranial nerves, while also commenting on the structural aspects.

Let us now discuss a few abnormalities that you are likely to encounter.

a. Palpebral fissure length - Hold a ruler across the eye's greatest horizontal axis from the medial to lateral canthus. At 40 weeks gestation the palpebral lengths are 1.85 +/– 0.13 cm (whites), 2.00 +/– 0.22 cm (blacks) or 1.95 +/– 0.20 cm (Hispanics). Local data in Indian children is not available but these figures should give you a rough guide of what to expect. Short palbebral fissures are found in the fetal alcohol, William's, whistling face syndromes and with microphthalmia.
b. Squint, ptosis–Discussed in neurological examination.
c. Eyepopping–When an examining light is removed, some infants show a transient widening of the palpebral fissure.
d. Colobomas (gap or discontinuity of a structure) of eyelids–Lower eyelid colobomas occur in Treacher Collins syndrome whilst those with upper lid defects occur in Goldenhar syndrome.
e. Excessive blinking–Eye strain, tic
f. Belpharospasm–Congenital glaucoma, corneal ulceration, conjuctivitis, keratitis
g. Upward slant of eyes–Down, Zellweger, Aarskog syndrome
h. Downward slant of eyes–Treacher-Collins, whistling face, cri-du-chat, Pfeiffer and 10p deletion syndromes
i. Hordeolum (stye), chalazion (meibomian cyst), haemangioma, dermoid cyst
j. Eyelashes–Absent in premature babies, Treacher Collins syndrome (inner 2/3 of lower lid). Long eyelashes can be inherited or are associated with chronically ill children and in those with Cornelia de Lange syndrome. Pediculosis can occur in the eyelashes. Hypopigmented eyelashes (in non-Caucasians) occur with albinism and uveomeningitis.
k. Eyebrows–May be absent in premature babies and appears less in amount in cartilage hair hypoplasia and Hallerman-Streiff syndromes. Eyebrows are bushy in Hurler syndrome and meet in the midline (synophrys) in de Lange and Waardenburg syndromes. Hypertrichosis of eyebrows can be present with hypotrichosis of scalp in the Coffin-Siris syndrome.

l. Swelling around eyes–Slight puffiness of the eyes and dark circles may be seen in those with nasal allergy (allergic shiners).

m. Lid oedema–Conjunctivitis, pertussis, measles, infectious mononucleosis, acute nephritis

n. Epicanthus–A fold of skin extending down from the upper lid to cover the medial canthus of the eye may be noted in normal newborns and disappears in 1-3 months. Prominent epicanthic folds occur with Down syndrome, congenital ptosis and Pompe's disease. Epicanthic folds can also occur in a variety of syndromes include the cerebro-hepatorenal, cri-du-chat, de Lange, fetal alcohol, fetal hydantion, leopard, Mobius, Noonan, Turner, Smith-Lemli-Opitz, Patau, Williams and Potter syndromes.

o. Spacing–Spacing between the eyes are estimated, but to confirm hypertelorism (wide spacing) or hypotelorism (close spacing), you should take measurements. The interpupillary distance is the best indicator of ocular hypertelorism (with the exception of the Waardenberg syndrome). It is hard to measure interpupillary distance particularly in infants. You may obtain special graphs to plot the distance between inner and outer canthi in different ages.

You could think of ocular hypertelorism as putting a third eye between the eyes. Some causes of hypertelorism are: Apert, Aarskog, Sotos, cerebrohepatorenal, chromosome 4p deletion, cri du chat, Crouzon, di George, fetal hydantion, Noonan, orofaciodigital, whistling face, Williams and Turner syndromes. Ocular hypotelorism occurs in arhinencephaly, cyclopia and holoprosencephaly.

p. Tearing–Epiphora (excessive tearing) is found is conjunctivitis, corneal ulcer, nasolacrimal duct obstruction, allergic reaction and exophthalmos. Absence of tears occurs in the familial dysautonomia syndrome.

Table 2.29: Conjunctival lesions

- Subconjunctival haemorrhage–pertussis, trauma, toxic shock syndrome, haemorrhagic diseases, Henoch Schonlein purpura, post normal delivery in neonates
- Conjunctivitis–infective, allergic, phlyctenular
- Conjunctival xerosis–vitamin A deficiency
- Pinguecula–elevated, yellowish lesion that extends from the outer canthus: occurs in Gaucher's disease.
- Pterygium–triangular membranous fold (whose apex involves the cornea, the base being continuous with the conjunctiva) is often the result of exposure to wind, dust and sun
- Epibulbar dermoids–Goldenhar syndrome

q. Conjunctival lesions–You should look for the following lesions given in Table 2.29.

r. Sclera–Sclera of infants and young children are normally bluish. Pathological states with blue sclerae are the following: Osteogenesis imperfecta, congenital glaucoma, Russel-Silver syndrome, Ehlers-Danlos syndrome, Marfan syndrome, melanin deposits (naevi/freckles).

s. Cornea–The cornea in newborn infants has a diameter of 9-10 mm. Megalocornea (>13 mm) occurs in hereditary abnormal eye enlargement and congenital glaucoma. The cornea is normally clear but can be clouded in a number of metabolic disorders like Hurler, Morquio, Scheie and Maroteaux-Lamy syndromes, GM1 gangliosidosis, mannosidosis, mucolipidosis, tyrosinosis as well as in interstitial keratitis (congenital syphilis). Corneal ulceration is a feature of keratomalacia (vitamin A deficiency) and herpes simplex (dendritic ulcer). Loss of corneal sensation occurs with familial dysautonomia. A ring called the corneal arcus is often present by age ten in those with familial hypercholesterolaemia. The Kayser-Fleischer ring associated with Wilson disease is characteristically different (Table 2.30). It is unilateral or bilateral, complete or incomplete, golden brown or greyish-green ring at the limbus of the cornea. KF rings may also be seen in some familial cholestatic syndromes and in chronic active hepatitis with cirrhosis. It may not be obvious to the naked eye and you, therefore, should use a slit lamp to visualize this.

Table 2.30: A few corneal abnormalities

Megalocornea	Corneal Arcus
Clouded	KF ring
Ulceration	
Loss of sensation	

t. Lens–Any opacity of the lens is called a cataract. A red fundal reflex surounds the opaque density if the cataract is not complete. Congenital cataracts are associated with TORCH infections, galactosaemia, homocystinuria, hypoparathyroidism, aspartyl glycosaminuria, osteopetrosis, Refsum syndrome, cerebro-hepato-renal syndrome, Marfan syndrome, incontinentia pigmenti, trisomies and the Smith Lemli Optiz syndrome. Cataracts can be inherited as an autosomal dominant condition. Radiation therapy, hypoparathyroidism and long-term steroid use are also common offenders.

u. Retrolental membranes–Retinopathy of prematurity, persistent hyperplastic primary vitreous, persistent pupillary membrane, retinal dysplasia.

v. Uveal tract–The only part of the uveal tract that you can see is the iris. Isolated abnormalities of the iris are rare in children and you should, therefore, consider in your mind the following pathologies given in Table 2.31.

w. Retina (Chap. 6).

x. Strabismus, diplopia, opsoclonus, nystagmus (Chap. 6, page 104-107).

Table 2.31: Iris abnormalities and pathologies

1. Ciliary infection – usually associated with uveitis and iridocyclitis. The iris may also appear dull and discoloured and sluggishly reacting. Slit lamp shows keratitic precipitates and cloudy appearance of the aqueous humour. Common conditions are pauciarticular juvenile chronic arthritis, tuberculosis, inflammatory bowel disease, Reiter disease, sarcoidosis and Vogt-Koyanagi-Harada syndrome.
2. Hypopigmented iris in albinism, Chediak Higashi syndrome
3. 'Salt and pepper' speckling of the iris (Brushfield spots) in Down syndrome
4. Iris nodules (Lisch nodules) in Neurofibromatosis
5. Heterochromia–Hetrochromic iridocyclitis of Fuchs, Waardenburg syndrome
6. Iridodonesis (quivering movement of the iris)–Homocystinuria, Marfan's syndrome
7. Iris coloboma–Autosomal disorder, trisomy 13, focal dermal hypoplasia, CHARGE associations, Wolf-Hirschhorn syndrome
8. Aniridia–Autosomal dominant, association of Wilm's tumour, Rieger anomaly

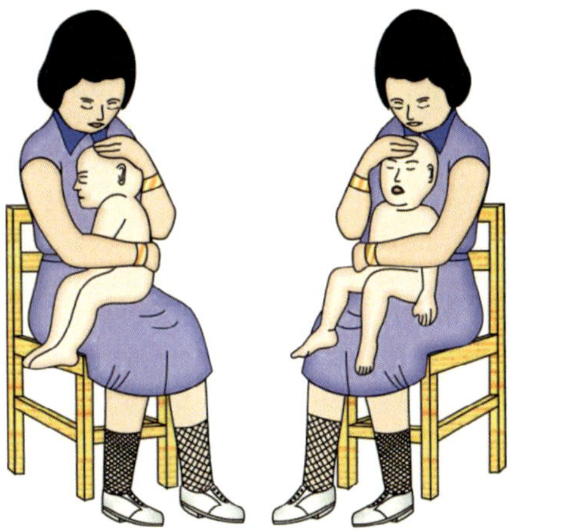

Fig. 2.9A: Position for examination of ear and throat

Ears (Fig. 2.9A)

1. Hearing - See section on neurology
2. Pinna - In the premature infant the cartilage is not fully developed. The pinna lies flat against the scalp with only slight incurving of the superior part at 33-34 weeks gestation. By 36 weeks gestation, the pinna springs back after folding. Incurving occurs in two-thirds of the ear by 38-40 weeks gestation. The anatomic landmarks of the fully developed ear pinna are shown in Figures 2.9A and B.

The external ear is often abnormal and "simple" in the dysmorphic child (Figs 2.9A and B). There may also be structural changes

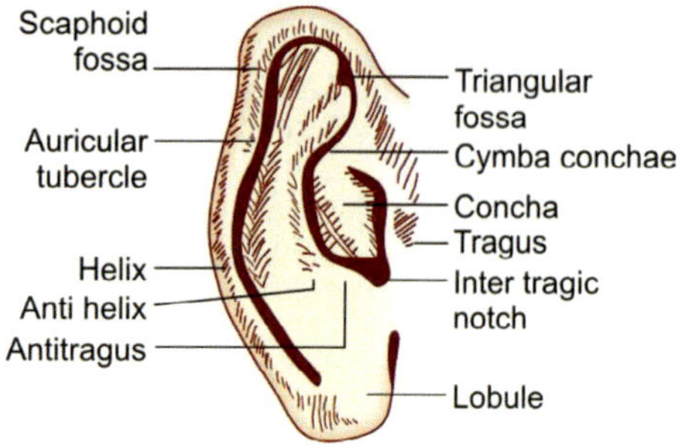

Fig. 2.9B: Anatomic landmarks of fully developed ear

around the ear that make it appear abnormal. Mastoiditis, lymph node enlargement and haemorrhage (Battle sign) from basal skull fracture are some examples. In the pinna itself, observe for the following:

a. Low set ear – Consider a plane connecting the medial and lateral canthi of the eyes. The insertion of the ear to the scalp lies normally on the same plane. The top of the ear is about 1/10 (of the height of the pinna) above a horizontal line drawn from the medial canthus. The ears may appear to be low-set (when in fact they are not) when the neck is short, cranial vault is high, the mandibular ramus is short or the auricles are rotated. In Down syndrome, the child has low-set small ears. The following table gives you some causes associated with low set ears (Table 2.32).
b. Prominent ear – Occurs in Fragile X syndrome, Potter syndrome (low set, large, floppy ear), lop ear (loss of superior crus, antihelix).

Table 2.32: Causes of low set ears

- Trisomy syndromes
- Apert syndrome
- Camptomelic dwarfism
- Noonan syndrome
- Turner syndrome
- Hallerman-Streiff syndrome
- Di George syndrome
- Fetal hydantoin syndrome

c. Pre-auricular papillomas or tubercles – Commonly these are due to maldevelopment of the first branchial arch. These can be isolated or occur as part of the Goldenhar syndrome.
d. Congenital aural fistulas – Usually isolated but can give rise to recurrent meningitis if leading into the cranium.
e. Darwinian tubercle (small prominence or thickening along the posterior segment of the helix near the tip of the auricle)–normal children, Marfan's syndrome.
f. Microtia–Treacher-Collins, Goldenhar syndromes.
g. Linear indentations of the ear lobes (or anterior/posterior lobule) - Beckwith Wiedemann syndrome.
h. Notched ears - Di George syndrome.

3. *Tympanic membranes and external auditory canal:* No examination is complete without visualizing the tympanic membranes. First you have to restrain the child so that he/she does not get hurt when you insert the auroscope. Sit the child (facing sideways) on the mother's lap. Ask her to put one hand over the child's head and forehead to hold him/her down on her chest. Instruct her to put the other hand across the child's chest to restrain him/her. Once you are satisfied with the arrangement, insert an auroscope to see the tympanic membrane (Fig. 2.10). In newborns and infants, the direction of the ear canal is upward whereas in older children it is downward and forward. Hold the pinna of the ear by the fingers of one hand and gently pull up and back in older children and downward in infants. Before inserting your auroscope, make note of the following observations:
   - External otitis
   - Foreign body
   - Cerumen
   - Herpes-zoster lesions
   - Discharge

It is useful to hold the handle of the auroscope between the thumb and index finger, rather like a pen. Insert the earpiece of the auroscope whilst manipulating the pinna to get a good view of the tympanic membrane (Fig. 2.10). Do the same with the other side. A sketch of the normal tympanic membrane is shown in Figure 2.11.

Normally the ear dum is slightly concave and translucent (pearly grey or ground glass in infants). Slight injection along the drum periphery may be noted normally and slight generalized erythema is normally induced by crying. Describe the tympanic membrane with reference to the points given below (Fig. 2.11).

i. Continuity of the membrane–Intact/ perforated
ii. Normal or dull in colour (otitis media with effusion)
iii. Loss of light reflex–Inflammation
iv. Membrane bulging and convex (pus, blood, air in middle ear) or retracted (Eustachian tube obstruction)
v. Bubble or air–Fluid column behind membrane (otitis media with effusion).

If you have a pneumatic auroscope, gentle squeezing of the bulb will allow observation of the mobility of the membrane in response to positive pressure. Similarly, releasing the bulb allows evaluation of the response to negative pressure. The tympanic membrane moves inward with positive pressure and outward with negative pressure. Fluid in the middle ear, scarring or adhesions impede drum mobility. A retracted drum usually does not move inward with positive pressure, but it moves somewhat outward with negative pressure. A hand held instrument that measures stapedial reflex (and gives graphical trace of tympanic compliance) is often of use. Normal reflex appears as a sharp conical curve, whilst an effusion makes it look flat.

Nose

The size and shape of the nose may give many clues to diagnosis. Here are some examples (Table 2.33):

Table 2.33: Different shapes of nose
1. Small nose–Down's syndrome, trisomy 18, Apert's syndrome
2. Misshapen nose–Normal newborn, cleft lip
3. Large nose–Seckel dwarf, 13q deletion syndrome
4. Depressed bridge of nose–Chondrodystrophy, cleidocranial dysostosis, congenital hypothyroidism, Conradi syndrome, cranio-metaphyseal dysostosis, Down syndrome, Hurler syndrome, Larsen syndrome, osteopetrosis, syphilis
5. Low nasal bridge with short, upturned nose–Fetal alcohol, fetal hydantoin
6. Small nose and anteverted nares–Aarskog syndrome
7. Hypoplastic alae nasi and broad nasal tip–Infant of diabetic mother (with femoral hypoplasia)
8. Thin beak like nose–Progeria, Apert syndrome, pyknodysostoiss, Hallermann-Streiff syndrome, Pfeiffer syndrome, Rubinstein Taybi syndrome, Saethre-Chotzen syndrome
9. Rudimentary nose (proboscis-like)–Holoprosencephaly.

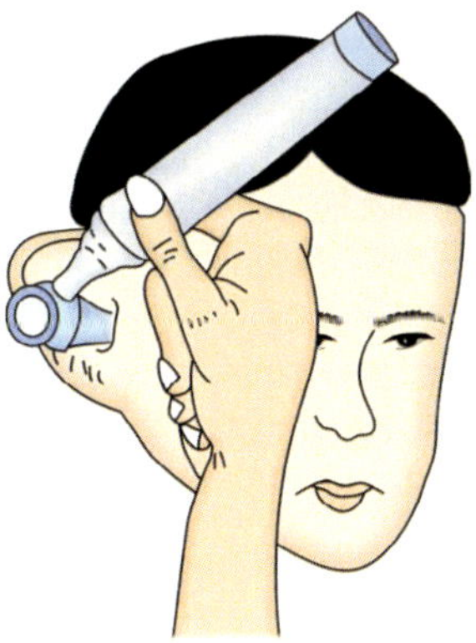

Fig. 2.10: Examination of ear by auroscope

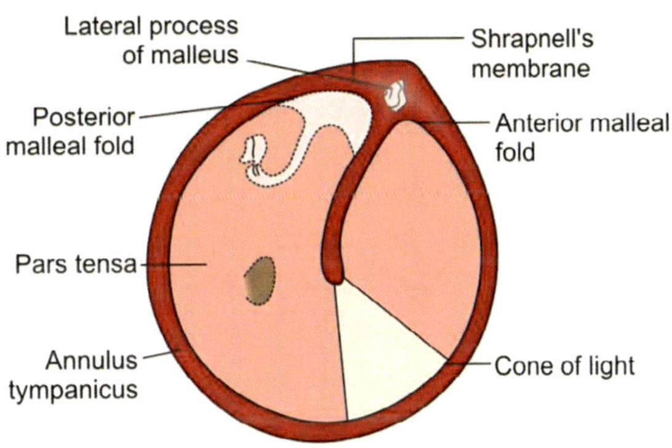

Fig. 2.11: Diagram of tympanic membrane

Tilt the tip of the nose and look for foreign bodies, swelling, purulent or bloody discharge, nasal obstruction, septal deviation and perforation. Nasal poyps are associated with cystic fibrosis. Choanal atresia is a condition where there is no patency of the nasal passage. If you suspect this in a newborn baby, pass a firm catheter first through one nostril and then through the other and demostrate the patency. Another way to check for nasal patency is to use the back of a metal spoon. Hold the back of a clean spoon (preferable cold) against the nostrils. If the child is breathing through the nostril, there should be condensation moisture on the metal surface. If you suspect nasal obstruction, look for signs of the CHARGE association.

Mouth and Pharynx

Inspection of the oral cavity and pharynx is usually unpleasant for young children and should be done quickly and with minimal discomfort. Some examiners prefer to leave this till the end of the examination, which is reasonable. First you may ask to see the teeth. Next instruct the child to open the mouth widely and protrude the tongue. If the pharynx is not visible, use a tongue depressor for a better view. In the infant who keeps his mouth highly closed, you should wait until he relaxes his clenched jaws or cries. Make sure you restrain the child during the examination. Good intra-oral lighting is essential. If you suspect epiglottitis, do not attempt to examine the pharynx, as it will precipitate laryngeal spasm and respiratory arrest (Fig. 2.9B).

At the beginning of the chapter, we discussed a "system" for the general survey and you will remember that examination of the mouth comes at the end. This is not to say that this should be done in haste or in cursory fashion. The mouth and pharynx holds many important clues to assist your diagnosis.

1. Size–Assess the size of the mouth in relation to the size of the face and other structures. A large mouth is said to be part of Morquio's and Beckwith syndromes. A wide mouth with prominent lips occurs in the fetal hyndantion syndrome. A fish mouth (downturned corners) appearance is associated with idioathic hypercalcaemia and the Russell-Silver syndrome. Small mouths are associated with Hallermann Streiff, oropalatodigital and whistling face syndromes.
2. Sucking and swallowing–This is more of relevance in the newborn baby. Babies at 34 weeks gestation start sucking and swallowing, albeit rudimentarily. At 36 weeks they are considered to have a mature suck and swallow reflex. At this time, about 30 rapid sucks are followed by one swallow. Infants with oropharyngeal incoordination due to neuromuscular impairment feed slowly and often choke. You will note that preterm infants in the neonatal intensive care unit need to be tube fed for considerable lengths of time. These infants need further time to establish satisfactory breast or bottle feeding. In term infants, botulism can impair sucking and swallowing and lead to pooling of saliva.
3. Drooling of saliva–Little salivation occurs in the newborn infant and is minimal until 2-4 months of age. Newborns with excessive mucus and saliva coming out of the mouth suggests oesophageal atresia. Infants commonly drool if they have an upper respiratory tract infection or they are teething. Be wary of drooling in the child with other serious problems–cerebral palsy, familial dysautonomia, Wilson disease, acute epiglottitis, scorpion stings, organophosphorus poisoning, peritonsillar abscess and foreign body in airway or oesophagus. The reverse of drooling is xerostomia due to decrease in salivary flow. This occurs in Sjogren, Mikulicz and uveoparotid syndromes.
4. Sucking pads–A fullness of the cheeks anterior to the masseter muscle occurs in malnourished children.

5. Mouth breathing–Adenoidal hypertrophy, nasopharyngeal obstruction.
6. Risus sardonicus–It occurs in some children with tetanus, in which the corners of the mouth are pulled outward and downward and the lip is stretched across the upper incisors to produce a sardonic grin.
7. Congenital cry facies–This occurs due to absence or hypoplasia of the depressor anguli oris. One corner of the mouth fails to move downward and outward, and is noticeable especially when the child cries. The lateral part of the lower lip may feel thinner on the involved side.
8. Bad breath (halitosis)–Common causes are poor oral hygiene, caries teeth, dry mouth, tonsillitis, nasal foreign body, sinusitis, adenoidal hypertrophy, Vincent stomatitis, enteric fever and lung abscess.
9. Circumoral pallor–Newborns, scarlet fever.
10. Lips–Note if any of these problems are present.
    - Large lips–Ethnic, Hurler's syndrome, angio-neurotic oedema
    - Cleft lip/palate
    - Pits or fistulas
    - Sucking pad/tubercle–Middle of the upper lip in normal newborns
    - Fusion of lip to underlying gum–Chondroectodermal dysplasia
    - Short philtrum–Di George, orofacio digital, Williams syndromes
    - Long philtrum–Femoral hypoplasia, gangliosidosis, Aarskog, Hurler, fetal alcohol and hydantoin syndromes
    - Cheilitis (drying, wrinkling, cracking, scaling of lips)–acute febrile illness, chapping, contact sensitivity
    - Angular stomatitis–Riboflavin deficiency
    - Perleche (fissuring, scaling, maceration, crusting of the angles of the mouth) - candida or streptoccal infection
    - Rhagades–Moist, radiating lesions about the corners of the mouth, found in congenital syphilis
    - Erythema–Kawasaki disease, herpes simples gingivostomatitis, mucositis from chemotherapy (dactinomycin, daunorubicin)
    - Cherry coloured lips and mucous membranes-carbon monoxide poisoning.
11. Buccal mucosa: Note the following when examining the oral mucosal lining (Table 2.34).
12. Gingivae:
    - Congenital epulis - In newborns, this is a benign, pedunculated, smooth, soft tissue growth arising from the gingival edge
    - Unerupted molars appear pale or colourless
    - Pearly white retention cyst - may persist for months in infants
    - Abscess - periapical abscess occurs at the base of the tooth, either in lingual or labial positions
    - Hypertrophy–Hydantion therapy, mouth breathers, poor dental hygiene
    - Gingivitis–neutropaenia, acute monocytic or myelomonocytic leukemia.

Table 2.34: Examination of oral mucosa
• Dehydration–Dry, little saliva
• Thrush–White, raised, membranous patches that resemble milk curds on the buccal surfaces, lips, tongue and pharynx. The patches are removed with some difficulty and leave mucosal lesions slightly oozing with blood. Chronic oropharyngeal candidiasis occurs in HIV, T-cell disorders, type 1 autoimmune polyglandular syndrome and severe combined immunodeficiency.
• Stomatitis–Commonly in cytotoxic chemotherapy, chronic granulomatous disease, Vincent stomatitis, herpes simplex and cyclic neutropaenia
• Aphthous ulcers–Inflammatory bowel disease, unexplained
• Diffuse erythema–Kawasaki disease
• Red erythematous spots–leukaemia, thrombocytopaenia, Forscheimer spots (rubella), trauma
• Koplik spots–First appearing on the buccal mucosa opposite the lower molars, they appear as greyish or bluish-white opalescent specks surrounded by a light red, blotchy areola.
• Bullous eruptions–Epidermolysis bullosa, pemphigus vulgaris, Steven-Johnson syndrome

13. Palate: The palate is a good site to look for pallor and jaundice. Petechiae may be present in immune thrombocytopaenia or leukaemia. Structural defects can be a cleft palate, high arch palate and cysts. Clefts are of four varieties. They can be:
    i. Limited to soft palate
    ii. Cleft extends through both the soft and hard palates up to the alveolar process
    iii. Soft and hard palates are both involved with a unilateral cleft of the alveolar process
    iv. Same as above but with bilateral alveolar clefts.

    Ask the child to open the mouth and inspect for a gap. In submucous cleft palate, there is no overt defect, but the midline of the palate feels thin on palpation. In newborns it is always preferable to examine the oral cavity digitally so as not to miss a small cleft. Cleft palate may occur as an isolated defect or as a component or the following syndromes: Trisomy 13, 18, mandibulofacial dysostosis, Wolf-Hirschhorn, orofaciodigital, velocardiofacial (submucous cleft) and Pierre Robin syndromes.

    High arched palate is a common occurrence in neonates who have been ventilated (with oral endotracheal tubes) for a considerable length of time. They are also said to be associated with mouth breathers, cerebral gigantism, Ehlers-Danlos, Marfan, Down and Treacher-Collins syndromes. Note that high arched or cleft palates can often be associated with other midline abnormalities such as septo-optic dysplasia (hypopituitarism).

    In newborns, small localised accumulations of epithelial cells or cysts are common on each side of the median raphe of the hard palate ('Epstein pearls') or along the alveolar ridge ('Bohn nodules'). When looking at the palate do also observe the uvula. A bifid uvula may be normal, or may occur with a submucous cleft palate or with Apert, di George, orofaciodigital and Treacher-Collins syndromes.
14. Tongue: The tongue seems large in congenital hypothyroidism, gylocogenosis type 2, Hurler syndrome, neurofibromatosis, Beckwith syndrome, haemangioma, lymphangioma and angioneurotic oedema. In contrast it is small in hypoglossal nerve lesions and in association with multiple cranial nerve palsies such as the Moebius syndrome. You should be vigilant for the following (Table 2.35).
15. Tonsils: Use a tongue depressor and have the child say 'aah'. Look for areas of pus

Table 2.35: Tongue – major abnormalities

- Dryness–Dehydration, mouth breathing
- Colour–Pale in anaemia, blue in cyanosis, purple in the Eisenmenger syndrome, magenta in Riboflavin deficiency
- Cyst–Thyroglossal cyst at the base of the tongue
- Pigmentation–Recent ingestion of coloured food and lozenges
- Coating (white, greyish or brownish-white)–Occurs in febrile illness such as enteric fever
- Strawberry tongue (raw red tongue with prominent fungiform papillae)–Febrile illnesses, scarlet fever, toxic shock syndrome, Kawasaki disease
- Black hairy tongue –A V-shaped brown to black area, anterior to circumvallate papilla, seen in haemophilia and purpura (hypertrophy of filiform papillae)
- Protrusion– Occurs in infants with mental retardation, Down syndrome, congenital hypothyroidism, puppet-like syndrome of Angelman and Nieman-Pick syndrome. In the neonate, a rhythmic protrusion of the tongue suggests intracranial haemorrhage or cerebral oedema. Tongue thrusting is often noted in infants who later demonstrate athetosis. In Syndenham chorea, the tongue is often undulating and cannot be held still on protrusion.
- Tremor–Werdnig Hoffman disease (fasciculations and atrophy of tongue)
- Fissures–Characterized by irregular fissures or grooves in a cerebriform or scrotal patern (Down syndrome)
- Geographic tongue–Annular smooth red patches with slightly grey margins. They begin posteriorly on the dorsum and spread anteriorly and laterally. They are usually of no clinical significance.
- Tongue tie (ankyloglossia)–Occasionally the frenum may be short and this appears as a notch at the tip of the tongue. True tongue tie is a rare phenomenon.

on the surface of the tonsils (streptococcal pharyngitis). A grey or yellowish membrane should indicate diphtheria, agranulocytosis, and infectious mononucleosis. Tonsils may be normally large due lymphoid tissue growth and may be mistaken for tonsillitis. Displacement of the tonsil to one side with painful swallowing occurs with peritonsillar abscess (quinsy). In Tangier disease, the tonsils are hugely enlarged, yellow-grey in colour and honeycombed in pattern.

16. Pharynx: The pharynx looks red in viral infections, bacterial pharyngitis or abscess. You may be able to palpate a smooth tense swelling in the lateral parts in a retropharyngeal abscess. Hyperplasia of the lymphoid folicles of the post pharyngeal wall occurs with recurrent pharngitis and adenoidal hypertrophy. The pharynx is usually swollen and congested with a cherry red epiglotis in epiglottitis (Fig. 2.9B).
17. Teeth: Count the number of erupted teeth. Although eruption of teeth follows a developmental pattern, much individual variation occurs. A guide to the eruption of teeth is given in Tables 2.36 and 2.37 (Figs 2.12A and B).

Rarely the newborn may present with natal teeth, usually mandibular central incisors. Natal teeth are attached to the gingival margin with little root formation or bony support. Supernumerary teeth on the other hand occur in the area of the maxillary central incisors and have bony support (demonstrated by X-ray). Natal teeth are associated with cleft palate, Pierre-Robin, Ellis-von-Creveld, Hallermann-Strieff

Table 2.36: Age of appearance of teeth

Primary teeth	*Age of appearance (months)*	*Secondary teeth*	*Age of appearance (years)*
Central incisors	6-7	1st molar	6
Lateral incisors	7-10	Central incisor	7
1st molar	12	Lateral incisor	8
Canine	18	1st premolar	9
2nd molar	24	2nd premolar	10
		Canine	11
		2nd molar	12
		3rd molar	18

Table 2.37: Number of teeth in different ages in boys and girls

Number of primary teeth	*Age in years*		*Number of secondary teeth*	*Age in years*	
	Boys	*Girls*		*Boys*	*Girls*
1	0.55	0.60	2	6.21	5.94
2	0.65	0.70	4	6.40	6.22
4	0.82	0.86	6	6.54	6.24
6	0.97	1.03	8	7.47	7.20
8	1.12	1.18	10	7.70	7.34
10	1.27	1.33	12	8.67	8.20
12	1.43	1.50	14	10.40	9.86
14	1.62	1.70	16	10.79	10.03
16	1.85	1.97	18	10.82	10.18
18	2.13	2.35	20	11.18	10.88
			22	11.47	10.89
			24	11.69	10.98
			26	12.12	11.66
			28	12.68	12.27

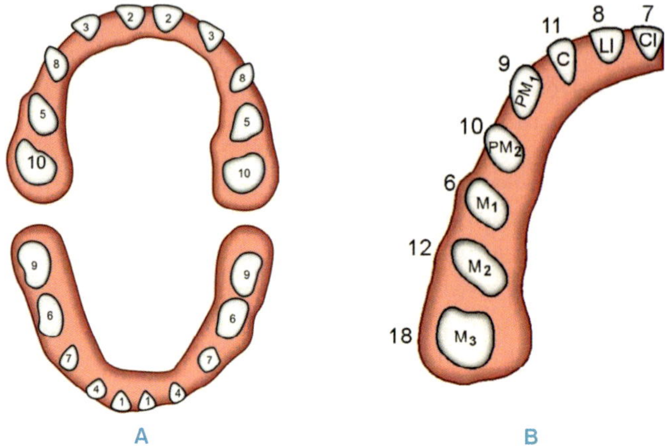

Figs 2.12A and B: (A) Primary dentition, (B) Permanent dentition (Left upper quadrant)

syndromes and pachyonychia congenita. Supernumerary teeth are associated with cleft lip and palate, Gardner, orofaciodigital, Hallermann-Streiff syndrome and cleidocranial dysplasias. Children with ectodermal dysplasia have poor dentition or conical central incisors.

Milk teeth are white in colour and have a smooth edge in contrast to permanent teeth which have an ivory (off-white) colour and a serrated edge. Black teeth are seen in children taking oral iron preparations. Yellowish discolouration is seen in those given tetracycline in infancy. Brownish discolouration with pitting and mottling occurs in dental fluorosis. Excess plaque formation over the teeth is due to poor oral hygiene. Brown teeth may also with amelogenesis imperfecta. Pink or reddish brown teeth occur with chronic porphyria. Caries teeth are extremely common and occur on the occlusal (biting) surfaces or on the contact surface between two teeth. Lesions may go deeper to reach the alveoli and may give rise to dental or periapical abscess.

Check the alignment of teeth–ask the child to bite down and then examine by separating the lips. The occlusal surfaces of the teeth should appose with good alignment with the posterior mandibular teeth slightly ahead of the corresponding maxillary teeth. Prognathism may occur as a racial trait. Protuberant spaced out teeth occurs in children with thalassaemia major.

Peg shaped teeth have notches on the distal border of the upper central incisors. They are classically seen in congenital syphilis. The Hutchinson tooth is shaped like the tip of a screwdriver, and also occurs in congenital syphilis. Mulberry molars have irregularly formed crowded cusps on a small occlusal surface.

The abnormalities can also be see in teeth. A few abnormalities have been show in Table 2.38.

Chest, abdomen: See relevant chapters in examination of respiratory and gastrointestinal systems.

Hands and Fingers

The examination of the hand provides a lot of information relevant to all systems. Look for the following in the hand:

i. Handendess–Handedness develops by 3 years of age but age variations occur. A

Table 2.38: Teeth – A few abnormalities

Black teeth	-	Oral iron tonic
Yellowish teeth	-	Tetracyclines
Brownish teeth with Pitting + Mottling	-	Dental fluorosis
Excess plaque	-	Poor oral hygiene
Brown teeth	-	Amelogenosis imperfecta
Pink/Reddish brown teeth	-	Porphyria
Hutchinson teeth/ Pegshaped teeth	-	Congenital syphilis

child with a consistent approach with one hand suggests a 'hemisyndrome'.

ii. Tremor–Essential tremor, Wilson's disease, anxiety, cerebellar disease, thyrotoxicosis, asterixis.

iii. Grasp–This reflects power of individual muscles. An ill-sustained grip is seen in chorea (alternate squeezing and relaxing).

iv. Size
- Small in achondroplasia, Down's syndrome, de Lange syndrome, Prader-Willi syndrome
- Large in gigantism, Sotos syndrome
- Long hands with arachnodactyly–Marfan syndrome, homocystinuria
- Macrodactyly–neurofibromatosis, Ollier disease, Mafucci syndrome, Proteus syndrome
- Shortening of digits–Down's syndrome, pseudohypoparathyroidism, Turner syndrome
- Digital hypoplasia of digits and nails (more on the ulnar aspect)–Fetal hydantoin syndrome.

v. Shapes of hand and fingers are given in Table 2.39.

vi. Colour changes
- Red–dactylitis, hand-foot-mouth syndrome, reflex sympathetic dystrophy, high output failure, liver failure
- Blue–cyanosis, Raynaud's phenomenon
- Yellow–Icterus
- Pigmentation–Addison's disease.

vii. Rash
- Macules–Erythema multiforme, viral rash, SLE, dermatomyositis
- Papules–Eczematous dermatitis, scabies
- Vesicles–Scabies, herpes simplex, molluscum contagiosum, staphylococcal scalded skin syndrome, burns, epidermolysis bullosa, congenital syphilis
- Nodules– Juvenile chronic arthritis, rheumatic fever
- Purpura– Meningococcaemia, Henoch-Schonlein purpura, Rocky-Mountain spotted fever.

Table 2.39: Shape of hands and fingers

- Syndactyly–Apert syndrome, Carpenter syndrome, focal dermal hypoplasia, Poland, Smith-Lemli-Opitz syndromes
- Polydactly–Chondroectodermal dysplasia, short rib-polydactyly syndrome, Lawrence-Moon-Biedl syndrome, Trisomy 13
- Aplasia of thumb/radius–Holt-Oram syndrome, thrombocytopenia-absent radii (TAR) syndrome
- Short broad terminal phalanges of thumb - Rubinstein-Taybi syndrome, Carpenter syndrome, Apert syndrome, Weaver syndrome, Peiffer syndrome
- 'Hitchiker' thumb–Diastrophic dwarfism
- Flexion of fingers with overlapping of digits–Trisomy 18
- Contractures–Insulin dependent diabetes mellitus with micro-vascular angiopathy, juvenile chronic arthropathy, mucolipidosis, Whistling face syndrome
- 'Policeman receiving tip'–upper branchial palsy
- Proximally placed thumb–Trisomy 22, diastrophic dwarfism, Cornelia de Lange syndrome
- Distally placed thumb–Trisomy 18, orocraniodigital syndrome
- Clinodactyly (incurving little finger due to shortening of the radial aspect of the middle phalanx)–Down syndrome, Silver-Russel syndrome, normal individuals.

viii. Dermatoglyphics

a. *Flexion creases:* Usually there are 3 palmar creases. When the two distal creases are fused and run as a single crease across the entire palm reaching the ulnar border of the palm, it is called a "simian crease" (Down's syndrome, 2-5 percent of normal children). A Sydney line (congenital rubella syndrome) is one in which the proximal crease runs across the entire palm while the distal crease is normally present (Fig. 2.13).

b. *Ridge arrangement on palms:* The ridges of the palm meet at certain places. These places where the individual ridge systems are confluent are known as triradii. Figure 2.14 shows the terminology of the triradii as a, b, c, d and t. The angle formed by joining the points a, t, d is known as the atd angle and is normally about 40°. In Down syndrome, the proximal point is shifted distally resulting in an obtuse atd

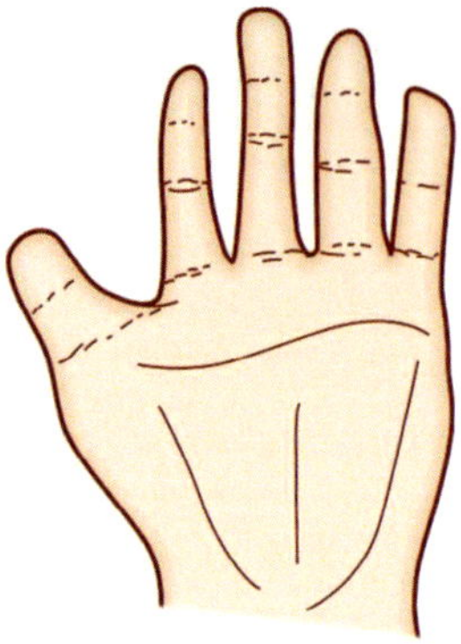

Fig. 2.13: Transverse crease (simian)

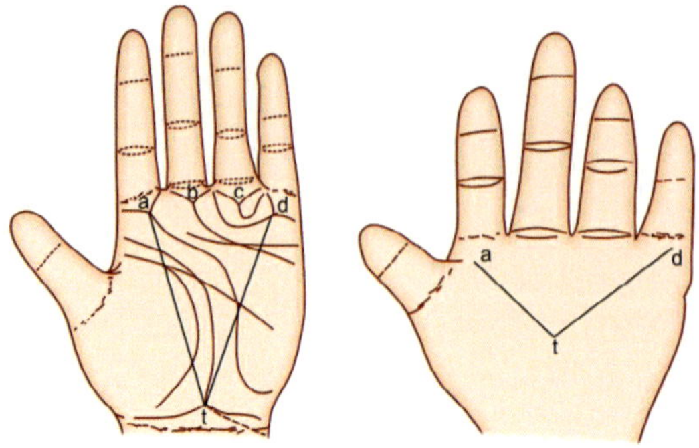

Fig. 2.14: Decrease of atd angle in Down's syndrome

angle. Other conditions with obtuse atd angle are Turner's syndrome and congenital rubella syndrome.

c. *Finger print patterns:* The characteristic patterns over the fingertips are loop, whorl, arch and combined. The usual distribution is - ulnar loop on little finger, radial loop on index finger, whorl or arch on the middle finger. Ulnar loops occur in Down's syndrome on all fingers. The congenital rubella syndrome is associated with a greater number of whorls whereas trisomy 18 children have more arches.

Joints

Joint problems in children are either primary or secondary. Common arthropathies in childhood are the juvenile chronic arthritis (JCA) group of joint disorders. Joints (and bones) are also involved in osteomyelitis, septic arthritis, trauma or malignancy. Systemic problems may present with arthropathy; some examples are rheumatic fever, collagen vascular diseases, leukaemias and septicaemia.

To examine the joint (usually a limb) in question, expose the arm or leg. You will look, feel and move the joint that you are examining (Table 2.40). First inspect the part of the limb from all around.

Table 2.40: Examination of joints - Inspection

- Swelling–Ill defined or well delineated
- Pain–painless or painful
- Redness–Local, widespread, any suggestion of abscess
- Scar–drain, muscle biopsy from adjacent area, intra-osseous needle introduction
- Muscle bulk around joint–normal, atrophy, contracture, hypertrophy
- Associated subcutaneous nodules–rheumatic fever
- Pallor–leukaemia, systemic infection
- Bleeding sites–Haemophilia
- Rash–Henoch-Schonlein purpura, Still's disease, systemic lupus erythematosus, dermatomyositis

Spinal pathology is not common with systemic conditions, although they can occur with the juvenile chronic arthropathies. Tuberculous disease of the spine is common, even in this day and age, and needs to be considered as a possible diagnosis. Look for scars, muscle wasting, scoliosis and kyphosis.

Palpate the joint on the affected site as well as the joint on the opposite side. Examination of the normal joint gives you a yardstick for comparison. Feel the temperature (warm in inflammation), and look for signs of tenderness. Is the overlying skin tense and shiny? This may indicate an acute inflammatory process. Are there any nodules to feel (rheumatic fever)? Is the muscle atrophied around the joint? If so is it localised to one area? If a joint is chronically inflamed over a period of time, the muscles may lose their function. Intra-articular steroid injection can give rise to local skin and muscle atrophy.

Move the joints passively unless the movement is too painful for the child. Establish the degree of unrestricted movement possible in that joint. Here are some joints that you will examine commonly (Table 2.41).

Table 2.41: Movements of the joints to be examined

1.	Interphalangeal and metacarpophalangeal joints of the hand–Handwriting, grip, button-unbutton shirt, tie shoelace, opposition of thumb to each of the fingers, thumb adduction, abduction
2.	Wrist–Extension, flexion
3.	Elbow–Extension, flexion
4.	Shoulder–Extension, flexion, abduction (lift your arms like the wings of an aeroplane or a bird), adduction, touch with both hands the small of your back
5.	Neck–Extension (look up at the ceiling), flexion (touch the chin on your chest), sideways flexion (touch your chin on your left or right shoulder)
6.	Thoracic and lumbar spine–Flexion, extension (bend down to touch your toes, bend backwards)
7.	Interphalangeal joint of toes–Flexion/extension ("wiggle" your toes)
8.	Metatarsophalangeal joints–Flexion, extension of toes
9.	Subtalar joints–Inversion, eversion
10.	Ankle joint–Flexion, extension
11.	Knee joint–Flexion, extension
12.	Hip–Flexion, extension, adduction, abduction, circumduction

Check the joints above and below the joint that you have just examined. If you suspect an arthropathy, it is preferable to do a full examination of all the joints in the body, as outlined above. Is there a pattern emerging? How many joints are affected? Oligoarthritis is usually involvement of four or less joints in the body. They commonly occur in girls and are associated with iridocyclitis. It is good to ask for a history of eye pain and lacrimation. If in doubt, you should send the child for a formal slit lamp examination by the ophthalmologists to check for uveitis.

Finally, establish the degree of mobility of the child. Does he/she use crutches or orthoses? What activities of daily living can he/she do? What is the degree of pain relief? How far can the child walk without pain?

Anthropometry

It is absolutely crucial to measure physical growth in all children. Growth is a sensitive marker of the well being of the child and may well be an indicator of an underlying illness. Growth (synonymous with height) may also be impaired as a primary process in which case you have to be aware of endocrine causes as well as genetic mechanisms. In this chapter, we shall deal with various anthropometric measurements like weight, height and head circumference.

Weight: This should preferably be measured by a beam type of weighing machine. Spring balances are not accurate and dependent on the elasticity of the spring which varies with the age of the machine and temperature of the environment. The measurement should be done with child wearing minimum clothing (ideally in the nude). The balance should be balanced first by bringing the lever to zero to see the oscillation of the fulcrum. The child is then put on the weighing machine and the levers are adjusted till the fulcrum is in the middle. The weight is measured nearest to 25 gm accuracy and recorded. Electronic weighing scales are accurate and easy to use and have replaced the cumbersome beam balance in many centres (Fig. 2.15).

For a quick calculation of expected weight from the age, the following formula may be used: weight in kg = (age in years + 4) × 2. This is a rough guide and does not take into account any interethnic variation. It is, therefore, essential to plot the child on a growth chart (preferably drawn from local data) and check on his/her pattern of growth.

The weight for age is a reliable indicator of the nutritional status of a child. The severity of

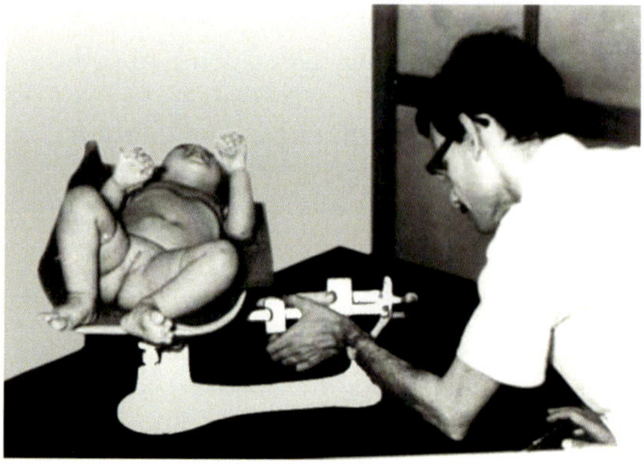

Fig. 2.15: Weight measurement in a beam balance

undernutrition can be assessed on the basis of the classification of the Indian Academy of Pediatrics: Grade I (71-80%), grade II (61-70%), grade III (51-60%) and grade IV (50% or less). Below is a table that gives the figures for grading of malnutrition for Indian children upto the age of 14 years (Table 2.42).

Length (Crown-heel length): The length is measured on a measuring board, with a fixed head piece and a movable foot piece that has wooden scales fixed to both sides. You will need at least one other person to help you do this. Make sure that the child is looking upwards when lying on the measuring board. Your assistant should check if the knees are perfectly extended and you can then flush the foot piece against both feet (Fig. 2.16).

Table 2.42: Grading of malnutrition suggested by the Indian Academy of Pediatrics (weight in kg)

Age	*50th percentile of NCHS Standard*	*Grade I*	*Grade II*	*Grade III*	*Grade IV*
Birth	3.4	2.4-2.7	2.1-2.3	1.7-2.0	1.6 or less
3 months	5.7	4.0-4.5	3.5-3.9	2.9-3.4	2.8 or less
6 months	7.6	5.4-6.1	4.6-5.3	3.9-4.5	3.8 or less
9 months	9.1	6.5-7.3	5.5-6.4	4.6-5.4	4.5 or less
12 months	10.1	7.2-8.1	6.2-7.1	5.1-6.1	5.0 or less
15 months	10.7	7.6-8.6	6.5-7.5	5.4-6.4	5.3 or less
18 months	11.4	8.1-9.1	6.9-8.0	5.8-6.8	5.7 or less
2 years	13.4	9.5-10.7	8.2-9.4	6.8-8.1	6.7 or less
2.5 years	14.6	10.4-11.7	8.9-10.3	7.4-8.8	7.3 or less
3 years	15.6	11.1-12.5	9.5-11.0	7.9-9.4	7.8 or less
3.5 years	16.6	11.8-13.3	10.1-11.7	8.5-10.0	8.4 or less
4 years	17.7	12.6-14.2	10.4-12.5	9.0-10.7	8.9 or less
4.5 years	18.8	13.3-15.0	11.5-13.2	9.6-11.4	9.5 or less
5 years	20.0	14.2-16.0	12.2-14.2	10.2-12.1	10.1 or less
5.5 years	20.7	14.7-16.6	12.6-14.6	10.5-12.5	10.4 or less
6 years	21.9	15.5-17.5	13.3-15.4	11.2-13.3	11.1 or less
6.5 years	23.2	16.5-18.5	14.1-16.4	11.8-14.0	11.7 or less
7 years	24.5	17.4-19.6	14.9-17.3	12.5-14.8	12.4 or less
7.5 years	25.9	18.4-20.7	15.8-18.3	13.2-15.7	13.1 or less
8 years	27.3	19.4-21.8	16.6-19.3	13.9-16.6	13.8 or less
8.5 years	28.6	20.3-22.9	17.4-20.2	14.6-17.3	14.5 or less
9 years	29.9	21.2-23.9	18.2-21.1	15.2-18.1	15.1 or less
9.5 years	31.3	22.2-25.0	19.1-22.1	16.0-19.0	15.9 or less
10 years	32.6	23.1-26.1	19.9-23.0	16.6-19.8	16.5 or less
10.5 years	33.9	24.1-27.1	20.7-24.0	17.3-20.6	17.2 or less
11 years	35.2	25.0-28.4	21.5-24.9	17.9-21.4	17.8 or less
11.5 years	36.7	26.1-29.4	22.4-26.0	18.8-22.3	18.6 or less
12 yeras	38.3	27.2-30.6	23.4-27.1	19.5-23.2	19.4 or less
13 years	42.2	[illegible]	[illegible]	21.5-25.6	21.4 or less
14 years	48.4	34.6-39.0	29.8-34.5	24.9-29.7	24.8 or less

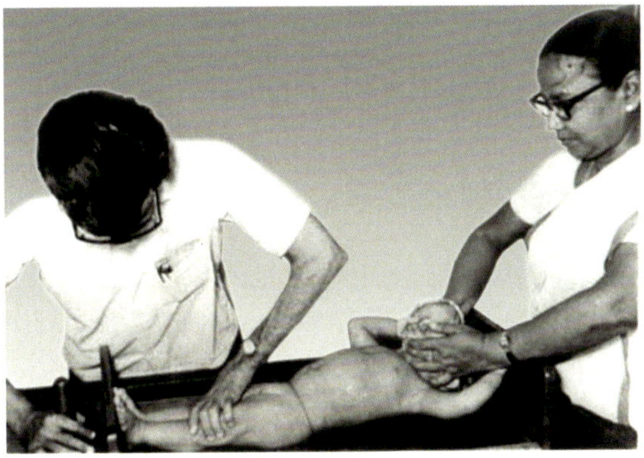

Fig. 2.16: Length measurement

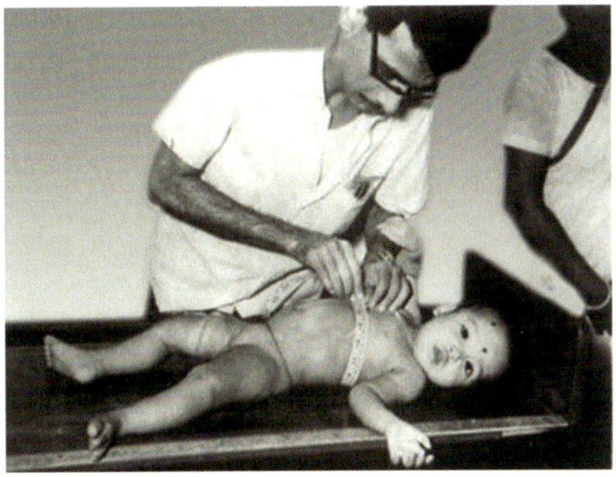

Fig. 2.17: Chest circumference measurement

In a child above the age of five years, it is better to take the same reading standing up. A stadiometer that has been calibrated should be used. Make sure that the child looks straight ahead with the lower margins of the eyes in the same horizontal plane as the external auditory meatus. Ask the child to "breathe in and stand tall." Use gentle upward traction over the mandibles to straighten the cervical spinal curvature. Ensure that the heels are not lifted from the ground. The head board can then be placed horizontally on the top of the head and the height measurement taken.

For a quick estimation of height/length, the following aide memoire is useful: Length at birth = 50 cm; length at 1 year = 75 cm; length from 2-12 years = (age in years × 6) + 77 cm. Remember this is only a rough guide and the best way to record the child's length is to plot it on a suitable growth chart.

Chest circumference: The chest circumference is measured ideally by a fibre glass tape; if not available, an ordinary linen measuring tape, standardized against a wooden scale from time to time, may be used. The tape is first laid stretched on the measuring board with reverse side upwards. The child is then put on the reversed tape on the measuring board. The tape is passed through the xiphisternal junction and surrounds the chest in that plane. The measurement is done midway between inspiration and expiration and recorded nearest to 0.1 cm. The tape should not be passed through the nipple line, as the nipple lines may be variable (Fig. 2.17).

Cranial circumference: The cranial circumference is measured by the same tape, and is passed over the supra-orbital ridges in front and that part of the occiput which gives the maximum diameter. Usually it is over the occipital protruberance, but not always. Therefore only the maximum diameter is to be considered. It is recorded nearest to 0.1 cm. Figure 2.18 shows the technique of cranial circumference measurement.

The usual head circumference at birth is 36 cm in boys and 34 cm in girls, but indigenous Indian values are probably 1 cm lesser. An easy way to remember the values for head growth in childhood is given in Table 2.43.

Table 2.43: Head circumference - Measurement

First 3 months	Growth 2 cm/month
Second 3 months	Growth 1 cm/month
Next 6 months	Growth 0.5 cm/month
At 1 year, head circumference	47 cm
At 2 years head circumference	49 cm
At 4 years head circumference	51 cm
At 11 years head circumference	52 cm

Mid-Arm circumference: The midpoint of the arm is first determined by passing the tape from the

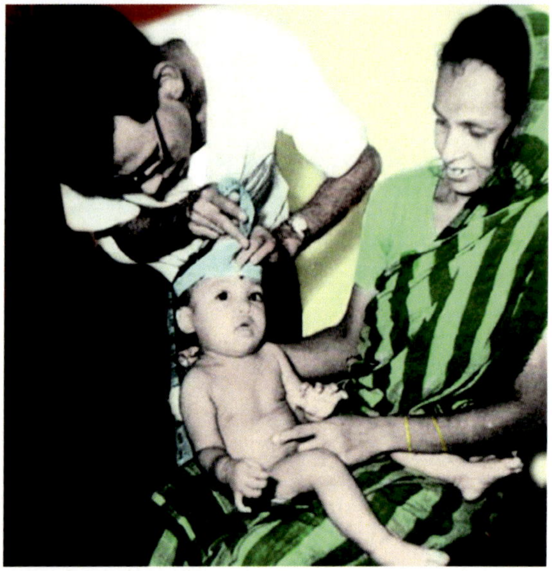

Fig. 2.18: Cranial circumference measurement

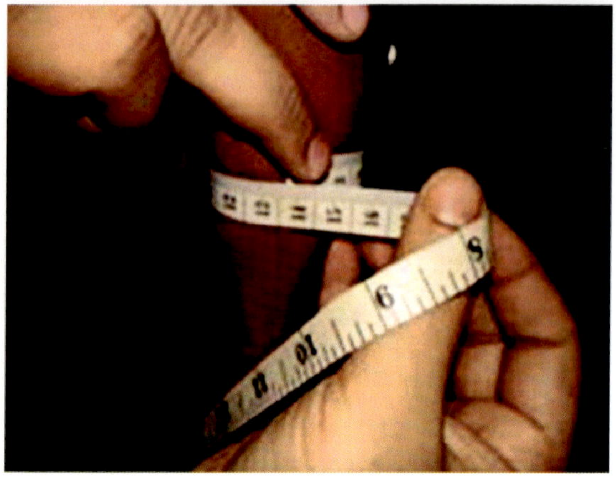

Fig. 2.19: Mid-arm circumference

acromial end of the clavicle to the olecranon process of the ulna. At the midpoint (half of the length of the arm) the circumference is measured by passing the tape around the arm in that plane. It is recorded nearest to 0.1 cm (Fig. 2.19).

Age Independent Anthropometry

a. *Mid arm circumference:* The midarm circumference is relatively constant between 16.5 cm to 17.5 cm in children 1-5 yrs of age and therefore this measurement may be considered as an age independent variable in that age group. Any child with an MAC less than 12.5 cm (< 5 yrs of age) is considered malnourished. It is a useful method of assessment of nutritional status. In a community setup, Shakir's tape is a replacement for MAC measurement. The red area (12.5 cm) denotes malnutrition, the yellow (13.5-12.5 cm) denotes impending malnutrition, while the green area (above 13.5 cm) represents children who are normal.
b. *Weight for height:* The degree of wasting can be measured by comparing the child's weight with the expected weight of a healthy child of the same height. Combinations of these measurements have been used to distinguish different types of malnutrition. Waterlow suggested that weight/height could be used to distinguish between malnutrition of recent origin (wasting) and malnutrition due to a considerable period of months. In chronic malnutrition the child is stunted, that is the weight-for-age and height-for-age are low. In acute malnutrition, height-for age is normal but weight-for age is low, and is called wasting. Thus, the weight and height measurements are useful together to understand the dynamics of malnutrition and enable us to distinguish between acute malnutrition and chronic malnutrition. In nutritional dwarfs, the weight/height is equal as there is chronic adaptation. The child may pass off as a normal child for lower age if the chronological age is not known.
c. *Quac stick:* Quaker's midarm circumference measuring stick is a height-measuring rod calibrated in MAC rather than height. Values of 80 percent MAC for height are marked on the stick at corresponding height levels. If a child is found taller than his arm circumference level on the stick, he is considered malnourished. The 'Quac stick' was devised in Mexico and has since been adapted in Africa and India.

d *Mid arm to head circumference ratio:* It is a simple and useful ratio to quantify malnutrition. A ratio 0.280 to 0.314 indicates malnutrition. Values between 0.250 and 0.279 denote moderate malnutrition, whilst those less than 0.249 indicate severe malnutrition.

e. *Quetlet's index:* It is based on the relationship between weight and height and is expressed as weight (kg)/height (cm) × 100. Normal values vary between 0.14 and 0.16. In gross malnutrition the value is less than 0.14.

f. *Mid upper arm to height ratio:* This is another useful indicator of nutritional status. A ratio of less than 0.29 indicates gross malnutrition, while the normal value ranges from 0.32 to 0.33.

g. *Bangle method:* This is another age independent anthropometric parameter where you slip a bangle with an internal diameter of 4 cm up the forearm. The bangle should be made to move up without squeezing the hands. In case the bangle slips over the elbow, malnutrition is said to be present. This is really an mid arm circumference that is meant for use in the community. Though simple to use, is not very reliable.

h. *Body mass index (BMI)*

$$\text{BMI} = \frac{\text{Weight (kg)}}{\text{Height (m)}^2}$$

This ratio is somewhat like the Quetlet's index. BMI represents adiposity in a child but does not discriminate between fat free (lean) mass and fat mass. However, in practice this is a relatively easy and reproducible tool to assess obesity. BMI values have been used to draw standardized percentile curves in children and adolescents. A child is overweight if the BMI is > 85th centile (NCHS). A BMI at or above 95th percentile for age is considered to represent obesity. You must remember however these are Western standards and unlikely to be suitable for application in the Indian context. Indians have a greater amount of fat than the BMI ratio suggests. In adult Indians, the World Health Organisation has lowered BMI cut-offs from 25 and 30 to 20 and 25 to represent overweight and obesity respectively.

The chief value of BMI is in the follow-up of obese children. You should be able to determine trend over time when plotted on a BMI centile chart. You may consider measuring waist circumference as an adjunct to quantify visceral fat mass. However, in obese children, measurements are rather erratic as it is often difficult to localize the point at which the tape should be passed. Ideally you should select the midpoint between the iliac crest and lower end of the ribs on either side. It is often difficult to palpate the iliac crest due to excess fat deposition.

i. *Ponderal Index (PI):* This is another index similar to BMI and is often used in defining IUGR babies.

$$\text{PI} = \frac{\text{Body weight (gm)}}{\text{Length (cm)}^3} \times 100$$

ii. *Sex Maturity Rating (SMR):* This is often missed out but remains an integral part of growth assessment of the child. It is important to be aware of the maturation of the secondary sex characters and their relation to physical growth. Examining the genitalia can be slightly awkward in the older child, so you should be duly sensitive and explain the procedure first. If the child disagrees to the examination, you could show him/her pictures depicting sexual development and ask him/her of the likely stage. The Tanner pubertal staging in children is given in Tables 2.44 and 2.45 (Figs 2.20A and B).

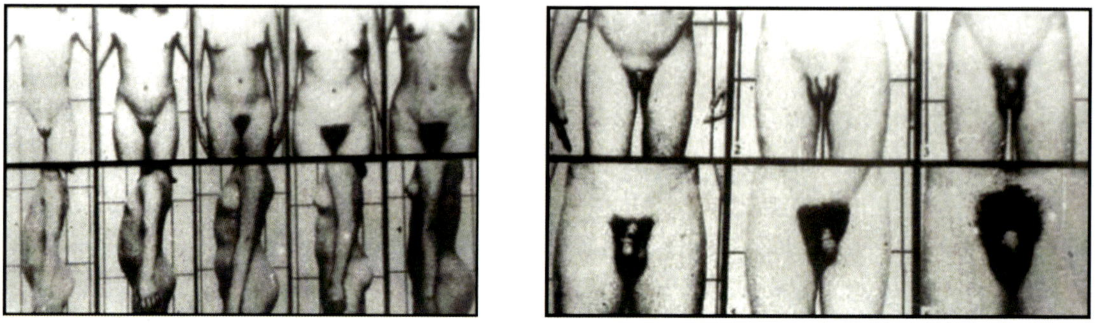

A B

Figs 2.20A and B: (A) SMR girls, (B) SMR boys

Table 2.44: Tanner pubertal staging–Girls

Girls		
Pubic Hair	*SMR*	*Breast*
Preadolescent	1.	Preadolescent
Sparse, lightly pigmented, straight, medial border of labia	2.	Breast and papilla elevated as small mound, areolar diameter increased
Darker, beginning to curl, increased amount	3.	Breast and areola enlarged, no countour separation
Coarse, curly, abundant but less amount than adult	4.	Areola and papilla form secondary mound
Adult feminine triangle, spread to medial thighs	5.	Mature; nipple projects, areola part of general breast contour

Table 2.45: Tanner pubertal staging–Boys

Boys			
Pubic Hair	*SMR*	*Penis*	*Testes*
None Preadolescent	1.	Preadolescent	
Scanty long, slightly pigmented	2.	Slight enlargement	Enlarged scrotum, pink, texture altered
Darker, starts to curl, small amount	3.	Longer	Larger
Resembles adult, amount less, coarse, curly	4.	Larger, breadth increases in size	Larger, scrotum dark
Adult distribution, spreads to medial surface of thighs	5.	Adult size	Adult size

3 EXAMINATION OF THE GASTROINTESTINAL SYSTEM

The gastrointestinal tract extends from the mouth to the anus. It is not just a passageway for food, but is also connected to an intricate set of secretory glands that control the processing, absorption and elimination of ingested material. The abdomen contains a large part of the GI tract and also other organs (kidney, adrenals, testes) that can be examined alongside.

You may divide the abdominal wall by imaginary lines into nine compartments. There are two vertical lines, each starting from the midpoint of the groin (femoral artery) on either side and passing upwards to cross the costal margin at the tip of the ninth costal cartilage. The two horizontal lines are called the subcostal and interiliac lines. They pass horizontally across the lowest points on the costal margin and tubercles of the iliac crests respectively. The four lines intersect and form nine quadrants: right and left hypochondria, epigastrium, right and left lumbar, umbilical, right and left iliac and hypogastrium or suprapubic. It is useful to know the quadrants as symptoms and signs relating to the abdomen can be conveniently localised (Fig. 3.1).

HISTORY

Ask the symptoms with regard to onset, evolution and response to treatment. Common symptoms of gastrointestinal disease are abdominal pain, bowel disturbances (diarrhoea, constipation), vomiting, distension, jaundice, anorexia and failure to thrive (Table 3.1). It is important to take a good history of the diet, more so if the child is not putting on weight. A number of the symptoms are subjective, so ask questions to clarify your doubts. Some mothers will complain that their child does not eat, where in fact the child is thriving well. There are also those who find it difficult to provide proper nutrition but maintain that their child is eating "all the time." You could ask what the child likes to eat instead of "what the child eats everyday." Do not appear to be threatening, as this will rarely give you the right answers. Build on the rapport to ask, "How many times a week can

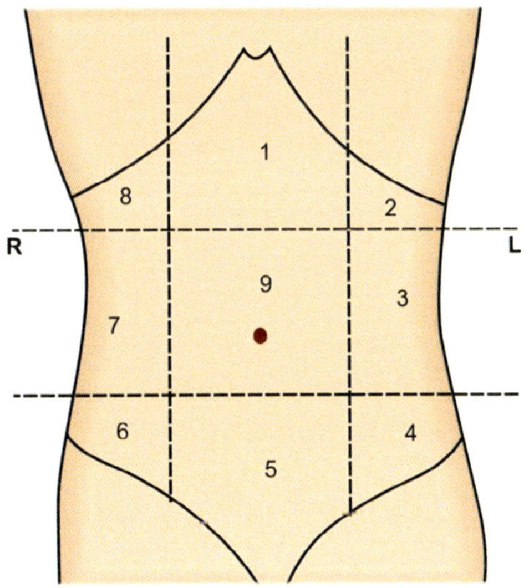

Fig. 3.1: Compartments of the anterior abdominal wall: 1. Epigastrium, 2. Left hypochondrium, 3. Left lumbar region, 4. Left iliac fossa, 5. Hypogastrium, 6. Right iliac fossa, 7. Right lumbar region, 8. Right hypochondrium, 9. Umbilical region

you afford to give him this.", Or "where do you get your milk and eggs from?" Once you are sure of a clear dietary history, put down an average diet and work out the calories and protein from such a diet. Refer to the chapter on nutritional values to work out if the diet is appropriate.

Table 3.1: Chief complaints of gastrointestinal system

- Abdominal pain
- Bowel disturbance — Diarrhoea / Constipation
- Blood in stool
- Vomiting, jaundice
- Abdominal distension
- Loss of appetite
- Weight loss

Pain

Abdominal pain is an important part of gastrointestinal symptoms. Unfortunately visceral pain is rarely well localized and may be misleading. Common causes of acute tummy aches are gastroenteritis, appendicitis, urinary tract infection, gastritis and peritonitis. Functional causes of abdominal pain are common and difficult to differentiate from organic aetiology (Table 3.2). Look up the section on pain (history) for a fuller description.

Table 3.2: Common causes of abdominal pain

- Gastroenteritis
- Appendicitis
- Urinary tract Infection
- Gastritis
- Peritonitis
- Functional

Diarrhoea/constipation

Disturbance of bowel movement results in diarrhoea or constipation. Diarrhoea is an excessive loss of fluid and electrolytes in stool. Dysentery is described as frequent passage of stool mixed with blood and often associated with tenesmus and urgency. Diarrhoea may be caused by gastroenteritis, systemic infection, food poisoning, milk protein intolerance, coeliac disease, giardiasis and disaccharidase deficiency. First ascertain that the stools are truly 'loose'. Is the stool so watery that it trickles down the side of the child's legs? Are the motions oily, sticky and floating on water? The latter suggests malabsorption. Is there blood in the stool? What is the consistency? Are there any undigested food particles, as in children with toddler diarrhoea?

Constipation is the relative increase in consistency, decrease of frequency or difficulty in passing motions. Children may be constipated due to a poor diet. The bowel often loses its habit to 'go' everyday. There are potentially more serious causes—Hirschprung disease, hypothyroidism, cerebral palsy, hypokalemia, hypercalcaemia, vincristine ileus, narcotic drugs and coeliac disease. Enquire about the number of times the child will open his bowels. Is the motion rock solid? Do they cause bleeding? Is there tummy ache associated with this? Do you think that there is secondary faecal soiling?

Blood in Stool

Parents are often alarmed when the child has blood in the stools. Often it is a mucosal tear of the anal or rectal mucosa. Bleeding per rectum is a common association of gastroenteritis, mostly bacterial. Do think of worrying conditions like intussusception if there are other symptoms. Amoebic dysentery is common in the slightly older population. Inflammatory bowel disease and coeliac disease are not very common, but not all that rare either. More often than not, you will end up with no clear diagnosis. In such situations it is best to be pragmatic. If the child in unwell and has diarrhoeal stools, look for signs of intussusception and infection. If the child is very well in himself, eating and drinking and without abdominal tenderness, then it is reasonable to wait and watch. The mother may rush to the doctor alarmed at the sight of blood in stool. Here is a list of the causes of gastrointestinal bleeding in an infant or child (Table 3.3).

Table 3.3: Causes of gastrointestinal haemorrhage

Common
- Acute bacterial gastroenteritis
- Swallowed maternal blood (newborn)
- Amoebic dysentery
- Food poisoning
- Hookworm infestation
- Intussusception
- Anal fissure
- Cow's milk protein intolerance
- Lymphonodular hyperplasia

Rare
- Necrotising enterocolitis
- Volvulus
- Meckel's diverticulum
- Coeliac disease
- Inflammatory bowel disease
- Stress ulcer
- Coagulation disorder

Vomiting

The child who is sick may have problems with his/her gastrointestinal tract or any other systemic disorder. You could have vomiting along with the diarrhoea of gastroenteritis. Equally the child may vomit when given cytotoxic chemotherapy. Or there may be vomiting along with retching shortly after the irritation of a cough spasm. Bile stained vomitus signifies obstruction below the ampulla of Vater. There are exceptions to this – often children who are vomiting at frequent intervals bring up a little bile as part of normal regurgitation into the stomach. A bloodstained vomitus (haematemesis) is due to swallowed maternal blood, epistaxis, ruptured varices as in extrahepatic (or cirrhotic) portal hypertension or stress ulcers. It is useful to note the child's age - some conditions present at certain ages and their knowledge will allow you to home you on the right cause. Here are some causes of vomiting as per age group (Table 3.4).

Table 3.4: Common causes of vomiting

Neonate
Swallowed air (inadequate burping), gastro-oesophageal reflux, the 'mucusy' baby, systemic infection, gut dysmotility in the premature infant, intestinal obstruction, adrenal hyperplasia

One-month baby
Congenital hypertrophic pyloric stenosis, systemic infection, metabolic disorder, gastro-oesophageal reflux, duodenal atresia

Older child
Gastroenteritis, drug side effects, gastritis, appendicitis, urinary tract infection, hepatitis, raised intracranial pressure, cyclical vomiting, migraine, chronic renal failure, inborn errors of metabolism, bleeding varices

Appetite

Quite a few alimentary disorders produce anorexia. The child who is unwell will find it difficult to eat or drink. Debilitating conditions like tuberculosis and kwashiorkor are associated with a poor appetite. Some causes can be related to the treatment offered. Drugs like metronidazole or chloroquin take away the desire to eat. The child may be emotionally stressed to have an appetite. On the contrary, children may have a rather good appetite if they have ascaris infestation, uncomplicated marasmus, receive corticosteroid treatment or have hypothalamic disorders.

Fever

Common causes of pyrexia with gastrointestinal problems are: viral hepatitis, parenteral diarrhoea, malaria, kala-azar, and liver abscess. Evaluate fever as in the section in general survey.

Potbelly

This is a common complaint of parents who suppose that the child is suffering from a 'liver' disorder. A potbelly contour in toddlers is common and normal (unless examination reveals organomegaly, ascites) and therefore the patients must be reassured. The appearance is secondary to the exaggerated lumbar lordosis in children of this age.

Jaundice

In newborns physiologic jaundice is common. Be aware of other causes of neonatal icterus. If jaundice is prolonged to the second week, ask yourself the question if there is a surgical cause that is being missed. Obstructive jaundice occurs with biliary atresia, intrahepatic biliary paucity, Alagille syndrome, prolonged parenteral nutrition, choledochal cysts and congenital hypopituitarism. Unconjugated jaundice is common in the breast fed baby. Hypothyroidism, galactosaemia, sepsis, urinary tract infection, prolonged intestinal stasis and haemolysis are other common causes.

In the neonate the appearance of jaundice according to the age in days may sometimes be helpful in making a diagnosis (Table 3.5).

Table 3.5: Causes of jaundice in neonatal period

Day 1	Rhesus or ABO incompatibility
Day 2	Crigler Najjar syndrome, early physiological jaundice
Day 3	Physiological jaundice, early sepsis
Day 4	Sepsis
Day 7	Neonatal hepatitis, biliary atresia, galactosaemia

In the older child, ask for the onset, progression and presence of features of obstruction (clay coloured stools, skin itching, dark urine). What drugs did the child have? Is there a close contact with viral hepatitis? What is the sleep pattern of this child? Is the child sleeping more during the day and waking up at night? Has the child been behaving in an odd way? The last few symptoms are related to developing hepatic encephalopathy. Jaundice is common due to haemolytic anaemia, viral hepatitis, Wilson disease and Indian childhood cirrhosis. Look for the signs of fulminant hepatic failure if you have spotted jaundice.

Weight Loss

It is a feature of the body's negative energy balance. Malabsorption (persistent diarrhoea, coeliac disease, protein losing enteropathy) is a recognisable cause but first exclude inadequate nutrition. Most children who are not thriving well are undernourished both from poor quantity and quality of food. Some children find it difficult to eat from loss of appetite. Some have systemic diseases like tuberculosis, chronic haemolytic anaemias or worm infestation that siphon off the body's energy stores. Malignancy can lead to cachexia if nutrition is not dealt with adequately.

The term failure to thrive (FTT) is used commonly to denote that the child fails to grow normally up to his/her full potential. Quantitatively the child should be moving away from his/her growth centile and possibly have had crossed two major centiles (i.e., 75th, 50th, 25th). If the child is progressing at the same rate on a lower centile, it does not count as FTT.

Examination

Start the examination doing a thorough general survey. It is important to know the state of anaemia, clubbing, jaundice and vital signs. Examine the mouth and pharynx carefully for ulcers, bleeding, dental hygiene and any distinct pathology. Offer the older child a glass of water to drink. Observe if there is a problem with deglutition. Come down to the neck and search for dilated veins, scar marks from previous central lines and spider naevi. You can now proceed to examination of the abdomen. Note your findings under the following headings: inspection, palpation, percussion and auscultation.

It may seem easier to you to have a method of examination – the so-called "**system.**" Here is one way: inspect the abdomen while the child lies on the bed. You ought to be positioned on the right side of the child. While the child lies on his back, do the palpation, fluid thrill and percussion for shifting dullness. You need to turn the child on to one side for the fluid to drain down to that side. If you choose to turn the patient on to his left, you will have a good view of the back. Use this opportunity to inspect the back and palpate for renal angle tenderness. You can also feel the spine and make suitable comments. Finish doing the shifting dullness test. Lay the child back again and complete your examination with auscultation and examination of the hernial orifices. Offer to examine the genitalia – be gentle with the child when you are doing this. Do not offer to do a per-rectal examination (unless you suspect Hirschprung disease) as it does not add on to the already existing information. Some consider it unpleasant, and therefore it is best avoided.

a. Inspection

Ideally you should expose the abdomen from just above the xiphisternum to the mid-thigh. You should inspect the abdomen not only from the anterior, but also from the posterior and both sides.

- Visible peristaltic waves—Gastric outlet obstruction, malrotation of gut, duodenal stenosis, adrenal insufficiency, prune-belly syndrome
- Superficial abdominal veins—They are normal in infancy but may be pathological in the older child if they appear distended and engorged. The normal direction of venous flow is away from the umbilicus, both below and above it and the same pattern is exaggerated in portal hypertension (Fig. 3.2). Select a straight vertical segment of a vein with no tributaries in that segment, one below and one above the umbilicus. Place two fingers horizontally, side by side, on the vein above the umbilicus. Move the lower finger away thus emptying part of the vein. Remove the lower finger if there is filling from below, the vein should fill up easily. If filling from above, the vein should remain empty during this procedure. Now do the same procedure, this time removing the upper finger. If the blood flow is away from the umbilicus, the vein will remain relatively empty. If the blood flow is toward the umbilicus, the vein will distend quickly. This gives a fair idea of the direction of venous filling around the umbilicus. Remember to test for veins below the umbilicus as well (Fig. 3.2). Venous filling is from below upwards in the lower half of the abdomen in inferior vena cava and hepatic vein obstruction. In extrahepatic portal obstruction the veins in the lateral flank are more prominent.
- Shape—There is no 'normal' shape of the abdomen. An abnormally scaphoid abdomen in a newborn suggests diaphragmatic hernia. If the tummy appears full and distended, the following may be the possibilities: fat, fluid, flatus or faeces. Localised distension may suggest appendicular lump, a tumour from the abdominal wall, a 'phantom' tumour (poliomyelitis) or distended urinary bladder. Look also for the change of shape with breathing. In the newborn it is normal for the abdomen to bulge with inspiration. In the older child this may suggest weakness of the diaphragmatic muscles of respiration.
- Scars—The presence of scars may tell you about previous surgical procedures. A scar in the right iliac fossa is likely to be due to appendicectomy. Midline longitudinal scars are from exploratory laparotomy or other major abdominal surgery. A small scar over the epigastrium may mean a previous pyloromyotomy. A big scar over the right hypochondrium could be from a Kasai procedure or a hepatic transplant. Search for lateral and posteriorly placed scars of renal operations. They may be associated with scars of renal transplants in one of the iliac

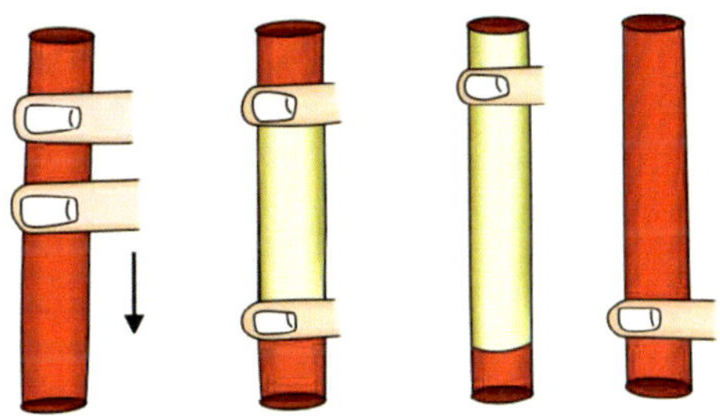

Fig. 3.2: Method of detection of blood flow in veins

fossae. You should also look carefully at the umbilicus. This may reveal a scar from a previous gastroschisis repair. It is sometimes difficult to spot the cosmetic scar of a pyloromyotomy performed through an umbilical approach.

- Umbilicus—Normally the umbilicus is slightly retracted and inverted and placed at the centre of the abdomen. If everted, an umbilical hernia may be present. You can confirm this by feeling an expansile impulse over the swelling when you ask the child to give a short cough. The following are some of the abnormalities that you might find:
  i. Omphalocele: It is a defect of the umbilical ring, containing liver and intestines and covered by peritoneum and amnion. Associations are the Beckwith-Weideman syndrome, trisomies and other congenital gastrointestinal, genitourinary and cardiac anomalies.
  ii. Gastroschisis: This is a paraumbilical, full thickness abdominal wall defect, usually a few centimetres in diameter, usually to the right of the umbilicus and between the recti. There is evisceration of bowel through the defect. Note that the umbilicus and umbilical cord are present to one side of the defect.
  iii. Delayed separation of the umbilical cord: Causes can range from local sepsis, leukocyte adhesion defect and prolonged stay of umbilical artery catheters.
  iv. Single umbilical artery: The normal distribution of vessels at birth is one vein and two arteries. Single umbilical artery can be an isolated finding or else associated with renal and other congenital anomalies.
  v. Diastasis/divarication of the recti: Commonly occurs in infants and small children.
  vi. Patent omphalomesenteric (vitello-intestinal) duct: May present as a weeping umbilical granuloma. In infants with patent urachus, urine may leak from the umbilicus.
  vii. Omphalitis: Characterised by a red, warm, moist periumbilical inflammation with or without a foul, purulent discharge.
  viii. Prominent venous circulation around the umbilicus: Collateral circulation may be associated with localised venous hum and thrill, portal hypertension and splenomegaly.
- Oedema, erythema and tenderness of abdominal wall–Necrotising enterocolitis, perforation of gut, peritonitis
- Local lesions–Abscess, haemangioma, burns
- Striae–White striae with sudden weight loss, purple striae with Cushing syndrome
- Fullness of flanks–Hirschprung disease
- Paradoxical respiration–Diaphragmatic palsy
- Epigastric pulsation–Thinly built individual, right ventricular hypertrophy, tumour overlying the abdominal aorta
- Hernial sites–Inguinal, femoral, umbilical
- Hydrocele–Hydrocele of the tunica vaginalis of the testis is a fluctuant smooth or tense swelling. The swelling in the scrotum shows positive transillumination. A hydrocele at birth is benign and goes away on its own.
- Hydrocele of the cord–Here the swelling is above the testis or in the inguinal canal but is not reducible, unlike a hernia
- Examination of the genitalia (Chap. 3, page 66).
- Anything else that may be obvious – stoma (ileostomy, colostomy), nasogastric feeding tube, gastrostomy feeding tube, drain, peritoneal dialysis catheter.

b. Palpation

There are two very important aspects to a good palpation. One, you should make the child feel relaxed so as to avoid muscle guarding. Two, you should look at the child's face to see if there is a response indicating tenderness. Palpate lightly to start with, and then proceed to deep palpation, if necessary. Make sure you have your fingernails trimmed, your hand is warm, and the child is comfortable. Palpate with the cushion of the fingers rather than the tips. Do not poke or hurt the child as it may cause resentment if a tender area exists. Palpate all the other sites first before you turn your attention to the area of tenderness. Approach gently and reassure the child when you do this. Sometimes children can be 'ticklish' and that makes examination difficult. Place the child's hand on the abdomen and your hand on top and use this combination for palpation. It is useful to perform a logical routine in palpating the abdomen. Here is a scheme you could follow:

- Start in left iliac region, go anticlockwise to end in the suprapubic region (first light then deep palpation)
- Palpate for left kidney, spleen, right kidney, liver and urinary bladder. Palpate deeply for retroperitoneal structures in the abdomen. Do also palpate the groins and examine the genitalia.

Technique

Sit down on the right side on the child. The only exception is when you palpate for a pyloric lump in congenital pyloric stenosis. It is best to palpate from the left with the left hand. You should talk to the child and allay all anxiety. The more cooperative he or she is, the better for the examination. Remember that palpation is not a test of force and will not yield anything substantial if you have to 'restrain' a child by force. Let the child lie on the bed in his/her own preferred position. There is no need to flex the hips so as to relax the abdomen. It helps to a cover for the lower part of the tummy, especially the genitalia. Children can often be put off if examined completely in the nude (Figs 3.3A to E) (splenomegaly).

Keep the fingers of your right hand straight with slight flexion at the metacarpophalangeal joints. For a left handed individual, you are permitted to stand to the left of the child and use your left hand. Gently palpate each quadrant noting for rigidity, tenderness or obvious lump (Figs 3.3A and B).

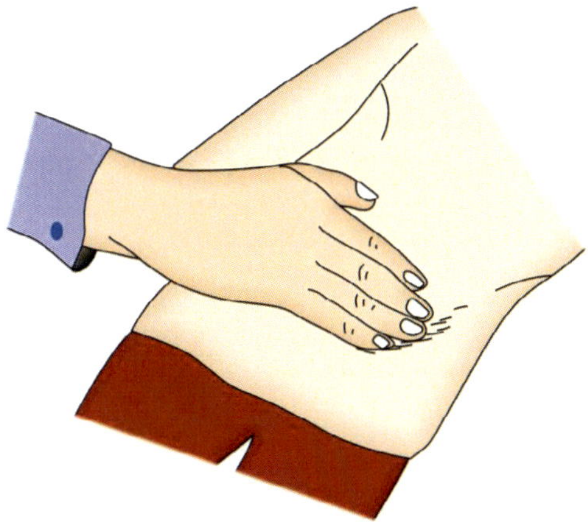

Fig. 3.3A: Correct method of superficial palpation – hand should be held flat and moulded to abdominal wall without any dipping or poking

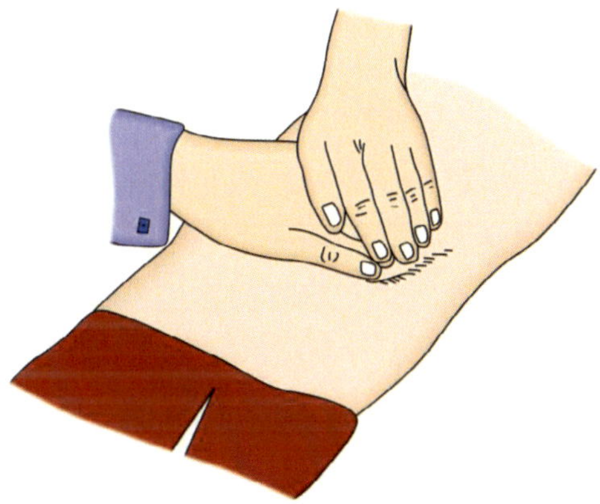

Fig. 3.3B: Deep palpation of abdomen

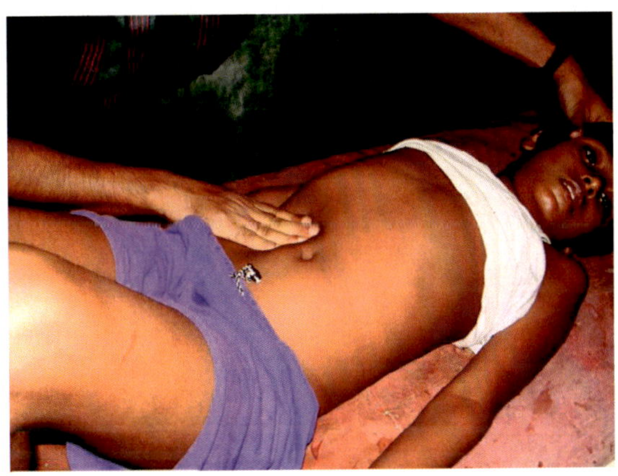

Fig. 3.3C: Palpating of liver

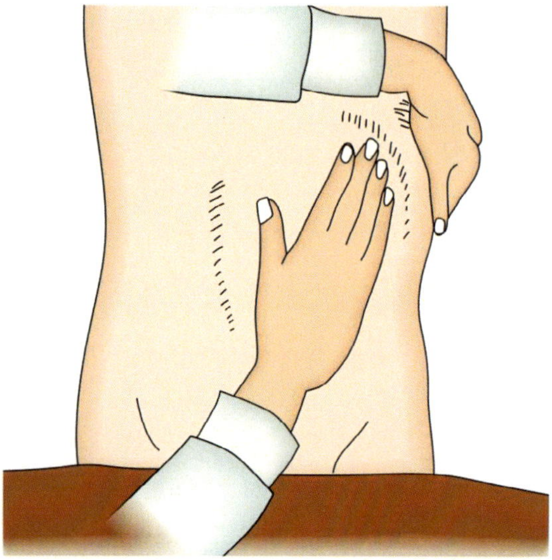

Fig. 3.3D: Classical method of palpation of spleen

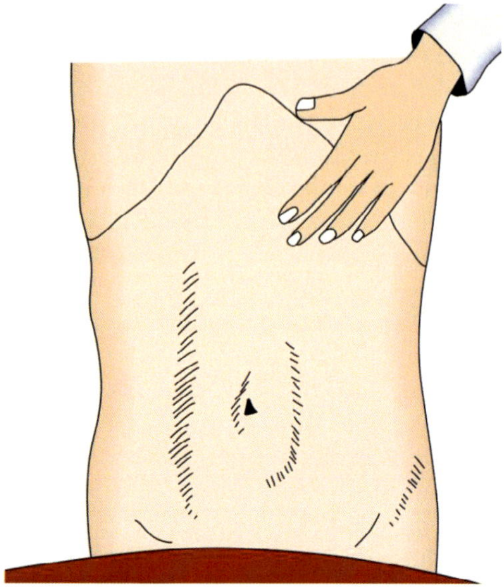

Fig. 3.3E: Alternate method of palpation of spleen

Left kidney (Figs 3.3F and G)

Place the right hand anteriorly in the left lumbar region whilst placing your left hand posteriorly in the left loin. Ask the child to draw a deep breath in and press the left hand forwards and right hand backwards. If the left kidney is enlarged it is bimanually palpable and can be pushed from one hand to another (ballotable).

In the newborns the lower pole of the kidney may normally be palpable.

Spleen

The spleen has to be enlarged to three times the normal size to be palpable below the left subcostal margin. Once the spleen has appeared in this position, it enlarges down towards the

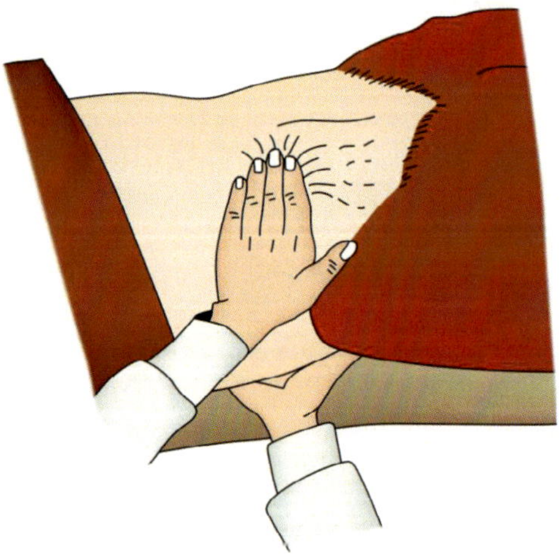

Fig. 3.3F: Palpation of left kidney from same side

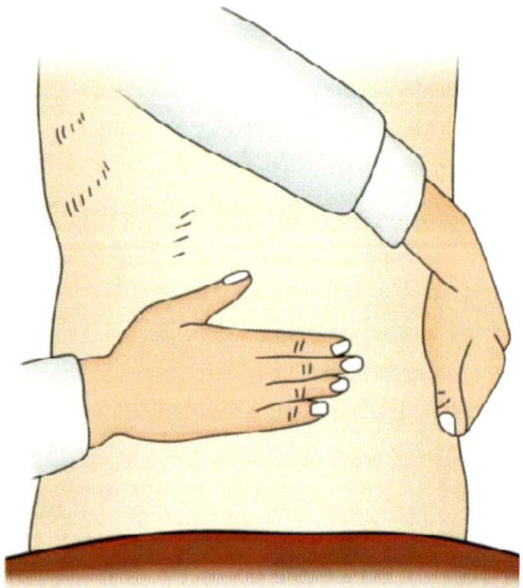

Fig. 3.3G: Palpation of left kidney from opposite side

right or left iliac fossa. Place the flat of the left hand over the lower ribs postero-laterally. Place the flat of the right hand on the anterior abdominal wall in the right iliac fossa and palpate upwards to the left subcostal arch. All the while, ask the child to breathe deeply (if he/she can cooperate). With your left hand support the rib cage so that the spleen may appear more prominent. Repeat the palpation starting from the left iliac fossa in the same way. Make sure to palpate below the left subcostal arch in both lateral and medial parts. If the spleen is palpable, it should come and touch your hand as a soft or firm swelling during the phase of inspiration.

It is sometimes difficult to appreciate the feel of a 'just palpable' splenomegaly. You may try Short's manoeuvre to feel the small spleen. Turn the child to the right lateral position and put the left hand on the left lower ribs. Place the flat of the right hand lightly over the abdomen below the left subcostal arch. As the child breathes deeply the spleen tip should just touch the tip of the fingers. In another method you may sit on the left side of the child and place your right palm over the left subcostal arch with the fingers resting lightly on the abdominal wall: the spleen should come and touch your fingers, if it is palpable. Practise examining for the spleen on all children and after a while you will get used to the feel of a soft, small spleen (Figs 3.3D and E).

A percussion technique is also used to detect splenic enlargement. Percuss over the anterior axillary lines in the lower intercostal spaces (normally resonant). If the spleen is enlarged, you will find dullness in inspiration and resonance during expiration.

A large splenomegaly is easy to identify – it is hard and will have anterior notches. There may, however, be confusion between a very large spleen and large kidney mass. Watch out for the following features to distinguish an enlarged spleen from a kidney. It has to be said that these features are not absolute and there may still be doubt at the end of the examination. An ultrasound examination is the best way out to differentiate the two (Table 3.6).

Table 3.6: Difference between splenic and renal mass on palpation

i. A notch in the lower medial border
ii. Not bimanually palpable
iii. Dull on abdominal percussion (band of colonic resonance over kidney)
iv. Upper border cannot be felt (one cannot 'get above it')

Complete the examination of the enlarged spleen by listening for a splenic rub (perisplenitis). Whilst examining the liver on the right side, bear in mind that the child may have situs inversus and associated polysplenia. Therefore, it is good practice to examine the liver and spleen as a whole before drawing your conclusions.

Here are some common causes of splenic enlargement (Table 3.7).

Table 3.7: Splenomegaly – Causes

- 'Normal' children – 15 percent newborns, 15 percent children, 10 percent adolescents
- Infectious diseases (typhoid fever, malaria, tuberculosis, kala-azar, infectious mononocleosis, endocarditis, septicaemia, brucellosis, toxoplasmosis, HIV)
- Haematological disorders (haemolytic anaemias, extramedullary haematopoiesis as in thalassaemia, osteopetrosis)
- Neoplasms (leukaemia, lymphoma)
- Infiltration and storage diseases (Niemann Pick, Gaucher disease, mucopolysaccharidosis, histiocytosis)
- Congestion (portal hypertension due to cirrhosis, or extra-hepatic causes, congestive cardiac failure)
- Cyst (congenital or acquired)
- Other–lupus erythematosus, juvenile chronic arthritis
- Pseudosplenomegaly (elongated splenic mesentery, enlarged left lobe of liver)

Right Kidney

Palpate for the right kidney in the same manner as the left. Place the flat of the right hand horizontally in the right lumbar region anteriorly. Push upwards with the left hand in the right loin and ask the child to breathe deeply. Press down the right hand and feel the lower pole of the kidney if it is palpable. Renomegaly is present in hydronephrosis, polycystic kidneys, Wilm's tumour, trauma to the loin and renal vein thrombosis. You may have trouble delineating a liver mass from a kidney swelling. In general you should be able to feel the liver edge. The kidney appears as a deep-seated structure and more rounded in its feel. However, confusion may well remain if either is excessively enlarged.

Liver

You normally palpate the liver margin in the right subcostal region. That is assuming that the child does not have situs inversus. Make yourself comfortable first and sit on a couch on the right side of the patient. In the two handed technique, place the flat of both hands side by side below the right subcostal region, fingers pointing towards the ribs. Ask the child to breathe in deeply. At the height of inspiration (as the liver is pushed down) press the fingers firmly inwards and upwards. The liver border, if palpable should rise beneath the fingers (Fig. 3.3C).

Alternatively place the flat of the right hand parallel to the right costal arch. The liver edge is then felt against the radial border of the index finger. Press lightly in the right hypochondrium if the liver border is indistinct.

Check the lower border of liver dullness. Percuss over the lower part of the chest wall on the right side from above downwards. The normal dullness appears in the 4th-5th intercostal space. An enlarged liver may have a higher upper border of liver dullness. It also helps to percuss for the liver over the abdomen. If there is a suspicion of hepatomegaly, you may percuss in the subcostal region with resultant dullness.

In ascites of considerable size, the liver is palpated by the 'dipping' method. Thrust the tips of fingers quickly but gently into the abdomen so as to feel the organs below when you are displacing the ascitic fluid below your hands. In neonates and young children, you can palpate the liver if you place the palm of the right hand at the subcostal area and allow normal respiration. The liver, if enlarged, will touch your palm.

Measure the liver edge in centimetres from the subcostal margin. In children the normal liver edge can be felt up to 2 cm below the ribs. In newborns, a liver edge of up to 3.5 cm may be normal. Measurement of 'liver span' is a useful concept and takes account of enlargement both upwards and downwards. Percuss the upper border of liver dullness and mark that point. Mark the lower edge of the liver in the right midclavicular line in the abdomen. Now join these two points and measure the distance to give you the liver span.

Below is a table showing average liver span at different ages (Table 3.8).

Table 3.8: Average liver span

Age (years)	*Span (cm)*
1	6
2	6.5
3	7
4	7.4
5	8
12	9

Table 3.9: Points to note in a palpable liver

- Liver span
- Consistency
- Movement with respiration
- Surface
- Edge
- Tenderness
- Pulsation
- Upper margin of liver dullness
- Bruit
- Gallbladder

Note the following in a palpable liver (Table 3.9).

i. Is it abnormal? Measure the liver span and have an estimate.
ii. Consistency – hard, firm or soft
 Soft—Congestive cardiac failure, infective hepatitis, malaria
 Firm—Lymphoma, chronic haemolytic anaemia, repeated malarial attacks, amoebic hepatitis, fatty liver, Indian childhood cirrhosis
 Hard—Malaria, myelofibrosis, metastasis
iii. Movement with respiration–normally mobile 1-3 cm with respiration

iv. Surface–smooth (congestive cardiac failure, malaria, kala-azar, viral hepatitis) or irregular (malignancies, metastasis, nodular cirrhosis)

v. Edge – a firm liver has sharp margins, a soft liver has rounded margins

vi. Tenderness–infective hepatitis, perihepatitis, congestive cardiac failure, amoebic hepatitis

vii. Pulsation–haemangioma, tricuspid stenosis (presystolic) tricuspid incompetence (systolic)

viii. Upper border of liver dullness – lowering occurs in hyperinflation (bronchiolitis), right sided pneumothorax, gas under diaphragm (perforated viscus, pneumoperitoneum) and cirrhosis (shrinkage). The upper border may be raised in amoebic liver abscess, subdiaphragmatic abscess, right-sided pleural effusion and basal pneumonia.

ix. Bruit–hepatitis, arteriovenous malformations, haemangioma.

x. Left lobe–palpate in the epigastrium to outline the left lobe of the liver. Riedel's lobe, a congenital variant of the right lobe, results in a tongue shaped process, best felt in the epigastrium.

xi. Gallbladder–a smooth, globular swelling moving with respiration (mucocele, choledochal cyst).

Urinary Bladder

Distension of the bladder may be evident on inspection (swelling in the hypogastrium), percussion or palpation. In childhood the bladder is an intra-abdominal organ and this means that the bladder is more easily palpable than in the adult. A bladder of considerable dimension may be confused with some other suprapubic lump. A spontaneous voiding or catheterisation will easily distinguish the two. Here are some causes of bladder distension: postoperative period, posterior urethral valves, encephalopathy, neurogenic bladder dysfunction, transverse myelitis and Guillain-Barre syndrome (Table 3.10).

Table 3.10: Causes of bladder distension

- Post-operative period
- Posterior urethral valve
- Encephalopathy
- Neurogenic bladder
- Transverse myelitis
- GB syndrome

An exostrophy of the bladder is characterised by the absence of an abdominal wall over the bladder area with complete or partial exposure of the bladder mucosa. An exostrophy of the cloaca is characterised by a stoma or prolapsed terminal ileum over the opening of the colon (accompanied by an omphalocele).

Retroperitoneal Structures

Use both hands to palpate deeply. Feel the aorta, retroperitoneal lymph nodes, faecal masses and deep-seated masses. Retroperitoneal lumps may be due to tumours arising from the peritoneum, kidneys, adrenals, or lymph nodes. It may help to have the child on all fours in a crawling posture. You can then palpate the abdomen from below – retroperitoneal structures may be better defined this way.

Points of Tenderness

The Mc Burney point in the right iliac fossa is a point on the outer two-thirds of a line joining the umbilicus and the anterior superior iliac spine. Tenderness at this point is said to be associated with appendicitis. Children generally have right iliac fossa tenderness (rather than a typical Mc Burney point localisation) as a sign of appendicitis. Be wary of appendicitis presenting in many different ways. Retroperitoneal appendicitis is particularly notorious for getting missed out. Examine for rebound tenderness if there is a suspicion of appendicular inflammation. Press on the abdominal wall and release your hand quickly. If the child has peritoneal involvement, he/she will feel pain when the hand is released. Guarding is also a sign of inflammation of the peritoneum. Whilst palpating the tummy you will have noticed a rigidity of the muscles on that side. This is the body's natural mechanism to contain inflammation. Get the child to turn the face away and give a short cough. Where does it hurt? Is it over the right iliac fossa? Ask the child to blow out his tummy like a balloon and watch for his reaction. He will fail to do so if there is a degree of peritonitis. In advanced cases of acute inflammation, pressure on the left iliac fossa may cause pain in the right lower quadrant (Rovsing sign). Flexion and internal rotation of the right thigh may also cause abdominal pain (obdurator sign).

You should remember that there could be many other causes of right iliac fossa pain other appendicitis. They may be gastroenteritis, urinary tract infection, constipation, typhlitis (inflammation of caecal wall), twisted ovarian cyst and inflammatory bowel disease.

Examine other parts of the abdomen for tenderness – the left iliac fossa, right and left renal angles, epigastrium and subcostal region. Left iliac fossa pain may be related to gastroenteritis, amoebic dysentery or constipation. Renal angle tenderness could mean perinephric abscess. Epigastric tenderness may be a result of gastritis. Similarly duodenal inflammation or cholelithiasis may be responsible for pain in the right subcostal region.

Groin

Inspect the groins and palpate the inguinal canal for any expansile impulse on coughing. Perform this test in the supine and later in the standing position. Palpate the femoral artery on two sides (see section on pulse) and along the artery for enlarged inguinal nodes. The presence of inguinal lymph nodes is normal in barefoot children. There may also be small cuts and scratches in the foot or the leg and cause the nodes in the groin to be prominent.

Male Genitalia

A full term newborn male should have a well-formed penis and scrotum. The urethra opens at the tip of the penis, which is normally cylindrical. A physiological phimosis is a normal finding. Small, white epithelial pearls or inclusion cysts may be transiently present on the distal portion of the prepuce in the newborn. Pearly white papules are often normally present on the adolescent penile corona in 1-5 rows and are not to be confused with venereal warts.

The scrotum is highly pigmented in the newborn. This is due to the surge in testosterone in the perinatal period. Both testes should be located in the scrotal sac (unless premature) each measuring about 1 cm in length. A hydrocele is often present at birth that disappears spontaneously. In the adolescent growth spurt, the testes and penis increase in size and secondary sexual characteristics mature to that of the adult (see sex maturity staging).

Note the following abnormalities while examining the penis:

i. Enlargement of penis (with or without testicular enlargement)–Precocious puberty (gonadotrophin dependent or independent).
ii. Micropenis–Micropenis is an abnormally small penis, the stretched length of which deviates from the mean by more than 2.5 SD. The full term neonate has a mean penile length of 2.5 cm. Retract the penis is measure along the dorsum to the top of the glans penis without including the foreskin. Causes of small penile length are hypogonadotrophic hypogonadism (Kallmann syndrome, Prader-Willi syndrome, congenital hypopituitarism, septo-optic dysplasia), rudimentary testes syndrome, 3 beta hydroxysteriod dehydrogenase deficiency congenital adrenal hyperplasia, 5 alpha reductase deficiency, partial androgen insensitivity, gonadal dysgenesis, and Noonan syndromes.
iii. Erection–Transient erection of infancy, priapism (local irritation, urethritis, urethral or bladder calculi, spinal cord lesions, sickle cell disease, leukaemia, Fabry disease).
iv. Chordee–Refers to abnormal ventral curvature of the penis as in hypospadias

v. Hypospadias–Urethral meatus opens on the ventral surface of the penis. The meatus may be near the glans or anywhere on the ventral surface of the penis and rarely in the perineum (glandular, penile, peno-scrotal, perineal). Hypospadias may occur alone or as part of undervirilisation in congenital adrenal hyperplasia, or the Smith-Lemli-Opitz or Denys-Drash syndromes.

vi. Epispadias–Urethral opening on the dorsal surface of the penis.

vii. Stenosis of urethral meatus–observe the urinary stream for impedance or deflection (in posterior urethral valve obstruction, the stream is lost and urine often comes out in drops)

viii. Meatal redness–Local trauma, diaper dermatitis, Stevens-Johnson syndrome, Kawasaki disease.

Next examine the scrotum and testes for any of the following defects:

i. Hernia – Check for:
   a. Impulse on coughing, reducibility (unless obstructed)
   b. Hernial sac in relation to pubic tubercle (lateral and below–femoral; medial, and above–inguinal)
   c. Contents - bowel gurgles, omentum feels soft and doughy
   d. Exclude other causes
      - Hydrocele, cyst of epididymis
        - can get above swelling, transilluminant
      - Undescended or ectopic testes
        - empty scrotum on that side
      - Saphenous varix
        - swelling disappears on lying down, venous hum
      - Aneurysm of femoral artery
        - expansile pulsation
      - Psoas abscess
        - Fluctuant, may be compressible from below to appear in iliac fossa
      - Inguinal lymph node
        - Search for source for site of infection in feet, legs, thigh, scrotum, perineum and perianal region.

ii. Torsion of the spermatic cord–Swelling and ipsilateral bluish or erythematous discolouration of the involved side with pain and tenderness. In the young infant, the only evidence may be an erythematous, warm, tender groin mass.

iii. Orchitis–Following viral fever (Coxsackie, mumps, rubella) the scrotum appears swollen, painful and tender and the skin red and shiny.

iv. Leukaemic infiltration–Firm swelling, with or without pain.

v. Epididymitis–Painful, red scrotum with thickened tender epididymis.

vi. Torsion of the appendix of the testis or epididymis–Sub-acute onset or sudden pain and oedema of the scrotum. A 'blue dot' discolouration may be visible through the skin and a tender mass may be palpated near the superior pole of the tests. The testis itself is non-tender.

vii. Henoch-Schonlein purpura–scrotal oedema, bleeding into scrotum, acute severe testicular pain and swelling along with other classical features.

viii. Varicocele–In pubertal boys, appears as a 'bag of worms'; increases on standing and reduces with recumbent posture.

ix. Undescended testes–Palpate for absence of testes in each side of the scrotum. Frequently the testes in a newborn are in the inguinal canal and so examine the root of the scrotum for lumps. Most undescended testes are of the migratory or retractile types (well-formed scrotum with testes that cannot be felt). Such testes may be pulled down gently into the scrotum. Another method is to have the child sit cross-legged so that the cremasteric reflex is inactivated and testes are not retracted upwards. Testes that cannot be palpated in the scrotum or in the inguinal canal may be intra-abdominal or absent. Search for ectopic sites above the superficial inguinal ring, in the femoral area, at the base of the penis or in the perineum.

x. Small or absent testes–Congenital anorchia, rudimentary testes syndrome, post radiation, Noonan syndrome, Klinefelter syndrome, XX males, Kallmann syndrome, Biedl-Bardet syndrome, and constitutional delay of puberty.
xi. Macro-orchidism–(testicular volume larger than that expected for age) Fragile X syndrome, tumour.
xii. Unilateral testis–Mixed gonadal dysgenesis, undescended testis, unilateral anorchia, atrophy.

Female Genitalia

It is easier to inspect the female genitalia rather than do a digital vaginal or rectal examination. The intact hymen makes a formal examination unlikely. In the adolescent girl, you sometimes can feel the cervix and uterus by doing a bimanual abdomino-rectal examination. This is rarely indicated. Examination of the genitalia is a traumatic experience for the child and needs a lot of prior preparation. Do not do a genital examination unless there is a definite indication. In this age, it may be better to perform invasive internal examination only under general anesthesia. Nevertheless, do not delay preliminary examination in instances where it is clearly indicated - child abuse, Lichen sclerosis or vulvovaginitis. Explain to the child and the parents and reassure them. Remember to have a female attendant at all times. The smaller child is best kept on the mother's knee.

Sit in front of the mother and support the child's feet on your knees. Place the soles of the feet together to abduct the thighs. Now spread out the labia majora to expose the labia minora, urethral meatus, and vagina. Forward retraction of the labia majora usually permits visualization of the hymen. Observe for:

i. Secondary sexual development (see pubertal staging).
ii. Personal hygiene, lice, scabies.
iii. Vaginal discharge – Whitish/blood stained discharge is common up to the first week of life. Discharge in the older infant can be from non-specific vaginitis, bacterial vaginosis and pinworm infestations.
iv. Erythema–Trichomonas, candida infection, toxic shock syndrome, trauma, vulvo-vaginitis.
v. Vesicles–Herpetic vulvovaginitis.
vi. Cyst, caruncle, prolapse of urethra
vii. Foreign body.
viii. Clitoris–Small (gonadal dysgenesis, hypopituitarism), large (precocious puberty with virilisation).
ix. Imperforate hymen.
x. Condyloma acuminata–Filiform, clustered, soft lesions in the perineal and genital areas.
xi. Sarcoma botyroides–Moist, grape like fleshy masses at the vulva
xii. Examination for sexual abuse–Abrasion and bruising of thigh, genitals, scarring of fossa navicularis, injury to posterior fourchette, tear of labia minora.

Anus and Rectum

Rectal examination is distressing to the child – Be gentle and reassuring. Make the child lie in the left lateral position and inspect the anal opening for:

i. Meconium–The normal newborn should have passed meconium by the first day. Passage of meconium through the vagina suggests a rectovaginal fistula.
ii. Location–In congenitally malformed rectum, the location may be far too forward, close to the genitalia.
iii. Pinworms or segments of tapeworm close to the anal opening.
iv. Rectal prolapse–The prolapsed rectum appears as a bright red tube like protrusion with or without a history of blood in the stool. Causes are constipation, chronic diarrhoea, cystic fibrosis, urinary obstruction, pertussis, malnutrition, spinal cord lesions, polyps and hypothyroidism.
v. Anorectal fistula–These fistulas develop from perianal abscesses and open on the perineum near the anus.

vi. Anal fissure–This may be an important cause for unexplained crying in infants. There may be a history of bright red blood on the stools. A fissure near the muco-cutaneous junction may not be evident unless the knees are curled well into the chest and a good light used. Sometimes a speculum may have to be used for lesions not seen on external inspection.

vii. Bruise, tears, laxity of sphincter suggests sexual abuse.

viii. Perianal cellulitis–It is characterised by a sharp demarcated, intensely red erythema of the perianal tissues.

To perform a per-rectal examination in the young child, it is best to use the little finger. In older children you may use the index finger. Put a generous amount of lubricant on the gloved finger and place the pulp of the finger (not the tip) flat on the anus, and press firmly and slowly in a slightly backward direction. After initial resistance, the sphincter relaxes and the finger is passed into the anal. Rotate the finger through 360° and feel the anatomy of the rectum. Instead of putting the child in the left lateral position, you may put him in a lithotomy position. Examine for the following.

a. Anorectal stenosis–A ring or diaphragm about 1.5-2 cm above the anus. In imperforate anus, the proximal rectal pouch ends blindly somewhere above the skin. The site is revealed by dimpling or increased pigmentation of the skin (but not always). This may occur alone or as part of the VATER association (vertebral defects, anal atresia, tracheo-oesophageal fistula with oesophageal atresia, radial and renal dysplasia) or the cat's eye syndrome (ocular coloboma, pre-auricular tags or pits, congenital heart disease, ocular malformation).
b. Anal papillae–Small smooth rounded anal tags.
c. Intussusception–A mass resembling the uterine cervix may be palpable.
d. Tenderness–Right sided tenderness may occur in appendicitis or pelvic abscess.
e. Tone of sphincter –
   - Lax sphincter–Myelomeningocele, spinal cord injury
   - Grips finger–Hirschprung disease is typically associated with a loaded rectum. The anal sphincter grips the finger; on release there is explosive passage of flatus and faeces.

Percussion

Use the same technique as for percussion of the chest. This time you need to percuss over the liver, spleen, bladder and other masses. More importantly shifting dullness by percussion is used to test for free fluid in the abdominal cavity.

Shifting Dullness

Lay the child supine after making sure that he/she has passed urine recently. Palpate the abdomen for liver and spleen to avoid percussion over a lump and thereby receiving the wrong information. Percuss from below the xiphisternum downward till the maximum point or resonance is reached. At this point percuss laterally to one side from the midline till a point of dullness is reached. Mark the point and continue percussion in the same direction up to the lateral muscle wall to make that sure that the dullness is not localized. Ask the child to roll over and lie on the opposite side without taking off the pleximeter finger. Allow some time for the fluid to settle in the dependent position and percuss again. The note which was previously dull should appear resonant if ascites is present. Continue percussion from the flank medially till an area or dullness (previously resonant) is reached. Percuss as far as the hand would allow. This shows continuity of dullness. Repeat the same procedure for the other side (Figs 3.4A and B).

To detect minimal ascites, place the child in a knee-elbow position to ensure gravitation of fluid to mid abdominal position (puddle sign). Percuss from the lateral to the periumbilical area, where you will expect to find dullness. In

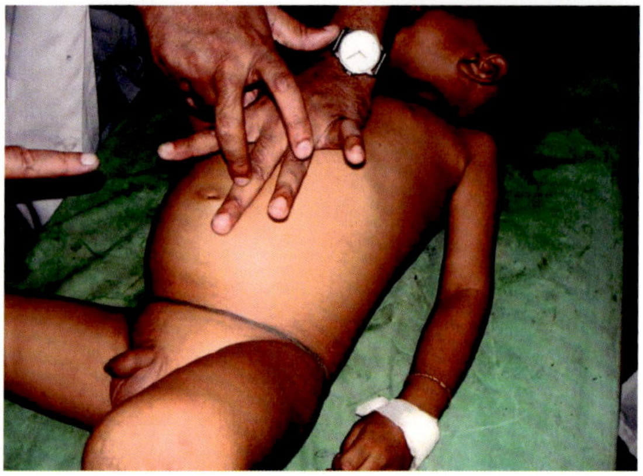

A

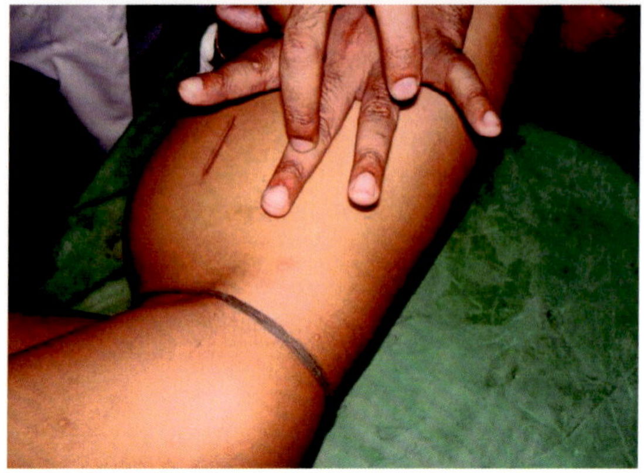

B

Figs 3.4A and B: Procedure to elicit shifting dullness

another method, the chest piece of the stethoscope is placed over the mid-abdomen and the abdominal wall is gentle tapped (or scratched) with the index finger from outside inward. A change of note is heard at the edge of the fluid pocket.

Fluid Thrill

Fluid thrill is present when the free fluid is gross and under tension. Lay the child flat on his back. Place one hand flat over the lumbar region of one side. Get an assistant to put the ulnar side of his/her hand firmly in the midline of the abdomen (the child's own hand will not suffice in this regard). Tap or flick the opposite lumbar region and feel the definite and unmistakable impulse on your hand in the opposite lumbar region. The purpose of the assistant's hand is to dampen transfer of the impulse through the fat of the abdominal wall (Figs 3.4A and B).

Hydatid Thrill

This is found during percussion of an enlarged liver or spleen. As the plexor taps the pleximeter finger, the scolices and hydatid sand in a cyst gets displaced. They come up again and touch the pleximeter soon after the tap.

Auscultation

Bowel sounds tell you if the intestines are moving normally. Place the diaphragm of the stethoscope firmly on the abdominal wall (usually to the right of the umbilicus) to listen for bowel sounds. Note in the process if the chest piece marks out an area of parietal oedema (indentation on the abdominal wall). Listen patiently and carefully to the bowels gurgling. Gastric peristalsis occurs about one in twenty seconds. The intestines in children move faster than this. Bowel sounds are excessive and exaggerated in acute mechanical obstruction. 'Sluggish' sounds occur in postoperative states, premature babies with slow gut motility or ileus and peritoneal inflammation. Listen for a few minutes before commenting on a 'silent' abdomen. Prolonged intestinal obstruction, generalised peritonitis, and paralytic ileus may give rise to this condition.

Use your stethoscope to listen to other sounds as well. You may detect a renal bruit from a renal artery stenosis or a venous hum over the epigastrium. It is common to auscultate a bruit in the iliac fossa in a child with a transplanted kidney.

4 Respiratory System

The respiratory system consists of the upper airway and the lower respiratory tract. The upper tract starts from the nose up to the larynx and includes the nose, sinuses and nasopharynx and larynx. The lower tract includes the trachea, bronchi, bronchioles and alveoli.

Before we proceed to the examination proper, it would be helpful to undersand a few anatomic landmarks. The bifurcation of the trachea corresponds in front with the lower border of the manubrium sterni (angle of Louis) and behind with the disc between the 4th and 5th thoracic vertebrates. The ribs are counted from the second rib downward. The second rib is that one whose costal cartilage articulates with the sternum at the angle of Louis (manubriosternal junction).

A line drawn from the second thoracic spine to the sixth rib in the mammary line represents the major interlobar fissure or the oblique fissure. On the right side, a horizontal line from the sternum at the level of the fourth costal cartilage, drawn to meet the line of the major interlobar fissure marks the boundary between the upper and middle lobes (minor interlobar fissure, transverse fissure) (Figs 4.1A and B).

To interpret a chest X-ray it is wise to know the anatomy of the bronchopulmonary segments. Most of the lower segments are situated posteriorly. The middle and upper lobes on the right side and the upper lobe on the left occupy most of the area in front. The axilla is that part in which all the lobes are accessible (Figs 4.2A and B).

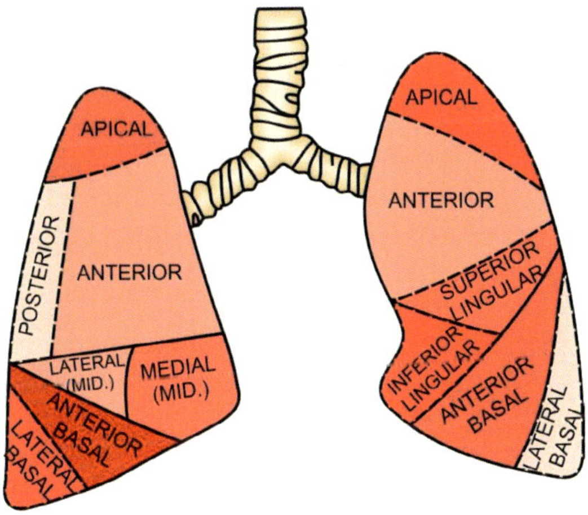

Fig. 4.1A: Respiratory segments supplied by segmental bronchi—anterior aspect

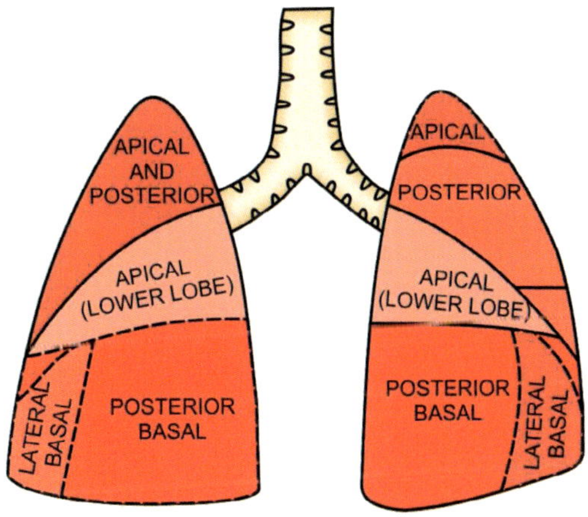

Fig. 4.1B: Respiratory segments supplied by segmental bronchi—posterior aspect

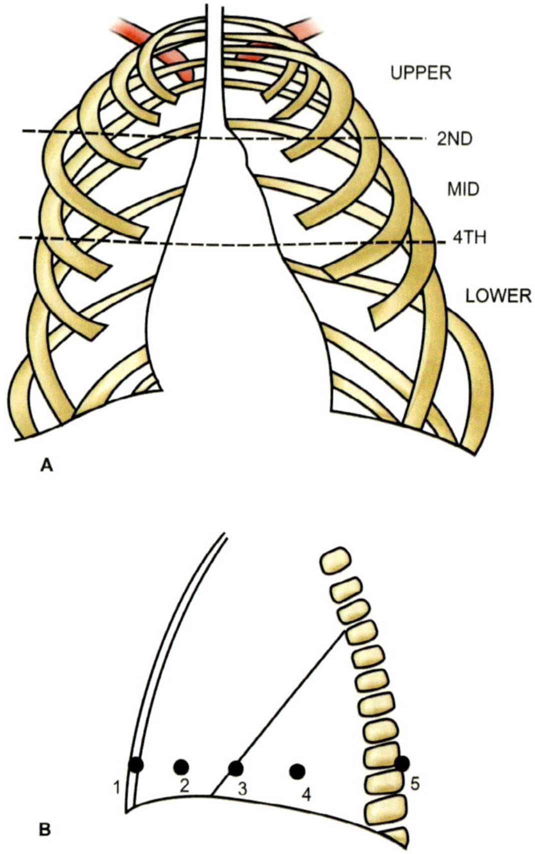

Figs 4.2A and B: The Upper, mid and lower zone of lung in X-ray chest: (A) PA view, (B) Lateral view

The upper border of the lung extends 2.5 cm (in the older child) above the medial third of the clavicle. The lower border on the midclavicular, midaxillary and scapular lines are at the 6th, 8th, 10th ribs respectively. The pleura extends to 2 spaces below and parallel to each of these landmarks.

History

Ask specifically for cough, sputum production, stridor, breathlessness (dyspnoea) and chest pain. You should make detailed assessments on each of the symptoms given below.

Cough

Infants do not have well-developed pathways for the cough reflex. For this reason their coughing is mostly ineffective. Expectoration occurs only after about 6 years of age; therefore, productive cough takes place only after that age. Enquire about the following:

- How long has it been present?
  A cough lasting for a few days may be due to coryza while a prolonged history would suggest pertussis or tuberculosis. There may be other causes of a persistent cough which are listed in Table 4.1.

Table 4.1: Different types of cough and their causes

Types of cough	*Conditions*
1. Loose, productive	Bronchitis, cystic fibrosis, bronchiectasis
2. Brassy	Tracheitis, habit cough
3. With stridor	Laryngeal obstruction, pertussis
4. Paroxysmal	Pertussis, cystic fibrosis, foreign body
5. Staccato (machine gun burst)	*Chlamydia* pneumonia
6. With vigorous exercise	Exercise induced asthma, cystic fibrosis, bronchiectasis
7. Tight (wheezy)	Reactive airways
8. Disappears with sleep	Habit cough, hysteria

- Worse at any particular time?
  A dry cough at night may be an early symptom of asthma. It is true however that all types of cough seem to be exacerbated at night. A cough, which is most severe on awakening in the morning, is often attributed to cystic fibrosis or bronchiectasis.
- Is the cough aggravated by dust, pollen or cold air?
  The increased reactivity of the airways seen in asthma and in some normal children after viral respiratory infections may present in this way. Severe coughing, whatever may be the cause may be followed by vomiting. In pertussis, a spasm of cough is followed by a characteristic forced inspiration through a narrowed glottis creating a 'whoop'

- Is there strong evidence to suggest asthma? Parents quite often ask this question if the child is wheezy for the first time. It is difficult to label a child as having "asthma" with the first few wheezy episodes. Look for associated clues which may turn the tables one-way or the other. A strong family history, maternal smoking in pregnancy and atopic illness in siblings tend to favour asthma. Eczema in the child also goes on to add to the atopic predilection. A reasonably good response to inhaled bronchodilators also seems to linked more to asthma than to viral wheeze.

Grunt

It is the body's protective mechanism of closing the glotttis during expiration to build up a positive end expiratory pressure. This protects the alveoli from collapse. Grunt is common in hyaline membrane disease, transient tachypnoea of the newborn and children with collapse-consolidation due to infection. The grunt signifies an increase in the work of breathing, and therefore, potentially serious in the older child.

Sputum

If the child can bring up sputum, ask for a description of the colour and consistency. Yellow or green sputum generally signifies lower respiratory infection but eosinophils in the sputum in asthma may also colour it yellow. Foetid sputum suggests foreign body inhalation or lung abscess.

Stridor

A predominantly inspiratory noise, this is caused by air being forced through a narrowed glottis and subglottic space. Stridor can occur acutely in laryngotracheobronchitis, acute epiglottitis, foreign body obstruction and diphtheritic laryngitis. A recurrent or persistent stridor occurs with laryngomalacia, allergic croup, papilloma, cyst, webs, abductor palsy, foreign body, tracheomalacia, thyroid enlargement, tracheo-oesophageal fistula, gastro-oesophageal reflux, Arnold-Chiari type II malformation and hysteria (Table 4.2).

Table 4.2: Causes of stridor

A. Acute	*B. Recurrent*
• Laryngotracheobronchitis • Acute epiglottitis • Foreign body obstruction • Diphtheritic laryngitis	• Laryngomalacia • Allergic croup • Papilloma, cyst, webs, abductor palsy • Foreign body • Tracheomalacia • Thymus enlargement • Tracheoesophageal fistula • Gastroesophageal reflux • Arnold-Chiary type II malformation • Hysteria

Haemoptysis

Blood in the sputum is haemoptysis. First be sure if it is haemoptysis or a haematemesis (or epistaxis). Haemoptysis is preceded by a bout of cough that brings up a small quantity of bright red blood. Haemoptysis in children may occur with bronchiectasis, lung abscess, pulmonary sequestration, idiopathic pulmonary haemosiderosis, pulmonary oedema, tuberculous cavity or a bleeding disorder (Table 4.3).

Table 4.3: Causes of haemoptysis

- Bronchiectasis
- Lung abscess
- Pulmonary sequestration
- Idiopathic pulmonary haemosiderosis
- Pulmonary oedema
- Tubercular cavity
- Bleeding disorder

Epistaxis

Epistaxis occurs with blood flowing freely usually from one nose (or both) without warning. Nose picking, trauma and foreign body are common causes. Other causes are adenoidal hypertrophy, allergic rhinitis, sinusitis, polyps, acute nasopharyngitis, paroxysmal cough (pertussis, cystic fibrosis), thrombocytopaenia, bleeding disorder, hypertension, and renal failure, angiofibroma and sometimes during menarche. When bleeding occurs at night the child swallows the blood and the epistaxis masquerades as a haematemesis (as he/she vomits) or melaena (blood in stools).

Dyspnoea

Dyspnoea is the subjective sensation of breathlessness or the awareness of the presence of breathing. Intermittent dypnoea may be due to asthma. Dyspnoea without an organic cause may present as the hyperventilation syndrome. In the smaller child and infant, look for tachypnoea, suprasternal or subcostal suction, chest retractions, cyanosis and audible wheezing.

Chest Pain

Pleuritic pain is sharp and stabbing (stitching) and is made worse by deep breathing or coughing. The pain is often severe but may be mild. The pain improves when an effusion develops to separate the inflamed surfaces. A constant severe pain may follow rib fractures. An aching pain may be due to spontaneous pneumothorax on the same side. Chest pain may arise as a cause of pain referred from the abdomen.

Physical Examination

The anatomical and physiological differences between the child and adult mean that there will be some differences in physical signs. The chest wall of the infant and young child is more compliant. This explains the signs of intercostal and subcostal recession seen during severe respiratory illness. The chest wall is also thinner and the distance between the stethoscope and bronchi smaller. Thus there is less alteration in the quality of breath sounds in each cycle. A number of signs may be variable in the small child. You may not hear crackles in a child with a consolidation. Conversely you may interpret conducted sounds from the throat as 'crackles'. Listen in when the child is not making upper airway noises. Do the sounds seem to come from a superficial source?

Inspection

a. Count the respiratory rate and comment on the rhythm and chararacter of breathing (see general survey). Look for signs of dyspnoea. Lift the tip of the nose to see the inside of the nostrils. Observe for a dull grey mucosa (allergic rhinitis), blood, foreign body and polyp.
b. Compare the size of the chest against the measurement of the head circumference. At birth, the head circumference is bigger than the corresponding chest size. The chest should overtake the head size at 6-9 months of age. If the head is bigger by the end of the first year, think of malnutrition and hydrocephalus. At birth (term baby) the chest circumference is 33 cm; that at one year is 48 cm and that at 3 years is approximately 52 cm. This is a broad generalisation. If in doubt, look up centile charts for head circumference to assess if the chest is truly small in comparison to the head
c. Look also at the shape of the chest. In infancy, the transverse diameter and the anteroposterior diameter of the chest are equal so that the chest appears round. After 2 years, the transverse diameter increases so that the appearance is transversely oval. A round chest in an older child is often due to chronic obstructive lung disease. Here are some abnormal shapes that you may come across.
   - Bulging precordium—left ventricular hypertrophy, complex congenital anomalies, pneumomediastinum
   - Intercostal bulging—large pleural effusion, marked expiratory effort
   - Retractions—mild retractions are normal; more marked retractions occur with atelectasis, pneumonia, bronchiolitis,

cystic fibrosis, asthma, laryngeal obstruction and choanal atresia. Inspiratory retraction of the sternum does not always signify insufficient pulmonary aeration but may be a normal phenomenon in small premature infants. Rib crowding may be present on the same side in collapse or fibrosis.

- Funnel chest (pectus excavatum) - characterised by depression of the sternum and costal cartilages. The defect usually begins in the 2nd intercostal region and becomes more prominent toward the xiphoid. They may be associated with absent pectoralis muscles, Marfan's syndrome, Noonan syndrome and in some normal children (Fig. 4.3).
- Pigeon breast (pectus carinatum) - characterised by a prominent, protruding sternum with vertical depressions along the costochondral junction lateral to the sternum. This deformity is found in patients with the rickets Morquio, Noonan and Schwartz-Jampel syndromes (Fig. 4.4).
- Harrison groove - a horizontal depression of the rib cage along the attachment of the diaphragm extending from the lower end of the sternum to the mid axillary line. It may be congenital or may occur as sequelae of rickets or severe chronic respiratory infection in early childhood.
- Barrel shaped chest - the sternum appears to be pushed out and the ribs more horizontal than usual. This occurs with chronic obstructive lung diseases (asthma, bronchopulmonary dysplasia).
- Narrow fixed thorax — occurs in asphyxiating thoracic dystrophy as part of a generalised skeletal abnormality.
- Rachitic rosary - rounded knob like prominences or beading at the costochondral junctions (rickets). This condition should not be mistaken for the normally palpable costochondral junctions in many normal infants (Fig. 4.7).

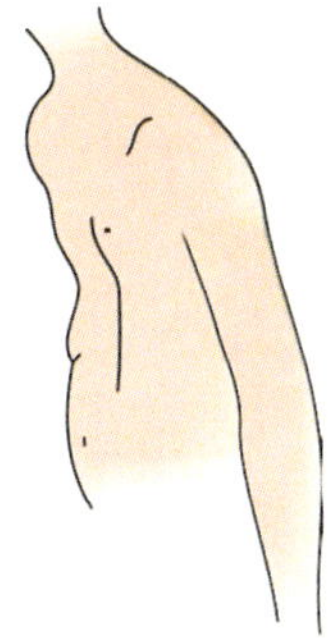

Fig. 4.3: Pectus excavatum

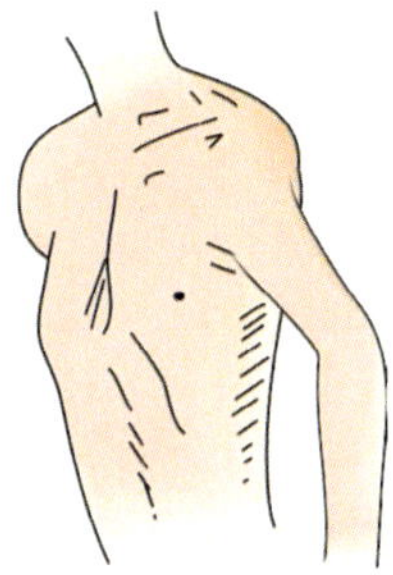

Fig. 4.4: Pectus carinatum

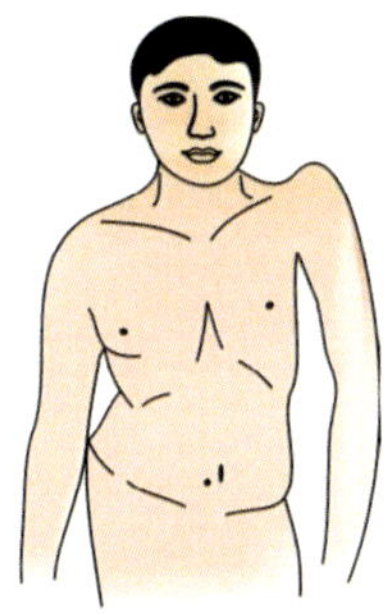

Fig. 4.5: Kyphoscoliosis

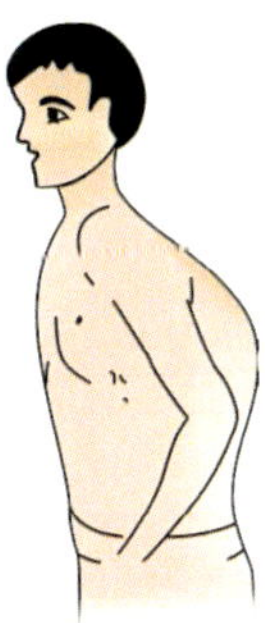

Fig. 4.6: Kyphosis

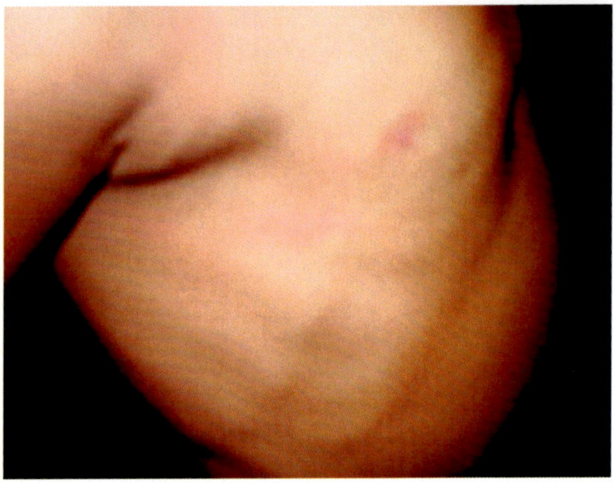

Fig. 4.7: Rachitic rosary

- Scorbutic rosary—This is characterised by a sharp edge like depression at the costochondral junction (scurvy).
- Agenesis or hypoplasia of pectoralis major and minor - this is accompanied by hypoplasia or absence of the breast and nipple (Poland's syndrome).
- Precordial pulsation—in states of hyperdynamic circulation (anaemia, left to right shunt, aortic regurgitation, mitral regurgitation), thin chest wall, pulmonary hypertension.
- Epigastric pulsation—right ventricular hypertrophy.

d. Scars—midline sternotomy scars indicate major cardiac surgery. They are often associated with scars around the xiphisternum and epigastrium (pericardial drains). Lateral thoracotomy scars indicate Blalock Taussig shunts, repair of patent ductus arteriosus, repair of coarctation and pulmonary artery banding. They may be present along with abdominal scars that suggest repair of diaphragmatic hernia or oesophageal atresia.

e. Movement of chest with respiration (see section of respiration under general survey).

f. Note features that are obvious – a Hickman central line or the button of a portacath, scars and chest drains. They may add up to give you the whole picture.

Palpation

a. *Chest palpation:* Feel a swelling for warmth, size, shape, tenderness and consistency. Bony tenderness resulting in sternal pain may be a feature of leukaemia. Tenderness of the chest wall may be due to injury, muscular (intercostal) pain, costochondritis, herpes zoster (pre-eruption) and pleurisy.
You can measure chest expansion measured at the nipple line between full inspiration and expiration. In the cooperative older child this should be at least 4 cm. You should examine the chest systematically for:
   - Swelling pain/tenderness
   - Trachea
   - Apex beat
   - Respiratory excursions
   - Vocal, rhonchial, friction fremitus

b. *Palpation of trachea:* This can be done in either sitting or supine positions. Align the head, neck and shoulders so that no one side is unduly prominent. Gently place the tip of the index finger in the suprasternal notch and extend slightly upwards to touch the trachea. Now move your finger to the right and left of the tracheal prominence. On each side of the trachea is a depression between the trachea and the sternomastoid. You will have to judge if the depression is more on the right or the left. If the finger indentation is more on the right, then the trachea is deviated more to the left (Figs 4.8 and 4.9). A slight deviation of the trachea to the right is within normal limits. Marked deviation to any one side signifies a pull (collapse, fibrothorax) to that side or a push (pleural effusion, pneumothorax empyema, lobar emphysema, tumour) to the other. Remember that a slowly developing effusion (tuberculosis) does not cause a mediastinal shift. An effusion low down or a small isolated collapse of a segment may not alter tracheal position.

c. *Cardiac impulse:* Refer to apex beat (cardiovascular system)

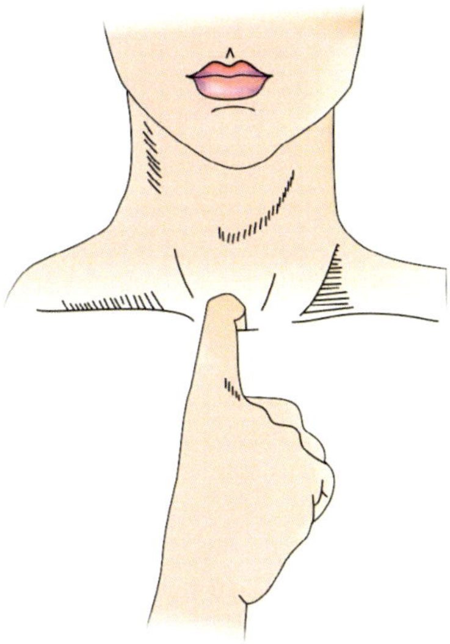

Fig. 4.8: Palpation of trachea conventional method

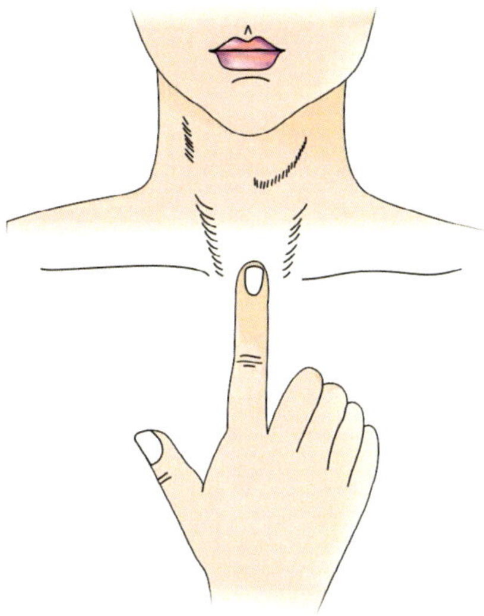

Fig. 4.9: Palpation of trachea easier method

d. *Asymmetry:* Palpate for asymmetry of excursion of movement. Lay the palms of the hands on the chest symmetrically on the posterior surface of the chest with the thumbs touching each other in the midline. In the upper part, the chest moves vertically. So if there is restriction of movement, the thumb on that side will have move less in a vertical direction. Now place the palms encircling the chest with the thumbs in the midline. This can either be done in the mammary and submammary area anteriorly or in the infrascapular area over the back. Note the lateral excursion of thumbs.

e. *Tactile vocal fremitus:* Place the palm of the hand in different areas of the chest and ask the child to say 'one-one' or 'ninety-nine'. You may use similar repetitive sounds in the local vernacular. Use the same hand in all the areas (do not use both hands simultaneously as the sensation in the 2 hands may be different). In increased vocal fremitus you should be able to feel distinct vibrations such that the sounds seem to be present just under your hand. You may also be able to detect palpable wheezing or a pleural rub with your hand. Increased vocal fremtus can be caused by consolidation and a big cavity with patent bronchus. A word of caution – these signs are unreliable in children and therefore do not jump to conclusions without corroborative evidence.

f. *Transillumination:* Darken the room and shine a bright light object (it is best to use a fibreoptic cold light source) on to the chest wall. The side of the pneumothorax in the neonate will show up transilluminant. This test is of little or no use in the older child.

Percussion

You should have a fair idea of which areas to percuss. The anterior aspect of the chest wall is divided into the presternal area and right and left anterior portions. Each side, left or right, is subdivided from above downward into supraclavicular, infraclavicular (up to 2nd rib), mammary (up to 5th rib) and infra mammary regions. On the lateral aspects, there are 2 areas, the axillary region (up to the 4th rib) and infra axillary region. Over the back on either side, the regions from above downward are supra-scapular, interscapular and infrascapular.

The basic technique of percussion for a right-handed clinician is as follows:

Place the left hand on the chest wall, palm downwards and fingers slightly separated, so that the second phalanx of the middle finger is precisely over the area to be percussed. The middle finger of the left hand is called the pleximeter finger. Press this finger down on the chest wall while all the other fingers are lifted up (so as to avoid dampening). The right middle finger is called the plexor. With the plexor, strike the pleximeter sharply at right angles like a hammer. The whole movement must be at the wrist joint and not at the elbow. Note also that as soon as the blow has been given, the striking finger must be raised. The blow should be no heavier than is necessary to elicit the resonance of the part being percussed and the wrist joint should move loosely (Fig. 4.10).

Percuss from above downward keeping the pleximeter parallel to the ribs (except for eliciting mediastinal dullness when the pleximeter finger is kept vertical and percussed from lateral to medial). Compare bilaterally for qualitative and quantitative difference of note. Percuss both the front and the back. There is no singular advantage of direct percussion over the clavicle and it is probably not worthwhile to do so (Figs 4.11A and B). Percussion in the child less than two years of age is of no great value – so do not spend too much time in tapping on a frightened toddler. It may be useful in the sick child to examine the anterior aspect of the chest in its entirety (movement, percussion and auscultation) before moving on to examine the back. This way you will not have to go backwards and forwards to complete your examination.

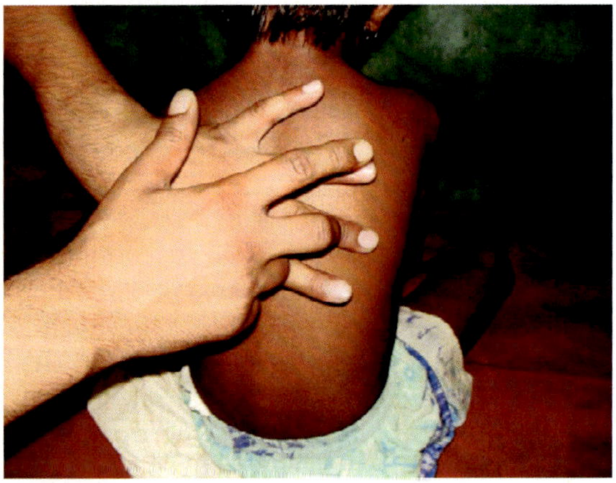

Fig. 4.10: Method of percussion

The principle of percussion is to set into vibration a body of air in a cavity of sufficient size and appropriate shape so as to produce a resonant noise. There is also a characteristic feeling in the pleximeter finger. The sound and feel of resonance over a healthy lung has to be learnt by practice. In general it is low pitched and clear in character.

The normal degree of resonance varies from individual and from region to region. The chest wall below the clavicle is thin and hence more resonant. The percussion over the scapulae is necessarily dull. The lower limits of lung resonance are determined in quiet respiration and light percussion. The lower border of the right lung lies in the mammary line at the 6th rib, in the mid-axillary line at the 8th rib, and in the scapular line at the 10th rib. On heavier percussion, the liver and diaphragm contribute to dullness two spaces higher up. On the left side, the lower border overlaps the stomach, so that there is a transition from lung resonance to tympanitic stomach resonance. The other areas

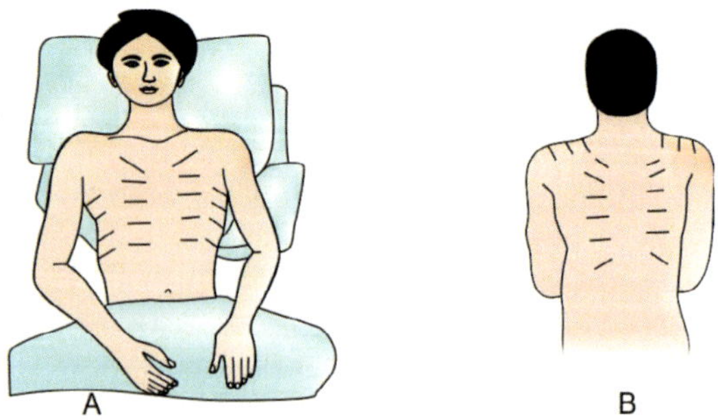

Figs 4.11A and B: Areas of percussion: (A) Front, (B) Back

are more or less similar to the corresponding areas on the right side.

Abnormal percussion notes are produced in diseased states and are given in the Table 4.4.

Table 4.4: Type of percussion note and the diseased state

Type	Interpretation
Tympanitic	Hollow viscus
Hyperresonant	Pneumothorax
Resonant	Normal lung
Impaired	Consolidation, collapse, fibrosis
Dull	Consolidation, collapse, pleural thickening, pleural effusion

Auscultation

It is difficult to auscultate the smaller child lying down. Most often he or she will resent having to lie on a bed away from the security of his mother's lap. It is therefore prudent to auscultate while the mother or father holds the child upright against the shoulder. You may find that you have to seize the opportunity and listen in when the child is quiet. The rest of the examination including palpation and percussion can come later.

Use the diaphragm of the stethoscope to listen representative areas anteriorly, posteriorly and over the axilla. Note the following on auscultation:

- Breath sounds–vesicular, bronchial, bronchovesicular
- Vocal resonance–bronchophony, whispering pectoriloquy, aegophony
- Added sounds–pleural rub, wheezes, crackles.

Breath Sounds

In infancy and early childhood the breath sounds are relatively louder and harsher than in older children and adolescents. Examine the breath sounds starting from the supraclavicular fossae and proceed downward one intercostals space at a time, comparing findings on both sides of the chest. Breath sounds are of normal intensity when inflating normally but will be reduced if there is localised airway narrowing, or if there is intervening pleural thickening. Breath sounds may be of increased intensity in children with thin chest walls. There are different types of breath sounds–vesicular, bronchial and broncho-vesicular. A brief description for each is given below.

1. Vesicular breath sounds are quiet, low-pitched rustling sounds. There is no pause between the end of inspiration and the beginning of expiration. When airway obstruction is present the expiration is prolonged.
2. Bronchial breathing sounds harsher and seems to arise from the larger airways. In conditions of collapse, consolidation or fibrosis, the breath sounds are transmitted to the surface through an intervening airless zone from the underlying large airways without attenuation. Listen with your stethoscope over the trachea to get used to hearing brochial breath sounds. The 'hollow' or 'tubular' character is more important than the loudness, as often the intensity can be diminished in overlying effusion. Historically bronchial breathing were classified into the following categories:
   - Tubular : high-pitched
   - Cavernous : low pitched (cavity)
   - Amphoric : high pitched, resembles the sound produced by blowing air across the mouth of a jar (tension pneumothorax, large superficial cavity with patent bronchus)

   It has to be said that there is very little to be gained by making such fine differentiation in a child who is probably crying and miserable. Nevertheless it helps to sharpen your clinical acumen and refresh your skills when you remember to look for such signs in cases of florid chest pathology.
3. The third variety of breath sounds is called bronchovesicular but in reality they are

vesiculobronchial in character. They are vesicular breath sounds with a more bronchial character during expiration. In a healthy child they are typically heard near the roots of the lung at the back or in the right infraclavicular region.

4. Vocal resonance (Table 4.5): This is like vocal fremitus except that you auscultate, not palpate over the chest. Normally when the child says 'one-one' or 'ninety-nine', you will not be able to perceive distinct syllables. In conditions where the resonance is increased, the sounds appear to originate from just under the chest piece of the stethoscope and the syllables are more distinct. In some situations, the vocal resonance seems to be nearer the earpiece (more intense) and is termed 'bronchophony'. A 'whispering pectoriloquy' is an increased resonance where the words spoken become clear and seem to be spoken right into the listener's ear. A high-pitched nasal intonation or bleating character (resembling the bleating of a goat) is called 'aegophony'. Do not spend too much time in evaluating the type of bronchial breathing. They are extremely subjective and more of academic interest than of real value.

Table 4.5: Vocal resonance and their causes

Vocal resonance	*Cause*
Diminished	Pleural effusion Pneumothorax Thickened pleura
Increased	
Whispering pectoriloquy	Consolidation Superficial big cavity with patent bronchus Collapse with patent bronchus
Bronchophony/ Aegophony	Consolidation above the level of pleural effusion

5. *Added sounds:* These are abnormal sounds that arise in the pleura or lung. Make sure that the sounds are not artefacts due to the chest piece rubbing over the skin. Make sure you do not auscultate over the clothes as this will not only be erroneus but will also mislead you with artefactual adventitious sounds. The various added sounds can be as follows:
   - Crackles
   - Pleural rub
   - Wheeze

a. *Crackles/crepitations:*

These are short, explosive sounds perceived as bubbling or clicking noises. When the large airways are full of sputum, a coarse rattling sound may be heard even without a stethoscope. It is a common idea that crackles are produced by air bubbling through moist secretions. This is the exception (pulmonary oedema) rather than the rule. Crackles are actually caused by sudden changes in gas pressure related to the sudden opening of previously closed small airways.

Expiratory crackles are low pitched, scanty and loud and may clear with coughing. They occur with airflow obstruction. Inspiratory crackles can be end-inspiratory and occur with pulmonary oedema, interstitial pulmonary fibrosis and resolving pneumonia. Late inspiratory crackles heard particularly at the bases indicate delayed airway opening (stiff lungs in interstitial pulmonary fibrosis) or oedema of the smaller bronchi (pulmonary oedema).

Fine crackles sound like the rustling of paper and are related to consolidation, acute pulmonary oedema or bronchopneumonia. Coarse crepitations are much louder and are heard in consolidation, lung abscess, bronchopneumonia and cystic diseases of the lungs. Bronchiectasis is responsible for coarse crepitations with a leathery creaking quality ('leathery rales'). In most situations it is important to be aware of the overall clinical condition and how your observations fit into a diagnosis. If you have an infant with a fluffy cough and diffuse crackles (more than wheezes), the likely diagnosis is bronchiolitis.

Crackles can be confused with pleural rub (see below) and with pharyngeal sounds. In the latter, the noise is heard without a stethoscope and a change of position or a cough will lead to disappearance of the sound.

b. *Pleural rub:*

A creaking, grating or rubbing noise, it is characteristic of pleural inflammation. It usually occurs with chest pain and may on occasion be palpable. A pleural rub occurs at the end of inspiration and the beginning of expiration when the surfaces of the visceral and parietal pleura are in contact. The inspiratory or expiratory components are distinct and separate in crackles. Unlike crepitations, the pleural rub does not change character with coughing.

c. *Wheezes:*

These refer to the older terminology of 'rhonchi' and are musical sounds associated with airway narrowing. A wheeze is chiefly expiratory (collapse of the smaller airways) but may also be inspiratory in more severe cases when the larger airways are also involved. In severe asthma the obstruction may be so great that air entry is very poor – in such cases, no wheeze is heard (silent chest).

A 'monophonic' wheeze is generated by localised narowing of a single bronchus (foreign body, endobronchial tuberculosis). 'Polyphonic' wheezes are particularly heard in expiration and are characteristic of diffuse airway obstruction (asthma, bronchiolitis). There is dynamic compression of the bronchi, which is accentuated in expiration when narrowing of the airway occurs. Some clinicians prefer to classify wheezes into sibilant and sonorous types. The former is said to be of high pitched, squeaky, and originates in the smaller bronchi. The latter is low pitched and originates in larger bronchi. This differentiation has no clinical significance from a management point of view.

d. *Other sounds:*

- Succussion splash: Affix the chest piece to the upper border of dullness in a suspected pleural effusion and shake the child to elicit splash of the fluid (hydropneumothorax).
- Coin test: Place a coin in front of the chest and tap with another coin and auscultate at an identical spot on the back. A loud bell like tinkle is audible in patients with pneumothorax.
- Friction test: Place the chest piece on the centre of the chest and rub your fingernail on on either side of the chest wall. The sound of scratching is heard well on the side having pneumothorax.
- Ewart's sign: Bronchial breathing may be audible over the left lower interscapular area in a patient with pericardial effusion (compression of left main bronchos leading to collapse).
- D' Espian's sign: There is bronchial breathing and increased vocal resonance in the midline over the back below the level of the 4th thoracic vertebra in case of a mediastinal mass.
- Hamman's sign (mediastinal crunch): Systolic crunching noises are auscultated over the left sternal border from 3rd to 5th interspaces in mediastinal emphysema with left sided pneumothorax.

Reconciliation

This is not part of the clinical examination but is crucial to formulating an opinion on the child's diagnosis. As you proceed through the various tests you will pick up signs that may be contradictory. Accumulate all your information and come to a decision as to the most likely diagnosis. Analysis of your findings will also mean that you have a list of differential diagnoses.

Clinicians work on a best-fit principle. Use the collected information and rationalise your thought on the possibilities. Now rank them according to the probability of occurrence. Here are some hints to help you along.

a. *Left pleural effusion*

Chest expansion	reduced on left
Trachea	shifted to right
Percussion note	stony dull
Breath sounds	absent or decreased
Added sounds	none
Vocal resonance	absent or decreased

b. *Right upper lobe consolidation*

Chest expansion	reduced

Trachea	central or slightly to right
Percussion note	dull
Breath sounds	bronchial
Added sounds	crackles
Vocal resonance	whispering pectoriloquy

c. *Collapse of right lower lobe*

Chest expansion	reduced on right
Trachea	central
Percussion note	dull lower right
Breath sounds	absent or decreased
Added sounds	none/crackles/wheezes
Vocal resonance	decreased/normal

d. *Large right pneumothorax*

Chest expansion	reduced on right
Trachea	shifted to left
Percussion note	hyperresonant
Breath sounds	absent or decreased
Added sounds	usually none
Vocal resonance	decreased

5 CARDIOVASCULAR SYSTEM

The cardiovascular system is a central feature in a good examination. Signs and symptoms pertaining to this system often depend upon the age of the child. You should therefore develop your skills of examination so that they can be suited to each age group. The more practice you get the better. With practice, you will not miss the subtle signs associated with neonatal cyanotic congenital heart disease or the older child with cardiomyopathy.

Dyspnoea is a measure of the child's subjective sensation of breathlessness. You will appreciate that the well child either plays or sleeps and rarely is inactive. The child who is quiet and lethargic is obviously unwell. For the older child, you could consider grading dyspnoea as one does for an adult (Table 5.1).

Table 5.1: Grading of dyspnoea (NYHA grading)

Grade I	Dyspnoea while performing heavy unaccustomed exercise (running)
Grade II	Dyspnoea while performing accustomed exercise (daily routine activity) and against gravity
Grade III	Dyspnoea on performing light work (going from one room to another)
Grade IV	Dyspnoea at rest (orthopnoea)

Background

Obtain a background to the child's presenting symptoms. Is there a family history of congenital heart conditions? Is a sibling affected with a similar condition? If a first degree relative is affected, the recurrence risk of congenital heart disease increases from a background 0.8 (2-6%). What was the antenatal scan result? Did the mother have any fever and rash during the first part of her pregnancy? If so think of rubella as a possibility.

Children with migratory joint pain, fever and skin nodules may have had rheumatic fever. What are the home conditions and sanitation facilities? Kawasaki disease may present with pyrexia, cervical lymphadenopathy, oral mucositis and rash. Have a low threshold for diagnosing this if you think the symptoms fit the criteria.

Cyanotic Spells

Ask for a history of cyanotic episodes. Does the child go "blue around the lips and mouth"? The parents may have noticed the excess colouring when the child was playing or crying. Breath holding spells may be confused with cyanosis due to congenital heart disease. Both are provoked by rapid (and deep) breathing. In the former, the cyanosis tends to appear somewhat later. In cyanotic spell, the child may adopt a typical posture in an effort to minimise blood supply to the heart, the so called "squatting" posture with hips and elbows flexed. This helps to constrict the arteries by increasing systemic resistance, and shunting off more blood toward the lungs. The posture also constricts the veins, thereby preventing excess venous return. There may be variations of the posture adopted during a cyanotic spell. In one variation, the child flexes the hips while resting on the mother's shoulders. In another, the child drops to the ground and curls up into a ball. The hypoxia associated with such an episode may trigger off secondary seizures.

EXAMINATION

Examination is based upon five principles - inspection, palpation, percussion, auscultation and 'reconciliation' (Table 5.2). The last is really not an examination, but rather an analytical overview of the findings. As with the other systems, you will find signs that seem to have variable interpretations in different situations. Use the best-fit principle to explain your examination findings.

No cardiovascular examination can be complete without a thorough general survey. Of particular note are the facial appearance, pulse, blood pressure, cyanosis, perfusion and neck veins. The regional examination is of crucial importance to proceed towards a correct diagnosis. You should use such background information to build a pen picture of your case. Remember that you do not necessarily have to be precise about the diagnosis in the cardiovascular examination and that it is acceptable to have a reasonable differential diagnosis list. Very often you will gather enough clues from the general survey and regional examination to make up this differential. You should never have the presumption that examination of the cardiovascular system is all about heart sounds. Auscultation is important but forms only a part of the whole.

Table 5.2: Scheme of examination
• Inspection
• Palpation
• Percussion
• Auscultation
• Reconciliation

1. Inspection of the chest wall – look at the chest for
   - Shape of the chest (Chap. 4, page 75)
   - Precordial bulge
   - Cardiac impulse
   - Scars (see section on respiratory system).
2. Palpation
   - Corroborate findings on inspection
   - Apex beat.

The apex beat is the down most and outer most point of definite cardiac impulse. To examine this, put the child lie on his back (or some consider sitting and leaning forward) and place the palm of the hand over the precordium on the left side. Put your hand also on the right side, otherwise you may miss dextrocardia. Localise the apex beat with the tip of a finger. Count the ribs starting from the sternal angle, which serves as a landmark for the 2nd rib. The space below is the 2nd intercostal space. Count down to the space where you have localised the apex beat and note the space. Next measure the horizontal distance of the apex beat from the left midclavicular line. In children up to 3 years of age, the apex is usually in the 4th intercostal space, outside the midclavicular line. In children aged 4-7 years, the apex is in the same (or in some on the 5th) space inside the midclavicular line. From 7 years of age, the position of the apex is 1 cm inside the left midclavicular line on the 5th space. The apex beat shifts further to the left if examined in the left lateral position, and is spread over an area of approximately 3 cm (Table 5.3).

The point of maximum cardiac impulse (MCI) is not the same as the apex beat. This can be helpful in determining the dominance of a ventricle–right or left. In left ventricular dominance, the MCI is close to or coincides with the apex. Those with right ventricular predominance have the MCI over the lower left sternal border.

- *Thrill*

A palpable murmur is called a thrill and transmits to the hand placed lightly over the chest, very much like the sensation of a purring cat. Thrills may be systolic or diastolic or both.

1. A systolic thrill in the left 2nd intercostal space is likely to be due to pulmonary stenosis, while a diastolic thrill means probable pulmonary regurgitation.

Table 5.3: Variations of the apex beat

a. Difficult to palpate or locate apex–Infants, obesity, pneumomediastinum, pericardial effusion, pleural effusion.
b. Cardiomegaly–Location of the apex beat more than 1 cm lateral to the midclavicular line in the 4th intercostal space in young children and outside the midclavicular line in the 5th space in older children.
c. Displaced apex–Cardiomegaly, dextrocardia, mediastinal shift.
d. Type of apex–Normal, left or right ventricular. The normal apex is one that is most difficult to define. It is located on the normal position and is akin to the right ventricular (RV) apex except that it is much less forceful. The RV apex is more out than down and may have a "tapping" nature. The LV apex is more down and is forceful in nature. Such an apex may be due to 'pressure overload' (aortic stenosis), which causes a forceful sustained heave, or due to 'volume overload' (aortic or mitral regurgitation) which results in an ill sustained impulse.

2. A to and fro thrill is the same area is possibly due to patent ductus arteriosus. That on the right may well be as a result of a Blalock-Taussig shunt.
3. A diastolic thrill in the left 3rd space suggests aortic regurgitation, whereas that situated over the apex suggests mitral stenosis. A systolic thrill in the apical region is suggestive of mitral regurgitation. A continuous thrill at the apex is probably due to mitral stenosis and regurgitation.
4. The thrill of aortic stenosis is palpated in the right 2nd intercostal space and is transmitted up to the carotid artery. **Remember, therefore, to put your finger over the left carotid artery every time when you search for a thrill. A thrill is always pathological; functional murmurs are never associated with a thrill.**

- *Parasternal impulse*

Place the ulnar side of your hand lightly to the left of sternum. The finding of a parasternal impulse indicates enlargement or hypertrophy of the right ventricle or left atrium. A similar test is to put the ulnar side of your hand over the left 2nd intercostal space. Such a sign indicates pulmonary hypertension. A left ventricular heaving apex beat with parasternal lift can be due to biventricular hypertrophy. You can grade parasternal impulse as:

Grade 1 :	Mildly lifts the hand, but can be obliterated
Grade 2 :	Lifts the hand but does not stay with it
Grade 3 :	Lifts the hand and stays with it

- *Other pulsations*
  - Suprasternal (coarctation of the aorta, aortic regurgitation, unfolding of aortic arch).
  - Left 2nd intercostal space (palpable second sound known as diastolic shock, due to pulmonary hypertension).
  - Right sternal edge (huge right atrium as in Ebstein disease).
  - Interscapular and infrascapular region (Suzman's sign in coarctation of the aorta).
- *Other relevant areas*
  - Palpate other relevant areas-joints in rheumatic fever, liver edge and pedal oedema in congestive cardiac failure, trachea and spine if the apex beat is displaced.

3. Percussion

Percussion of the heart is rarely done, as it does not add much to the clinical assessment. It may be hazardous in the child with cyanotic heart disease where it may dislodge an embolus. Dullness beyond the apex suggests pericardial effusion. In this condition the 2nd intercostal space is also dull in the lying position. This disappears as the patient sits up. In pulmonary artery dilation and pulmonary hypertension, dullness (Gerhardt's dullness) is present both in lying and sitting positions.

4. Auscultation

Auscultation for the beginner can seem frustrating, as you will often seem to have the incorrect findings. With practice and perseverance you will be able to train yourself to listen with growing confidence. You may have to improvise your examination to catch the child in a good mood. Use any trick you have up your sleeve to make sure that the child is not crying. Use distraction techniques using an interesting toy or a set of colours. Sometimes it is best that you go away and come back to examine when the child is sleeping. Over time you will be able to listen correctly, correlate with regional examination findings and draw appropriate conclusions.

The stethoscope used for auscultation should combine both a bell-type chest piece and a diaphragm. High-pitched sounds (1st and 2nd heart sounds, aortic diastolic murmur, systolic murmurs, opening snap) are heard well with the diaphragm. Low pitch sounds (3rd or 4th heart sounds, mitral stenosis murmurs) are best heard with the bell. Palpate the carotid artery as a time reference (systolic or diastolic) and also to check if there is any thrill.

It is best to auscultate all the areas of the chest first and then formulate an opinion of the quality and character of heart sounds and murmurs. There is little point in commenting on the heart sounds and murmurs in each individual area. Instead you should reserve your judgement for heart sounds and murmurs in the 'best heard' areas. For example, say, "the first heart sound is normal (you have listened to the mitral area), with mobile, close split of the second heart sound; there is a soft, grade 2/6 ejection systolic murmur best heard in the left second intercostal space, and this radiates through to the back". You should know which areas to auscultate and they are given in Figure 5.1 and Table 5.4.

Table 5.4: Areas of auscultation
i. Mitral area–corresponds to the apex beat
ii. Tricuspid area–lies just to the left of the lower sternum
iii. Aortic area–right of the sternum in the 2nd intercostal space
iv. Pulmonary area–left of the sternum in the 2nd intercostal space
v. Other areas–
• Back-murmur of collaterals (pulmonary atresia, coarctation of the aorta, Blalock-Taussig shunt)
• Abdomen-renal artery bruit (renal artery stenosis), bruit over transplanted pelvic kidney
• Carotids-carotid bruit (aortic stenosis)
• Liver–haemangioma, arteriovenous malformations
• Scalp–vein of Galen malformation

Heart Sounds

The events of the cardiac cycle are shown in the Figure 5.2. The mitral and tricuspid valves close to give the 1st heart sound. Next the aortic and

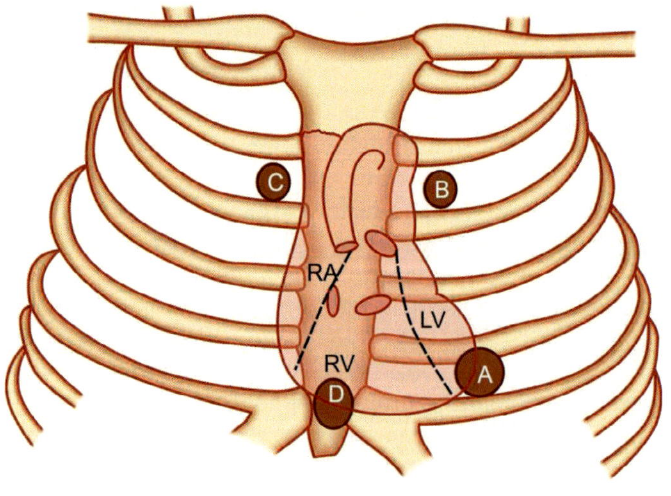

Fig. 5.1: Areas of auscultation of heart sounds (A) Mitral area; (B) Pulmonary area; (C) Aortic area; (D) Tricuspid area

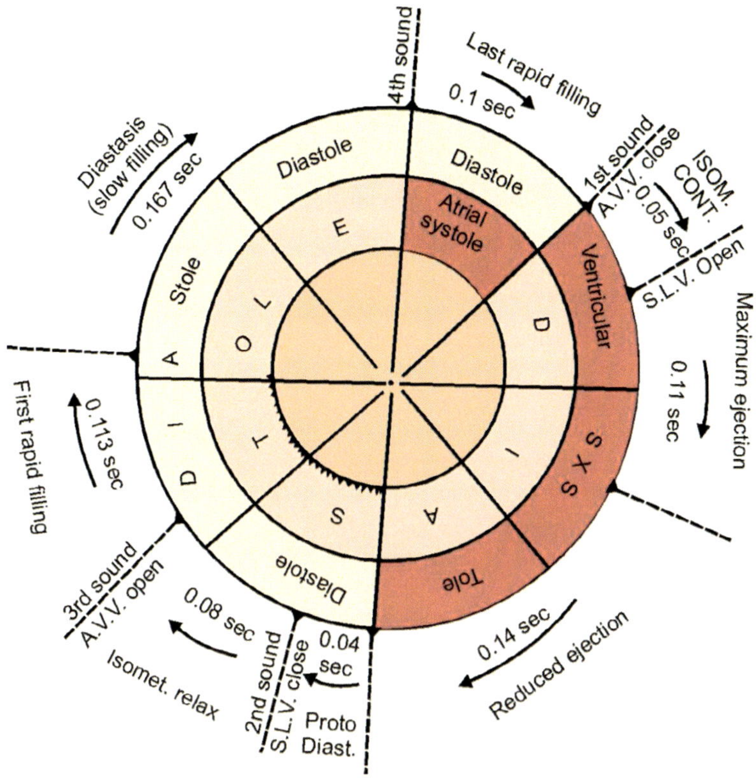

Fig. 5.2: Cardiac cycle

pulmonary valves open inaudibly. The closure of the aortic and pulmonary valves gives rise to the second sound. Closure of the pulmonary valves occurs after aortic valve closure because the pressure in the right ventricle is lower than the left. Soon after this the mitral and tricuspid valves open inaudibly. The first heart sound is short and sharp (hence the onomatopoiesis–'lup'); the second sound slightly low pitched ('dub') and is normally split (aortic and pulmonary components).

Record any deviation from normal as:

i. *Alterations in intensity:* This is rather a soft sign – use this in relation to other features of the disease. A loud first heart sound is normal in an infant with a thin chest wall but pathological in rheumatic mitral valve disease. Abnormally loudness is also a feature of tachycardia, short PR interval and mitral prolapse. Conversely heart sounds normally appear faint in the obese child, as well as in pericardial effusion.

ii. *Splitting:* The mitral valve closes slightly before the tricuspid valve and this gives rise to splitting of the first sound. The splitting is of a very short span of time and the human ear cannot detect the small difference. When audible, splitting of the first sound is not always a sign of heart disease. The chief importance lies in avoiding confusion with an atrial sound (S4). The first sound should be preceded by S4 and followed by an ejection click. It may difficult to define clearly which is which. Time the sounds with the carotid pulse - the S4 (low frequency, soft sound) appears just prior to the first heart sound (or the carotid pulse). Very often the click is accompanied by a murmur and appears relatively distant to the first sound.

The first heart sound is rarely split in the normal state. More commonly split is associtated with tricuspid stenosis, Ebstein's anomaly and right bundle branch block (RBBB).

Splitting of the second sound is much easier to understand because the two sounds (A2 and P2) are more widely separated. Splitting is best appreciated in the 2nd left intercostal space (P2 normally not audible in other areas). A physiological split is that in which A2 is followed by P2. Normally a split of 0.06 second during inspiration and 0.02 seconds (close split) in expiration is normal for a child.

During inspiration, blood is drawn into the thorax and the right ventricular stroke volume increases. The right ventricle has to account for an extra volume of blood. The duration of right ventricular systole therefore lengthens and P2 is slightly delayed. In inspiration, the left ventricular inflow falls due to a stasis in the pulmonary veins associated with a negative intrathoracic pressure. As left ventricular volume falls, the systolic time is shortened and A2 occurs earlier resulting in a split. The opposite mechanisms occur in expiration. Split heart sounds are better appreciated in the supine position.

Causes of *normal split* S2 are:

1. Delayed pulmonary closure
   a. Delayed electrical activation of RV (RBBB, LV ectopics).
   b. Prolonged RV mechanical systole (pulmonary stenosis).
   c. Reduced impedance of vascular bed (prolonged hangout interval) - ASD, idiopathic dilatation of pulmonary artery, mild pulmonary stenosis.
2. Early aortic closure
   a. Shortened LV systole (mitral regurgitation, VSD)

A reversed split or *paradoxical split* is one in which P2 occurs earlier than A2. Reverse splitting is caused by:

1. Delayed aortic closure
   a. Delayed electrical activation of LV (LBBB, RV ectopics).
   b. Prolonged LV mechanical systole (LV outlet obstruction).
   c. Reduced impedance of systemic vascular bed (post stenotic dilatation of aorta, PDA).
2. Early pulmonary closure
   a. Relative early activation of RV (Wolf-Parkinson-White syndrome)

The second sound may be heard as *single* (either A2 or P2 inaudible) or closely split in the following conditions:

1. A2 inaudible
   a. Calcific aortic stenosis.
   b. Synchronous with P2 in Eisenmenger's syndrome.
   c. Concealed by
      i. Loud P2 in pulmonary area (pulmonary hypertension).
      ii. Loud pansystolic murmur of MR/VSD.
      iii. Loud prolonged ejection systolic murmur (pulmonary stenosis).
2. P2 inaudible
   a. Diminished intensity (Fallot, tetralogy, pulmonary atresia, hyperinflation of lungs).
   b. Synchronous with A2 (Eisenmenger's syndrome).
   c. Concealed by systolic murmur (aortic stenosis).

A split that is easily heard is for all practical purposes a wide split. This is found in atrial septal defect (ASD) and partial or total anomalous pulmonary venous drainage (PAPVD/TAPVD). A wide split occurs in ASD because of RV overload and also an associated RBBB. This split is sometimes fixed if the ASD is large and the right atrium cannot distend further in inspiration to accommodate the enhanced venous return. Other causes of fixed split are severe right heart failure, pulmonary embolism and cardiomyopathy impairing RV function.

iii. *Third and fourth heart sounds*

These low frequency sounds are heard in diastole (after S2). You will be listening to a set of three beats, and when the heart rate is rapid, this seems like a gallop rhythm. A gallop with S1, S2 and S3 is known as a triple gallop. If the fourth heart sound is added, it becomes a quadruple gallop. Sometime the diastole is shortened and the third and fourth heart sounds coincide. This is known as a summation gallop. You will be hard pressed to distinguish the triple gallop from a summation gallop, but in the latter the amplitude is greater.

The 3rd and 4th heart sounds originate in the ventricles. The S3 occurs early in diastole at the time of rapid ventricular filling (0.15 second after S2). The S4 occurs later in diastole and is caused by a bolus of blood delivered to the ventricle by atrial contraction. An S3 occurs normally, in states of hyperdynamic circulation and abnormal LV filling (LV failure, MR, anaemia). An S4 is due to a stiff and non-compliant ventricular wall.

Listen to these sounds with the bell of the stethoscope and the child turned to the left lateral side. An S3 may be confused with a split S2. The differences between S3 and split S2 are given in Table 5.5.

Table 5.5: Differences between S3 and split S2

	Split	*S3*
Location	Pulmonary area	Usually apex
Intensities of components	Equal intensities	Different intensities
Interval between components	Short	Relatively long

Other diastolic sounds that may cause confusion are the opening snap of mitral stenosis and pericardial 'knock'.

- The opening snap (OS) is a high-pitched sound heard in mitral stenosis and is followed by the typical rumbling mid-diastolic murmur. A shorter A2-OS interval signifies a more severe obstruction. It is best heard slightly more parasternal to the apex, where the rumbling diastolic murmur is less prominent.
- The pericardial 'knock' in constrictive pericarditis is a loud but low frequency diastolic sound that is due to an abrupt stop in the phase of early diastolic filling.
- An ejection click is a sharp high-pitched sound heard immediately after S1. An aortic click (systemic hypertension, aortic stenosis, bicuspid aortic value) is best heard over the aortic area of the apex. A pulmonary ejection click (valvular pulmonary stenosis, pulmonary hypertension, tetralogy of Fallot) is best heard over the pulmonary area. A pulmonary click differs from an aortic click in becoming quieter or absent during inspiration (in contrast to all other right heart sounds).

Murmurs

Murmurs are audible adventitious sounds due to turbulent flow across a value or an abnormal communication within the heart. Listen to a murmur only after you are sure about the character of the heart sounds. Always comment on a murmur in conjunction with the heart sounds. For a start, define the murmur by type – systolic or diastolic. You can further qualify it as being ejection, long systolic, pansystolic, early diastolic, mid-diastolic or continuous. Grading a murmur is a measure that helps to compare the loudness. Intensity is useful for comparison in time in the same patient. Sometimes the intensity can give you an idea of the type of pathology. A loud murmur of VSD is due to a small opening (Maladie de Roger). A soft murmur of aortic regurgitation is due to a large opening. Check the grading in the section "intensity" of murmurs.

Do not automatically jump to the conclusion that a murmur signifies pathology. A number of children have murmurs without pathological significance. It is important to be able to distinguish between innocent and pathological sounds. Innocent murmurs (also called 'flow' or 'functional' murmurs) are commonly heard in the setting of fever, anxiety, infection and states of increased cardiac output (Table 5.6). It is easy enough to refer a child for an echocardiogram with any murmur. Remember that a diagnosis of an innocent murmur can often be made on clinical grounds. It is only when you are in doubt that you should proceed for further investigation.

Table 5.6: The clinical characteristics of such an innocent murmur
i. Usually soft (grade 1-2), ejection systolic
ii. Not associated with thrill
iii. Localised
iv. Often musical
v. Intensity increased by physiological manoeuvres that increase cardiac output
vi. No symptoms attributed to cardiovascular system

The most common innocent murmur is the medium pitched, vibratory (almost musical) Still's murmur. It is short and ejection systolic in character, and is best heard along the left mid and lower parasternal border. Innocent murmurs are almost always systolic. The typical innocent systolic murmurs are (Table 5.7):

Table 5.7: Example of innocent murmur
1. Vibratory systolic murmur (Still's murmur)
2. Pulmonary systolic murmur (flow across pulmonary trunk)
3. Peripheral pulmonary systolic murmur (common in neonates, thought to be branch pulmonary stenosis)
4. Systolic mammary soufflé
5. Supraclavicular/brachiocephalic systolic murmur
6. Aortic systolic murmur
7. Cardiorespiratory murmur

There are also a few innocent noises (though not strictly murmurs) that are biphasic or continuous. A venous hum is produced by turbulent blood flow in the jugular venous system. It is generally heard in the right side of the neck or anterior portion of the upper chest. Listen over the neck when the child is sitting up and head turned to one side. The hum should diminish in the lying position, and with light compression of the jugular veins. A mammary soufflé and cephalic murmur can also be continuous.

When listening to a murmur, you should be methodical in making your observations. The murmur has to be evaluated in the light of other findings and therefore a full description is helpful. Take note of the following (Table 5.8):

Table 5.8: What to note in a murmur
• Timing
• Character
• Intensity
• Conduction
• Behaviour with respiration
• Valsalva maneuver
• Positional changes
• Change with exercise
• Transient arterial occlusion

1. *Timing*

Palpate the carotid to say if the murmur is systolic, diastolic or continuous. Note whether the systolic murmur occurs throughout the systole and overlaps the first heart sound (pansystolic). Do you think that there is a diamond shaped configuration to the murmur, building to a peak in mid-systole (ejection systolic)? A long ejection systolic murmur occurs in moderately severe pulmonary stenosis. A pansystolic murmur occurs in conditions like VSD or mitral regurgitation. Differentiate the long systolic from the pansystolic by noting the distinct first sound and a small gap between S1 and the murmur (period of isovolumetric contraction) in the former. It's difficult to be absolutely certain if the murmur that you hear is ejection systolic or long systolic without an ejection character (that is different from a pansystolic murmur). Murmurs of pulmonary stenosis and that of a VSD (not typically pansystolic) can appear alike. The site should give you a clue – ejection murmurs occur in the 2nd intercostal space, while VSD murmurs are best heard lower down.

2. *Character* (Table 5.9)

Table 5.9: Characters of murmur differences from one another
• Low pitched rumbling–mitral stenosis
• Soft blowing, high pitched early diastolic decrescendo - aortic regurgitation
• To and fro (systolic component ends before S2, then diastolic component starts)–mitral regurgitation and stenosis
• Continuous (murmur 'spills' into diastole)– patent ductus arteriosus
• High pitched blowing murmur at apex radiating towards the axilla–mitral regurgitation
• Loud, rough, rasping ejection systolic murmur in aortic area–aortic stenosis
• Low pitched diastolic murmur at apex–Austin Flint murmur (severe aortic regurgitation due to opposing directions of blood flow across aortic orifice and mitral orifice)

3. *Intensity*

Murmurs vary from the very faint to the very loud. Auscultate the area having the maximum intensity and base your grade of the murmur according to the Table 5.10. Remember that the grading is for both systolic and diastolic murmurs. Therefore with dual murmurs, assign individual grades for each.

Table 5.10: Grading of murmur	
Grade 1	: soft, picked up only by trained ears
Grade 2	: soft, but clearly audible
Grade 3	: loud murmur, not associated with thrill
Grade 4	: loud murmur, associated with thrill
Grade 5	: very loud murmur, heard even when one edge of the stethoscope is lifted from the chest
Grade 6	: very loud murmur, heard even without a stethoscope

It helps to know that a heart without a murmur does not automatically mean that it is normal. Transposition of the great arteries, double outlet right ventricle, cardiomyopathy, arrhythmias and many other defects may cause serious haemodynamic disturbances without producing murmurs.

4. *Conduction*

Pulmonary and tricuspid valve lesions are generally well localized to their respective areas. Aortic and mitral murmurs however often radiate extensively. Localize the site of maximum intensity and then slowly 'inch' your stethoscope to other areas (axilla, back, second spaces). In this respect two terms are used (often interchangeably) - 'radiation' and 'conduction'. A murmur at two distinct points on the chest wall is 'radiated' from one to the other, if there is no drop of intensity of the murmur along a line joining the two. A conducted murmur is one in which there is drop of intensity progressively outward from the site of maximum intensity. The murmur of mitral regurgitation (MR) selectively radiates to the axilla and left infrascapular area of the chest. The murmurs of patent ductus arteriosus and pulmonary stenosis conduct to the back.

The murmur of mitral stenosis (MS) is localised to the apex. In MS, the blood flow during the murmur is from the left atrium to the LV (i.e., from the posterior to a relatively anterior site). Hence, the murmur is localised to the apex. An MR due to posterior chordal rupture also radiates anteriorly but that of an anterior chordal rupture goes posteriorly. Aortic systolic murmurs may be as loud (or louder) at the apex than they are in the aortic area. Systolic murmurs that radiate into the carotid arteries are usually aortic in origin.

5. *Behaviour with respiration*

Murmurs originating in the right heart increase with inspiration (Carvallo's sign in tricuspid murmur) and that of the left side decrease with inspiration.

6. *Valsalva maneuver*

Ask the child to blow against a closed glottis (as if trying to pass stool) so that intrathoracic pressure goes up. Most murmurs decrease in length and intensity except that of hypertrophic obstructive cardiomyopathy (HOCM) and mitral valve prolapse (MVP). Following release, right-sided murmurs return to control intensity earlier than left-sided murmurs.

7. *Positional changes*

Most murmurs diminish with standing. The two exceptions are HOCM and MVP. The reverse occurs with squatting. You may find that getting a child to stand up from the lying position (about 10 times or so, if the condition permits) will bring out a soft systolic murmur associated with the acute phase of rheumatic fever.

8. *Exercise*

Murmurs due to blood flow across normal or obstructed valves (PS, MS) become louder with both isotonic (free hand exercise) and isometric (handgrip, lifting weights) exercise. Murmurs of MR, VSD and AR also increase with handgrip exercise but that of HOCM decrease with the same.

9. *Transient arterial occlusion*

You can inflate blood pressure cuffs on both arms to a few millimetres of mercury more than the systolic pressure. This occludes the arteries bilaterally and raises peripheral arterial resistance. This procedure augments the murmurs of MR, VSD and AR.

Pericardial Rub

This is a characteristic high-pitched noise likened to the creaking made by compression of new leather. Pericardial rubs occur in systole (louder) and diastole and are still present when the respiration is stopped voluntarily. Pausing breathing is difficult in children and therefore not practical in the younger ones. Listen carefully to the heart sounds and the breathing at the same time. You will find that the rub is like a 'crunch' that occurs with every heartbeat. If you are careful enough, you will notice that the breathing is out of step with this noise. It is however more complicated when you suspect a pleuropericardial rub. The presence of a friction rub indicates contact of the inflamed layers of parietal and visceral pericardium. The development of an effusion separates the layers and eventually results in disappearance of the rub. Pericardial rubs signify pericarditis which is usually bacterial, or sometimes tuberculous. You may hear a rub in the immediate post-operative state or following rheumatic fever.

Other Areas of Auscultation

Auscultation need not be restricted to the chest only. In fact there are other places which also provide vital clues (Table 5.11).

Table 5.11: Areas of auscultation other than heart

i. Lung fields for basal crackles (pulmonary oedema)
ii. Systolic bruit over renal artery (renal artery stenosis)
iii. Systolic bruit over right or left iliac fossa (transplanted pelvic kidney)
iv. Pistol shot sounds over the femoral artery in patients with high pulse pressure (AR)
v. Distal diastolic murmur (AR) – press the femoral artery distally with the chest piece (proximal pressure causes systolic murmur); other 'peripheral' signs include head bobbing ('de Musset' sign), visible capillary pulsation in nail beds ('Quincke' sign), water hammer pulse, wide pulse pressure, dancing carotids ('Corrigan' sign), systolic pulsation of enlarged liver and spleen, pupillary changes with systole.
vi. Suzman sign (pulmonary atresia, coarctation of aorta)–continuous murmur of interscapular collaterals at inter and infrascapular region
vii. Systolic bruit over a thyroid (thyrotoxicosis)
viii. Murmur over an arteriovenous malformation (cirsoid aneurysm, caroticocavernous fistula)

Reconciliation

Gather all your information and try and make sense of everything. With any other system of examination, you could talk of the findings as you go about examining. In the cardiovascular system, it is wise to stand back and hold your breath for a minute. Reflect on the positive signs and symptoms. What important negative signs have you got? What is most plausible diagnosis? If you do not have enough evidence to narrow the diagnosis to a specific condition (which is certainly possible), be truthful and say that you would rather offer a differential only.

You may have other tools given to you at this stage. A chest X-ray may be made available to you. Corroborate clinical signs of heart failure (tachycardia, tachypnoea and hepatomegaly) with pulmonary plethora (pulmonary vascular shadows extending to more than the outer third of the lung fields) on the X-ray film. The same applies for an ECG as well. Look for evidence of right axis deviation and bundle branch block with a presumptive diagnosis of ASD.

In general terms you should not worry about the final diagnosis from your clinical examination. It is rarely possible (and unsafe) to be exact (like Ebstein disease or TAPVD) from bedside clinics alone. You should have a logical working diagnosis (usually the commoner ones) and a set of differentials. The group of congenital heart diseases is a good example of this principle. From your examination you should be able to say if the child has cyanosis with heart failure and therefore fits into the 'transposition physiology.' That is your diagnosis falls under the broad umbrella of conditions that have similar haemodynamics. Similarly the cyanosed child without heart failure has the 'Fallot physiology'. This pertains to a group of conditions with restricted blood flow to the lungs. Here is a logical approach to the congenital heart diseases. This approach takes into account three factors: cyanosis, heart failure and type of apex (right, left or combined ventricular preponderance) (Tables 5.12 to 5.14).

Table 5.12: Cyanosis with heart failure

a. Right ventricular (RV) predominance
   i. TGA
   ii. Double outlet right ventricle (DORV) without pulmonary stenosis (PS)
   iii. Single ventricle without PS
   iv. Hypoplastic left heart syndrome (HLHS)
   v. Ebstein disease with right bundle branch block (RBBB)
   vi. TAPVD
   vii. Porcictont pulmonary hypertension (PPHN)
b. Left ventricular (LV) or combined ventricular (CV) predominance
   i. TGA with VSD/PDA
   ii. Persistent truncus arteriosus
   iii. Complex defects with PDA (duct dependent circulation)
   iv. Pulmonary atresia with intact ventricular septum
   v. Atrioventricular canal defects

Table 5.13: Cyanosis without heart failure

a. RV predominance
   i. Tetralogy of Fallot
   ii. TGA with PS
   iii. Moderate to severe PS
   iv. Pulmonary atresia with VSD
   v. Eisenmenger syndrome
   vi. DORV with PS
   vii. TAPVD with obstruction
b. CV/LV predominance
   i. Tricuspid atresia
   ii. Persistent arteriosus with PS

Table 5.14: Heart failure without cyanosis

a. RV predominance
   i. Coarctation of aorta (till 1½ yrs of age)
   ii. Cor triatriatum
b. CV/LV predominance
   i. Myocarditis
   ii. Myocardial ischaemia (hypoxic ischaemia)
   iii. Anomalous coronary artery
   iv. Endocardial fibroelastosis
   v. Common ventricle with L - transposition
   vi. VSD, PDA critical AS

Cyanosis should set off alarm bells ringing – note the time of onset of clinical cyanosis. Early onset of cyanosis (first week) indicates one of the **'T'** diseases: TGA, TAPVC, tricuspid atresia, truncus arteriosus, total (critical) PS and tricuspid regurgitation with the Ebstein anomaly. The Tables 5.12 and 5.13 should help you provide a suitable model to fit your patient. However, bear in mind that other conditions also give rise to cyanosis. Do not discount the possibility of lung conditions (surfactant deficient lung disease) that may present as a cyanosed neonate. There may also be some complicated situations where your clinical judgement will not appear to follow any model You should keep an open mind about the occurrence of dual pathology in such cases. For example, a cyanosed child with the apex in the right side of the chest can have asplenia, methaemoglobinaemia (with dextrocardia) and situs inversus with cyanotic congenital heart disease.

The onset of heart failure may give you some clues to the aetiology.

a. Very early onset (**first few days**) presentation of heart failure is common to the following defects: asphyxia, sepsis, supraventricular tachycardia, AV fistula, myocarditis, anaemia, hypocalcaemia, congenital heart block, persistent pulmonary hypertension and tricuspid regurgitation (Ebstein anomaly).
b. Failure at the **end of the first week** may be due to HLHS, TAPVC, critical AS, PS, coarctation of aorta, truncus arteriosus, DORV without PS, AV canal defect, AV fistula, premature PDA, renal failure and hypertension, thyrotoxicosis and adrenal insufficiency.
c. Congestive cardiac failure can occur **at any time** with supraventricular tachycardia, cardiomyopathy and myocarditis.

There are some pieces of information that you will pick up as the natural history unfolds. They should be invaluable in formulating your final diagnosis. For example, a preterm baby who is fluctuating between saturations of the high nineties and dips down to the seventies without change of oxygen concentration is likely to have a shunt (ductus arteriosus or pulmonary).

A cyanosed child with a normal heart anatomy and reasonably mature lungs and needing high concentrations of oxygen may well have persistent pulmonary hypertension. The blood gase may give you a clue. It is likely in this condition to have low oxygen levels with normal or low carbon dioxide.

The 'hyperoxia' test has similar connotations. This is not done as a routine, but can often be useful in the setting of the ventilated neonate who has either a lung condition or a cyanotic heart disease. If you give a child 100 per cent oxygen for 20 minutes, the partial pressure of arterial oxygen should go up to 20kPa. If oxygenation is compromised, in conjunction with low or normal carbon dioxide levels, the likelihood of a heart lesion increases. For lung conditions like respiratory distress syndrome, oxygenation is poor and the carbon dioxide is also high. This test is more easily done when the child is ventilated and therefore you can ensure sustained 100 per cent oxygenation. You can do a variation of this test by holding a mask tightly over the face and using 100 per cent oxygen. 'Hyperoxia' is not commonly done and the information it provides can reasonably be obtained from collateral evidence. It is also a dangerous test – duct dependent circulations may deteriorate rapidly when given too much of oxygen. It is therefore standard practice to start the neonate on intravenous prostaglandin (to keep the duct patent) if congenital cyanotic heart defect is suspected.

6 NEUROLOGY

If you are new to children, examination of the nervous system can seem daunting. But given the right attitude and practice, you should gather the relevant information from your examination without too much trouble. There will always be relatively difficult cases - children who have severe communication disorders who will not understand what you say, or children who are too little to obey your commands. In such situations, observe what you can and then deduce logical (but limited) conclusions.

As in the general survey, it helps if you have a **system of examination** which you can apply for all children. There is no one universal fit, but a sequential system is good as a starting point. Once you gather experience, you may choose to do the examination in a different order. This is acceptable as long as you do not miss out any important step. Let us discuss a system of examination that you could start off with (Table 6.1).

Table 6.1: Scheme of neurology examination

1. Higher functions and speech
2. Examination of the spine, nuchal rigidity, shunts and scars
3. Cranial nerves
4. Gait, motor functions and cerebellum
5. Sensory system
6. Autonomic system

Higher Functions

It is best to talk to the child as in a general conversation. Find out the things that he can do and those he can not. It's good to ask some relevant questions about the development at this stage because it ties in very well. You could give the child a puzzle to solve or pictures to colour. Simple tasks give you a lot of information – so be on the lookout for clues. Whatever you do, judge the child in the following categories (Table 6.2).

Table 6.2: Higher function

- Consciousness
- Position of child
- Awarness of environment
- Response to stimuli
- Activity
- Behaviour
- Emotional stability
- Handedness
- Memory

Consciousness

The term consciousness is rather vague and has a wide spectrum. For the well child who is alert and running around, defining "full consciousness" is not a problem. It does get difficult when you have a child coming from the emergency with poor verbal response and intermittent moans. Scales have, therefore, been defined to do away with the confusion of words like 'coma' and 'stupor,' which are often used interchangeably. However, for the sake of completeness, 'coma' is a state in which a child is unable to be aroused and is completely unaware of self and surroundings even in the presence of strong physical stimuli. 'Stupor' is a state that simulates sleep and can be reversed by vigorous stimulation. The quickest and simplest way to assess the level of consciousness is to use the AVPU scale:

A = Alert
V = Responds to voice
P = Responds to pain
U = Unresponsive

This is a rough tool to judge the depth of coma in the child till the time a modified Glasgow Coma Scale (GCS) (Table 6.3) can be done. Children on the 'P' part of AVPU correlate to a GCS of about 8. The GCS is a handy yet comprehensive tool. The total maximum score is 15. The minimum for no response in any category (eye opening, best motor response, best verbal response) is 3.

It's good practice to record the GCS from time to time. A child's GCS will fluctuate and the trend can often be a useful clinical clue. When managing the child, treat the child, not the GCS. For example, an isolated GCS of eight or less does not always mandate that the child needs ventilation. If the child is post-convulsive and can maintain his airway, then it is reasonable to wait and watch. Always remember to check the child's blood glucose level if there is deterioration of consciousness before proceeding to any other examination. Hypoglycaemia is an emergency that is easily reversible.

Position of the Child

Comment on the way the child lies on his/her bed or chair. The bed may be padded with side rails for the immobile child. There may be a wheelchair, which he/she uses for moving around. The child may be sleeping upright with a backrest if he/she has impending respiratory failure from ascending peripheral neuropathy. Children who have meningitis may not like to be handled and are generally irritable. They can lie with their eyes tightly closed and head turned away from the light. In severe meningeal irritation and in tetanus, the child is in opisthotonus with the occiput burrowed into the pillow. A floppy neonate with poor tone lies helplessly in a position called the 'pithed frog'

Table 6.3: Glasgow Coma Scale

Eye opening		
Score	> 1 year	< 1 year
4	Spontaneous	Spontaneous
3	To verbal command	To shout
2	To pain	To pain
1	No response	No response
Best motor response		
Score	> 1 year	< 1 year
6	Obeys	Spontaneous
5	Localizes pain	Localizes pain
4	Flexion withdrawal	Flexion withdrawal
3	Abnormal flexion(decorticate rigidity)	Abnormal flexion(decorticate rigidity)
2	Extension(decerebrate rigidity)	Extension(decerebrate rigidity)
1	No response	No response
Best verbal response		
Score	> 1 year	< 1 year
5	Orientated, converses, appropriate words	Smiles, coos, babbles
4	Disoriented, confused	Irritable
3	Inappropriate words	Cries to pain
2	Incomprehensible sounds	Grunts, moans to pain
1	No response	No response

posture. A child with decerebrate rigidity shows extension of the lower limbs, the upper limb in extension at the shoulder and elbow and the forearm pronated. In decorticate rigidity, the lower limbs are in extension, the shoulders in external rotation, but the elbows flexed and the thumb adducted into the palm.

Awareness of the Environment

How does the child interact with the environment around him/her? Does he/she communicate with you or the parents? Does he appear to watch his/her toys or the television with interest? Children with moderate learning difficulties will change expression at something of their interest. Those with encephalopathy will take no notice of the surroundings. Be wary of the child with severe visual impairment—he/she will not appear to take notice of any visual cues that you may use. Look for a blank stare and roving nystagmus in such a child.

Response to Stimuli

A child who is verbally communicating is obviously responding to the stimuli around him. For those who with poor verbal communication, you will have to try other stimuli, for example an interesting toy. Watch for behaviour changes (like a cry or a smile) in response to the stimulus. Once you have demonstrated responsiveness, ascertain if that is age appropriate. Children between 15-24 months often have stranger anxiety and are afraid of being handled by new faces. An autistic child does not make contact with the examiner and regards objects as if detached from humans. A child with a painful condition of the bones or joints (osteomyelitis, juvenile chronic arthritis, scurvy) does not like being handled.

Activity

How active is the child and is there a restriction in his movements? Is there any clue to suggest that the functional activity of the child is compromised? Is this is in keeping with your overall impression of the child? Are the higher functions at odds with the degree of disability? If so, is there a physical reason for disability – limb paralysis in cerebral palsy, poliomyelitis or joint inflammation.

Behaviour

You should get a feel for childhood behaviour at different ages. You are really looking for gross differences from normal. The child of two will normally say 'no' to every question you ask him/her (it is therefore prudent in the two year old to say 'do this,' rather than ask 'can you do this'). A child of five or six is socially interactive and plays with his/her mates. The child who is not should make you worry about autism or Asperger syndrome. The child with impulsiveness and short attention span may have attention deficit hyperactivity disorder. Note also the shy and withdrawn boy or girl who may have suffered neglect in his/her family.

Emotional Stability

This is useful to gauge the age appropriateness of the child's mental state. Emotional instability occurs in children with learning difficulties, where the overall intelligence performance is below par. Children with behavioural disorders like conduct disorder or oppositional defiant disorders often have associated emotional problems. Child abuse, be it in the past or the present, may adversely affect the child's mood and behaviour.

Handedness

Dominance of a hand is governed by the dominant cerebral hemisphere. For right-handed individuals, this is on the left side of the brain. Sixty percent of left-handed children have also their dominant centres in the left. Handedness develops over the first year and is prominent at three years. The child will draw a circle with his right or left hand consistently.

Hand preference in the early months should make you suspicious of a hemi-syndrome. This may be a subtle feature of hemiplegia from intrauterine events.

Memory

Memory can be either short term or long term. Test for short-term memory by giving the child a set numbers (say 1, 2, 3) and asking him to repeat it forwards, then backwards. The backward repetition is more affected in organic brain disorders. For long-term memory, ask the child to give his address, his school and the names of his friends, and also some past incidences that the child should remember (like festivals or birthday parties). You may see failure of long-term memory with degenerative brain disorders.

You could at this juncture test for intelligence, but this is best left for the clinical psychologists. Intelligence Quotient (IQ) testing is rigorous and is time consuming. There are some scales in use—Wechsler, Stanford-Binet, Peabody vocabulary and Bayley scales, to name a few. Very few of these tests are standardized for use in Indian children.

Speech

The conversation will provide good clues if the child has a speech problem. You should have made out from the history if the child has a hearing problem. Hearing impairment can impede the development of speech. Therefore, when talking to the child, make allowances for possible hearing failure. Note if the child is wearing a hearing aid (sensorineural deafness). As you talk and listen to the child, tease out the following components:

a. Absence or presence of speech
b. Quantity of speech—age appropriateness
c. Quality of speech—volume, phonation, articulation, content, rhythm.

You should have a fair idea of the normal development of speech. The infant says 'ma ma,' 'ba ba' without meaning at seven to eight months of age. He will have one word with meaning at age one. At fifteen months, he/she uses jargon and at eighteen months picks up on doll vocabulary. At two, he/she should put two words in a sentence and at two and a half understand the implications of prepositions like 'over' and 'under.' At three, speech comes on in leaps and bounds—he/she will have a good vocabulary and understand three step commands. At four the child is likely to tell you a story or detail the activity in a complex picture.

You should be on the look out for speech delay. Refer for audiology evaluation and consideration of speech therapy, if by:

12 months	-	no differentiated babbling or vocal imitation
18 months	-	no use of single words
24 months	-	single word vocabulary of less than 10 words
30 months	-	no evidence of 2 word combinations
36 months	-	no use of telegraphic sentences
48 months	-	no use of simple sentences.

The presence or absence of speech does not tell you the whole story. The quality of speech is equally important. Volume of speech is related to the amount of air pressure generated across the vocal cords. You could ask the child to blow out a lighted match at a distance of 5 cm or ask him to count from one to hundred.

'Aphasia' is disturbance of the ability to use language (not only speaking, but also writing and comprehension). Aphasia has been traditionally classified as motor (Broca's area), sensory (Wernicke's area), conductive (conductive fibres between motor and sensory areas) and nominal (angular gyrus). However each of the areas in the frontal, Rolandic, parietal, temporal and occipital regions subserve certain common functions. The disturbances in their functions are not just restricted to one site, and therefore anatomical delineation is not possible. It is best to describe the lesions as those of articulation, fluency, naming, repetition, reading and writing.

Phonation is a function of the vocal cords. Vocal paralysis may give rise to aphonia or dysphonia (bulbar paralysis). To judge articulation, content and rhythm of speech, listen to the child speak in long meaningful sentences. See how he/she interacts with his/her parents. Defects of articulation occur in cerebellar, pseudobulbar and bulbar lesions. In cerebellar dysarthria, the patient speaks slowly and deliberately, syllable by syllable, as if scanning a line of poetry. In pseudobulbar palsy, the pronunciation is slurred as if under the influence of alcohol. Bulbar palsy also causes nonspecific slurring. In cortical dysarthria there is irregular hesitancy in word production associated with orofacial apraxia. Fluency can be impaired in the child who has a stuttering problem.

Defects of articulation of individual words (depending on coordination and intelligibility) may results in lisping, rhotism and certain lexical syntactic disorders. In lisping the 'th' sound replaces the 's' sound. In rhotism, 'w' replaces 'r' ('wun' for 'run'). Children, when they start speaking, often have speech immaturities. Consonant deletions and substitutions like 'bue' for 'blue' and 'yow-yow' for 'yellow' are part of normal speech development. It is not normal, however, for a child to repeat the first syllable of a polysyllabic word ('gaga' for 'garage') at the age of three years. Also the use of back sounds, like 'k' instead of 'g' ('koe' for 'toe') is clearly abnormal at this age.

A child who has trouble understanding the language of others has problems in receptive language. Does the child respond to speech inconsistently? Does he have difficulty with abstract language? Does he often give inappropriate answers? Is there a lack of understanding of riddles and jokes? If there is a 'yes' then you have to watch out for communication disorders, perhaps the pervasive developmental conditions.

Examination of the Spine, Skull

Examine the spine at the beginning of the examination because it is a common tendency to forget doing this at the end. First look at the child from the back and note any obvious deformity – kyphosis, scoliosis or a combination. Is there a lump in the spine or an adjoining region? Run your hand down the curvature and feel for defects or any tenderness. Search for scars in the lumbosacral region – they may be from repair of a meningomyelocele. Next ask the child to bend down, as if to touch his/her toes. In postural scoliosis, there is exaggeration of a hump on the abnormal side.

Come up to the skull and feel for any lumps or patches of hair loss. There may be a scar from a surgical procedure. Ventriculo-peritoneal shunts are often hidden under cover of the hair. The same applies for a reservoir, if one has been put in.

It is important to test for nuchal rigidity in the child with suspected meningitis. Elicit neck rigidity by flexing the head upon the chest. Any resistance is suggestive of meningeal irritation. A frightened child may not allow movement of the neck, thereby confusing the examiner. In such cases, bring the child to the edge of the bed, and extend the neck over the edge. Then flex the head from extension to neutral. Limitation confirms meningeal irritation (Fig. 6.1A).

Kernig's sign tests for meningeal irritation is a slightly different way. Lie the child flat on the bed and flex the hip and knee to 90°. Then extend the knee further to 180°. In meningitis, due to irritation of the nerves and nerve roots, the muscles will go into spasm and prevent extension. Local injury to the spinal cord or muscles of the back may cause difficulties. To test the Brudzinski sign, flex the neck as you would to test neck rigidity. Flexion of the neck causes flexion of the hips and vice versa (Fig. 6.1B).

Another method to test minimal neck rigidity is to make the patient sit up with knees

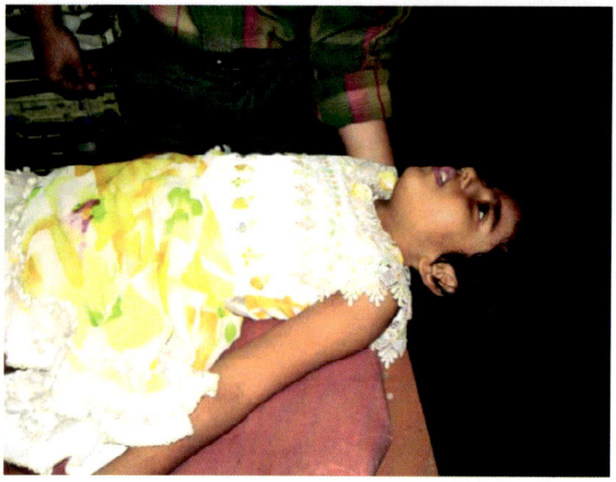

Fig. 6.1A: Examination neck rigidity

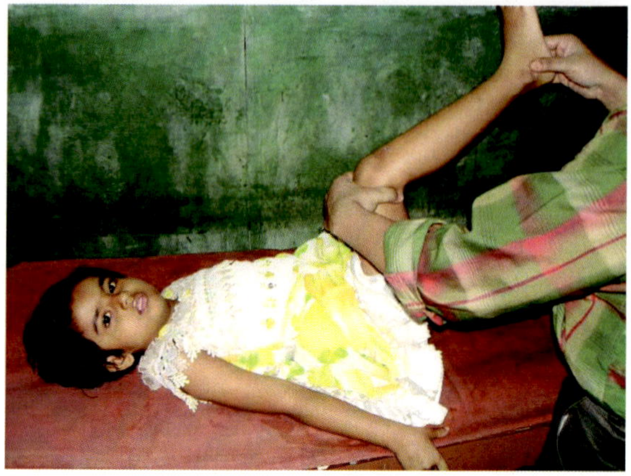

Fig. 6.1B: Elicitation of Kernig's sign

extended. The neck is then flexed. Normally flexion should be at least 45°. If minimal meningism is present, flexion will be limited to less than 45°. Bear in mind that these signs can only be elicited in the older child. In the toddler and infant, you may not be able to pick up the classic signs of meningism. In this age group undue irritability and reluctance to move may point towards a meningeal aetiology.

The "kiss the knee" test is another refined test for meningeal irritation. Put the child in the supine position and ask him to get up and kiss the knee on any one side. Make sure that he/she does not put his hands on the bed to do this. This maneuver puts the meninges on stretch and therefore a good test for minimal meningism. You can utilise this test in cases of viral meningitis and early poliomyelitis.

EXAMINATION OF THE CRANIAL NERVES

Olfactory

Anatomy

The receptors of the olfactory nerve, responsible for the sense of smell, are situated high in the nasal cavity. From these receptors, thin filaments pass centrally through the cribriform plate of the ethmoid to the olfactory bulbs, containing the second order of neurons. These neurons project to the olfactory area of the cerebral cortex (uncus and parahippocampal gyrus).

Test

It is not customary to test for smell in the younger child. You could ask the parents if they have noted any deviation from what is perceived as normal smell. In the older cooperative child inspect the nostrils first for nasal catarrh. Explain to the child what you are about to do. Ask him/her to close his/her eyes and sniff whatever substance if laid out in front. One nostril is tested at one time. Ask the child to name the odour. Use common aromatic substances such as oil of cloves or almonds, coffee, vanilla or even toothpaste or soap. Strong irritant odours are best avoided.

In 'anosmia', which can occur with head injury, the sense of smell is absent. It is important to test for anosmia in a child with delayed puberty (Kallman syndrome). 'Parosmia' is a rare abnormality in which pleasant odours seem offensive. Olfactory 'hallucinations', usually of an unpleasant nature, are characteristic of complex partial seizures in the aura stage.

Optic Nerve

Anatomy

The fibres of the optic nerve originate from the retina and pass back to the optic chiasm (Fig. 6.2). Here the fibres from the inner nasal half of each retina (representing the temporal field) decussate, whilst those from the outer temporal

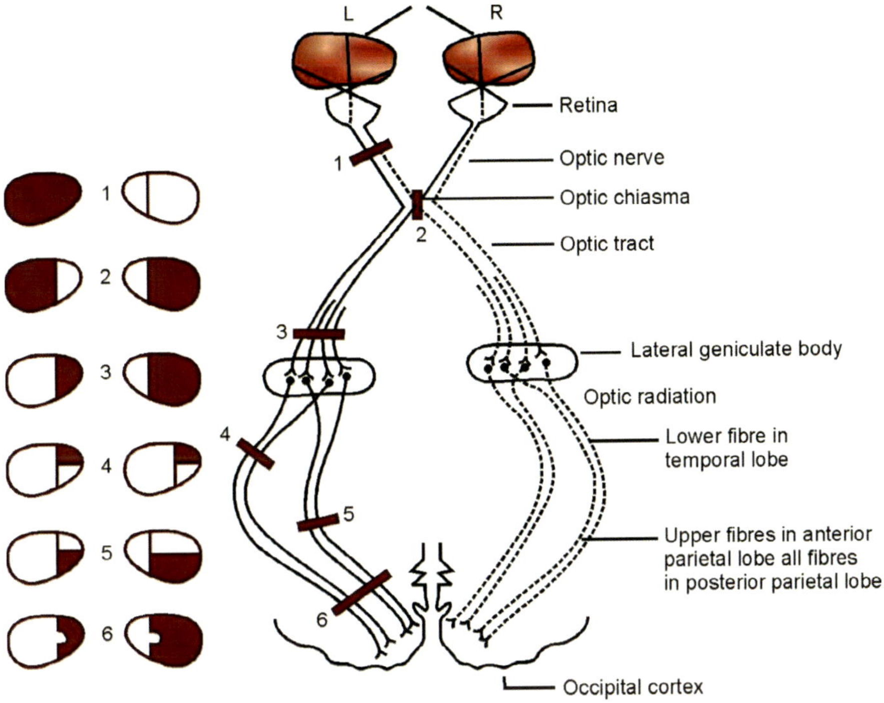

Fig. 6.2: Optic nerve pathway

half (nasal field) remain on the same side. The optic tract is formed after this chiasmal decussation and passes posterior to the lateral geniculate body of the same side. Some pre-geniculate fibres project to the superior colliculi. The optic radiation starts in the lateral geniculate body, goes backwards through the posterior limb of the internal capsule to the calcarine cortex of the occipital lobe. In the calcarine cortex, the left half of field of vision is represented on the right and vice versa. The most peripheral part of the visual fields is most anterior here. The macular area is represented at the occipital pole (Fig. 6.2).

Test

We discussed a method to examine the "eyes" as a whole in the section on general survey. This method will test for the optic nerve and also go on to test for the 3rd, 4th and 6th cranial nerves. To examine the optic nerve in isolation, you have to go through the following: cortical vision, acuity, colour vision, field of vision and fundoscopy.

Cortical vision: A child following a bright object of light usually has intact cortical vision. To show that a patient has intact cortical vision, one approach would be to make a gesture so as to poke the eye. In children after 10 months of age, this will provoke a blinking reaction. An inconsistent response suggests that vision is intact but its interpretation (e.g. parietal lobe lesions) is impaired. This is not a very sensitive test and one that can be perceived as menacing.

Acuity: The best way to test this is by using the Snellen chart, but this is only possible only in children who know their letters (usually those who are literate and above the age of six). Ensure that the room you are testing is adequately lit up, and that the distance from the chart to the child is exactly six metres. Ask the child to read from the top downwards. The letters of the alphabet are designed to subtend an angle at the eye. This can be translated into visual acuity by noting the number on the last line read by the child. This number appears on the denominator—for example 6/12 or 6/6.

For children between the age of three and six, a slightly different approach is used. The matching card letter test employs the same principle as the Snellen chart. However, it does not rely on the child's ability to identify letters. A chart with letters is positioned at three metres from the child. Make the child sit up on the mother's lap and give her a card with the same letters as they appear on the chart in the distance. Tell the child "show me the same" when you point to a letter on the chart – the child should point to the same letter on his/her card.

There are variations to this matching letter test. The system called STYCAR has single letters on the chart to match against. The Sonksen-Silver cards have lines of letters, and this tests the child's ability to differentiate letters in the periphery of the line (as opposed to test centrally). Children with amblyopia can be missed if only single letters are used. Normally, children are far-sighted up to six or seven years of age. A three-month infant has acuity of 6/60, whereas at one year it is 6/18.

Below the age of 2½ years, the STYCAR graded balls test may be used. Ten white balls are either rolled on a dark strip horizontal to the line of the infant's gaze at 3 metres, or mounted on sticks for presentation behind a dark screen. Near vision may be tested by placing small objects like 'hundreds and thousands' (cake dressings) on a piece of felt on a tabletop. See if the child reaches for them. You can get the child's interest in one of them and drag it along the felt. At one point let go of the object and carry your hand in a smooth line. Watch if the child follows your hand or stops when the object was released. You can do this test for infants under a year, but this is really is a test for visual behaviour not that of acuity. For slightly older children, you can use the "Kay picture" test, which aims to check acuity using standardised picture cards.

In the young infant, acuity is difficult to test but ophthalmologists use several methods. They are: follow face test, optokinetic nystagmus and test for fixation behaviour.

Field of vision: We discussed the method in the section "Eye" in general survey.

Colour vision: This may be judged by coloured objects or by using Holmgren's wools. A formal testing using Ishihara chart is only possible in the older child.

Examination of the fundus: To do this you need an ophthalmoscope. It consists of a head, handle and batteries. The numbers that appear on the head indicate minus lenses in the viewing aperture (red numbers or numbers with a minus in front) or plus lenses (black or plain numbers). Myopia in the patient's lenses is neutralized by the minus lens and hyperopia by the plus lens of the ophthalmoscope. At the top of the head is a control to give different kinds of beams. Two round apertures (one large, one small), a slit, a grid, and a red free filter are usually provided. The slit is used to determine convexity or concavity of retinal lesions (in whether they are raised from the surface or are indented). The red free filter is used to detect small aneurysms and haemorrhages.

Shine the widest beam of the ophthalmoscope at a distance of two metres. The circle of light will catch both the corneas. As a result, the corneal reflex and the pupillary red reflex are both visible at one sitting (Bruckner's test). Next use a +8 lens and focus the light to see any scars or deposits on the cornea. Change to +10 or +12, so that the iris becomes visible. Determine the edge of the iris, whether it is regular and rounded. Now move back to '0' and look for the red reflex. Try to focus the fundus and move from the periphery towards the optic disc, by following the vessels. The macula is situated approximately 2 disc diameters temporal to the disc.

In the fundoscopic examination, the following need to be looked at: optic disc, vessels, peripheral retina and macular area. The macula appears as a dark, yellow-orange area lateral to and slightly below the optic disc. A bright light reflex is present around the fovea. In infants, the optic disc is pale and grey, an appearance similar to optic atrophy in later life. Optic nerve hypoplasia can be diagnosed if the disc is less than half of the normal size. The macular light reflex is absent up to 4 months of age. The normal ratio of the calibre of the arterioles to that of the veins is 3:5.

Pulsation in the retinal veins (artery = central stripe, vein = darker) as they enter the optic nerve head indicates normal intracranial pressure (disappearance of venous pulsation is an early sign of papilloedema). The temporal (lateral) portion of the disc is frequently pale. A partial or complete brown or black-pigmented ring is commonly present around the disc border. The nasal (medial) edge of the disc may appear slightly blurred.

You may come across the following:

i. Retinal haemorrhages—Commonly in normal newborns (1/3 of vaginal deliveries), childhood physical abuse, haemorrhagic disorders, sickle cell disease, cardiopulmonary resuscitation, trauma, raised intracranial tension.
ii. Medullated nerve fibres (focal white patch with brush stroke appearance)—Normal, though myelination generally terminates at optic disc margin.
iii. Choroid tubercles—Elevated spots, often better visible on direct ophthalmoscopy, typical of tuberculous meningitis
iv. Retinal colobomas—Aicardi syndrome, trisomies, CHARGE association, Goldenhar syndrome, linear sebaceous naevus, focal dermal hypoplasia
v. Retinal laser burns—Retinopathy of prematurity, Coats disease
vi. "Cotton-Ball" areas—chorioretinitis, candida endophthalmitis
vii. Cherry red spot—GM1 gangliosidosis, Tay-Sach disease, Sandhoff disease, sialidosis, infantile Gaucher disease, Niemann-Pick disease, mucolipidosis type 1
viii. Lipaemia retinalis (milky white, pink, waxy appearance of retinal vessels)—Familial hypercholesterolaemia, diabetes mellitus
ix. Retinoblastoma—Unilateral or bilateral, gray or yellow-white, glistening vitreous mass
x. Rubella retinitis—Unilateral or bilateral involvement of the posterior pole, especially the macula with small, black, irregular masses or fine to gross pigmentary speckling.
xi. Retinal astrocytomas (glistening, nodular, mulberry—Like mass or oval, gray flat areas in the retina)–Tuberous sclerosis
xii. Retinal angiomatosis—von Hippel-Lindau syndrome.
xiii. Retinitis pigmentosa (degeneration, atrophy and pigmentation)—Laurence-Moon-Biedl syndrome, Refsum disease, neuronal ceroid lipofuscinosis, Cockayne syndrome, abetalipoproteinaemia, Kearns-Sayre syndrome, Hurler syndrome.
xiv. Exudative retinitis—Coats disease
xv. Papilloedema—Space occupying lesions (tumour, tuberculoma, abscess, haematoma), pseudotumour cerebri, encephalitis, meningitis, Guillain-Barre syndrome, hypertensive encephalopathy.
xvi. Optic atrophy —Primary (well-delineated rim of disc) or secondary (rim may not be well delineated), though the difference may not always be possible to distinguish on fundoscopy.

Oculomotor, Trochlear and Abducens Nerves

Anatomy

The external ocular muscles are supplied by the 3rd, 4th and 6th cranial nerves in the following fashion-all muscles (including sphincter pupillae and levator palpebrae superioris) are supplied by the 3rd nerve except the superior

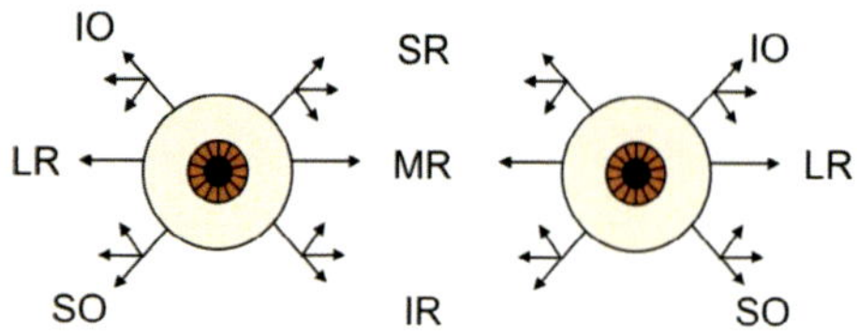

Fig. 6.3: Movements of extraocular muscles SR (Superior rectus); MR (Medial rectus); IR (Inferior rectus); SO (Superior oblique); LR (Lateral rectus); IO (Inferior oblique)

oblique (supplied by the 4th cranial nerve) and the lateral rectus (by the 6th cranial nerve). The medial rectus is the strongest of all the muscles—its function is to adduct the eye. The opposite function (abduction) is performed by the lateral rectus. The obliques act in the directions opposite to which their names suggest. Thus, the superior oblique depresses the eye (with adduction and in-torsion) while the inferior oblique elevates the eye (with abduction and ex-torsion) (Fig. 6.3) (Table 6.4). The nucleii of the 3rd, 4th, 6th cranial nerves are located in the brainstem at the level of the superior quadrigemina and extend as far caudally as the eminentia teres in the floor of the 4th ventricle. The nucleus of the 3rd nerve is the most anterior. Its rostral part (Edinger-Westphal nucleus) supplies parasympathetic fibres to the ciliary muscles and iris. Its caudal part chiefly supplies the extraocular muscles. The nucleus of the 4th nerve lies below the 3rd nerve nucleus. The 6th nerve nucleus is situated in the floor of the 4th ventricle at the level of the pons.

The 3rd nerves exits on the inner aspect of the cerebral peduncles between the superior cerebellar and posterior cerebral arteries, then passes forward to enter the lateral wall of the cavernous sinus. The 4th nerve emerges on the rostral part of the roof of the 4th ventricle. They decussate between their nucleii and emerge from the brainstem dorsally. The 6th nerve emerges between the medulla and pons after a long intracranial course.

Table 6.4: Movement of extraocular muscle

Muscle		Movement
Medial rectus	-	Adduction
Lateral rectus	-	Abduction
Superior oblique	-	Depression, abduction intorsion
Inferior oblique	-	Elevation, abduction extorsion
Superior rectus	-	Elevation
Inferior rectus	-	Depression

Test

We test the extraocular muscles (as in the chapter on "eyes" in general survey) by moving a finger or a torch (and asking the child to follow) in different directions—superior, inferior, medial and lateral. Note all the while the position of the eyes, the movements, any weakness, deviation, ptosis or abnormal motion.

Palsy of the 3rd nerve results in lateral and slight downward deviation of the eye. Palsy of the 6th nerve produces medial deviation of the affected eye. That of the 4th nerve produces little change at rest. There is slight upward deviation in the abducted position. The eye fails to move when abducted. This is often accompanied by a head tilt.

The 'setting sun' sign, a forced downward deviation of the eyes at rest with paresis of upward gaze, is an indication of raised intracranial tension. Here the pressure on the quadrigeminal plate causes impairment of the visual gaze centres. Normally this may be present in infants less than 4 weeks if the position of the head is suddenly changed. Normal newborns may show downward deviation of the eyes, skew deviation and intermittent opsoclonus (irregular chaotic oscillation of the eye in horizontal, vertical or oblique directions).

Squint

Squints are common in childhood and are broadly of two types: paralytic and non-paralytic. The paralytic lesions are those of the cranial nerves as described above. Non-paralytic squints are the result of abnormal pulling of the eyes in one direction. They may be manifest (tropia) or latent (phoria). They can result from refractive errors giving rise to accommodative esotropia (hypermetropes) or exotropia (myopes). Making a diagnosis of squint can be a challenge in the non-cooperative child. This is how you can test for manifest non-paralytic (concomitant) squint:

Sit the child on the mother's knee. In the older child, it's best to let them slouch as they sit. This puts the head in a fixed position. Have a tongue depressor with interesting stickers at both ends. These allow the child to engage his/her attention when trying to fix.

Use an occluder to cover one eye. Hold the object at a distance of 33 cm (and slightly tipped upwards) and ask the child to look at it. Move the object from side to side and make sure that he/she is actually looking at the object (the child should move his/her eyes along with your movement). Your concentration should be on the **uncovered eye**. Look for any movement inward (esotropia) or outward (exotropia) when the cover is removed. Repeat the test with the object at a distance of six metres.

To test for latent squint (phoria), you have to do the cover-uncover test. The idea is to cut off the binocularity of the eyes. This will allow the eyes to come to their natural position of rest. The cover-uncover test should be done quickly, but not too quickly for the child to lose focus of the object. There is, however, no great value in proving that the child has a latent squint – it needs no management.

Pupils

You have already noted the size and shape of the pupils and reactivity to light (direct and consensual light reflex) when examining the eyes. In infants less than 30 weeks gestation, pupils are large and there is no reaction to light. After 32 weeks gestation, light shone on one eye should constrict the pupil on that side (direct) along with constriction of the other pupil (consensual). The reverse happens when the light is removed. Approximately 12 percent of normal individuals have a slight but clinically evident pupillary inequality. Such physiologically unequal pupils react normally. The causes of unequal pupils are given in Table 6.5.

There are a few other tests that are mainly of academic interest. The cilio-spinal reflex is tested by pinching the skin of the neck and leads to dilatation of the pupils. In Bryne's reflex, pinching one lower extremity causes dilatation of the pupil on the other side.

Accommodation Reflex

We did not test for accommodation-convergence in our examination of the "eyes," but it is helpful to do so if focussing on the cranial nerves alone. Ask the older child to look at a distant object (theoretically infinity) and then bring a finger (without a menace) within the point of near vision and instruct him to look at it. The pupils become smaller on accommodating for a near object. The 'Adie' pupil is an abnormality characterized by poor pupillary constriction to light and loss of accommodation/convergence.

Ptosis

The upper eyelid margin comes down and covers more than 2 mm of the cornea. This is usually caused by a lesion of the third cranial nerve, but may also be due to other causes—congenital, myasthenia gravis and the Marcus Gunn pupil. In the latter, there is reflex elevation or closure of the ptotic lid in response to swallowing or movements of the jaw. Pseudoptosis may be due to inferior rectus palsy in which the eye is rotated upward giving the false impression of the eyelid covering the cornea. In such cases there is no obstruction to vision and so transverse furrows on the forehead (the child

Table 6.5: Causes of small and large pupil

Small	*Large*
Normal	Oculomotor palsy
Head injury	Fear, anxiety
Horner syndrome	Ipsilateral hippocampal herniation
Deep coma	Atropine medication
Organophosphorus poisoning	Drug toxicity

with ptosis tries to over-ride the defect by using his orbicularis oculi) are absent. Partial ptosis may be present in myopathies like myotonic dystrophy, myasthenia gravis. In Horner's syndrome there is ptosis with constricted pupils, anhidrosis and enophthalmos.

You should spot ptosis when you look at the child from a distance. Is the ptosis unilateral or bilateral? Bilateral ptosis suggests a more generalized disease such as myasthenia or myotonic dystrophy. Unilateral disease indicates local pathology—orbital cellulites, cavernous sinus thrombosis or a third nerve palsy. It may be difficult to detect ptosis in myasthenia unless the muscles are tired enough to droop. Use your pointed index and ask the child to look at the finger. Bring your finger up and then down and make sure that the child moves his eyes up and down in conjunction. After a few attempts, the child's eyelids may droop if he/she has myasthenia gravis.

Complete third nerve palsy results in ptosis, pupillary dilatation and loss of all movements (except lateral deviation). The eyes tend to rest in a lateral and downward direction. Partial damage to the third nerve, however, will not result in the full constellation of signs.

Proptosis

Abnormal protrusion of the eyeball is proptosis. Unilateral proptosis may be due to thyrotoxicosis, retro-orbital tumours, neuroblastoma, retinoblastoma, leukaemia, carotico-cavernous fistulae, cavernous sinus thrombosis, or orbital cellulitis. Bilateral proptosis (also called exophthalmos) may be due thyrotoxicosis, cavernous sinus thrombosis or histiocytosis.

Conjugate Movements of the Eyes

Doll's eye movements are normally present up to 10 days of age in the full term neonate, but there is little or no conjugation. The phenomenon refers to the apparent turning of the eyes to the opposite direction in response to rotation of the head. Besides neonates, it is also seen in coma and in conditions where optic fixation is impaired. In neonates, absence of Doll's eye response on one side indicates abductor palsy. Shortly after birth the eyes start getting conjugated and by two weeks of age, the infant will move his eyes towards light and fixate. Following movements are complete in all directions by four months. Depth perception based on binocular vision appears at 2-4 months.

Internuclear ophthalmoplegia (syndrome of medial longitudinal fasciculus) consists of paralysis of adduction of the contralateral eye on lateral gaze with nystagmus of the abducting eye and preservation of convergence.

Impairment or paralysis of movement of both eyes in one direction occurs in conjugate gaze paralysis. Paralysis of lateral conjugate gaze is characteristically found with lesions of the pons (Pontine Paramedian Reticular Formation or PPRF). Bilateral lateral conjugate gaze paralysis is caused by centrally placed pontine lesions above the level of the abducens nucleii. Upward conjugate gaze paralyses are associated with lesions in central midbrain, inferior thalamic region, or near the oculomotor nucleii.

In tonic conjugate deviation, the eyes are persistently turned to one side (usually toward the side of the lesion). Tonic conjugate deviation may also arise as a result of irritative cortical lesions (deviation toward the healthy side), which are usually accompanied by nystagmoid jerks to that side (a form of focal epilepsy). In the pons, irritative lesions are rare and a structural lesion causes deviation in the reverse direction (eyes towards the healthy side). Skew deviation of the eyes occurs in cerebellar diseases and lesions so the inner ear—one eye is directed upward and the other downward.

Nystagmus

These are involuntary movements of the eyeball that may be rhythmic or non-rhythmic. Less commonly, nystagmus is symmetrical with to and fro oscillation called 'pendular' nystagmus. Nystagmus may be in different directions—horizontal, vertical, rotatory or mixed. Fine nystagmus is where eye movement is less than

1 mm, while coarse nystagmus means movement more than 3 mm. Generally nystagmus has fast and slow components. You could grade nystagmus as: first degree (nystagmus on looking towards the direction of the fast component), second degree (moderate nystagmus in the medial position) and third degree (nystagmus on looking in the direction of the slow component) Table 6.6.

When you test for eye movement, you are also looking for possible nystagmus. Be cautious that nystagmus at the extremes of lateral gaze may be physiological. If nystagmus does happen, you should ensure that your finger is not any further than 45° from the centre. Remember also that nystagmus must be sustained for more than a few beats to be significant.

Nystagmus may also be elicited by caloric testing using warm and cold water. This is the principle of caloric testing for the semicircular canals in the inner ear. Vestibular nystagmus occurs only in one direction of gaze (away from the side of the lesion) and may be horizontal or rotational. Positional nystagmus occurs in benign positional vertigo, viral labyrinthitis and head injury. Central nystagmus results from brainstem disease. It may be in any direction including vertical. Up-beat nystagmus is associated with lesions in the floor of the fourth ventricle, pontine tegmentum and anterior cerebellum. Downbeat nystagmus is associated with extrinsic compression of the foramen magnum.

Nystagmus can be due to a cerebellar cause where it occurs towards the side of the lesion. Ataxic nystagmus occurs in internuclear ophthalmoplegia. See-saw nystagmus is found in parasellar tumours. Here as one eye rises and turns, the other falls and turns out. Pendular nystagmus is congenital and caused by poor visual acuity. This is characterised by absence of the rapid phase and the presence of slow searching movements.

Table 6.6: Nystagmus—Various types
A. Horizontal, vertical, rotatory, mixed
B. Fine nystagmaus, coarse nystagmaus
C. First degree, second degree, third degree
D. Upbeat nystagmus, Down beat nystagmus
E. Ataxic, pendular, see-saw

Diplopia

Whilst checking eye movements, it is helpful to ask the child if he/she "sees double." A false image appears in the direction towards which the paralysed muscle usually pulls. For example, in medial rectus palsy, diplopia is present on looking towards the nose. In inferior oblique paralysis, the direction will be upwards and inwards, whereas in superior oblique paralysis it will be downwards and inwards. Be wary of the child with mono-ocular diplopia. There are really very few causes to account for such a phenomenon. If there are no local lesions in the eye (like a lens subluxation), consider an element of functionality to the diagnosis.

Causes of diplopia are: Space occupying lesion of the brain, refractory errors, Guillain-Barre syndrome, Fisher syndrome, myasthenia gravis, pseudotumour cerebri, botulism, Sydenham chorea.

TRIGEMINAL NERVE

Anatomy

This is a mixed nerve having motor and sensory components. Those are three divisions of the fifth nerve-ophthalmic, maxillary and mandibular. The first two are sensory, the third has a sensory and a motor component (Table 6.7).

Test

a. Motor – Ask the child to clench the teeth and palpate over the masseters and temporalis muscles bilaterally. Ask him to open and close the mouth. A paralysis of one side will lead to a deviation of the jaw to the non-paralysed side when the mouth is open. Test the pterygoids individually by asking the patient to move the lower jaw to each side (which tests the opposite muscle).

Table 6.7: Trigeminal nerve

Branch	Sensory	Motor
Ophthalmic	Conjunctiva (except lower lid) Lacrimal gland Tip of the nose and skin over medial part of the nose Upper eyelids – forehead and scalp up to the vertex	None
Maxillary	Cheek, front of temple Lower lids, conjunctiva Side of nose Upper lip, teeth Upper pharynx, roof of mouth, soft palate	None
Mandibular	Lower part of face Lower lip Tongue, lower teeth part of ear salivary glands	All muscles of mastication except buccinator

b. Sensory – The sensory component (touch and temperature) may be tested in the individual regions supplied by the 3 divisions as shown in Figure 6.4.

c. Corneal reflex The sensation of the cornea is carried by the 5th cranial nerve while the 7th nerve mediates the effector response. It is not standard practise to test for corneal reflex and will not give you any more information than any of the other tests for the individual nerves involved. However for the sake of completeness, you could use a wisp of cotton and touch the sclero-corneal junction. Ask the child to look in one direction while approaching from the other (to avoid a visual blink reflex). This will cause a blinking action in both eyes. Test both sides. An easier (but crude) method would be to blow into the patient's eye, and notice the blinking.

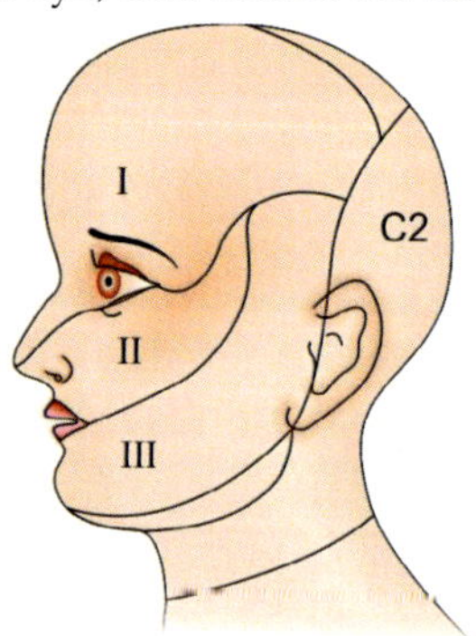

Fig. 6.4: Trigeminal sensory nerve distribution

d. Jaw Jerk–Ask the patient to open the mouth. Place your index finger at the tip of the mandible and tap gently with a percussion hammer. An exaggerated reflex indicates an upper motor lesion above the 5th cranial nerve nucleus.

FACIAL NERVE

Anatomy

The motor nucleus of the facial nerve is found in the pons medial to the descending nucleus of the 5th nerve. Efferent fibres loop round the nucleus of the 6th cranial nerve before leaving the pons on its lateral aspect. At the cerebello-pontine angle, it is joined by the nervus intermedius. The two then enter the facial canal and then onto the geniculate ganglion. The nervus intermedius carries taste sensation from the anterior 2/3 of the tongue via the lingual and the chorda tympani nerve. The afferent fibres have their cells of origin in the geniculate ganglion and terminate in the upper medulla. From the geniculate ganglion, secretory fibres pass via the petrosal nerves to the lacrimal glands (Fig. 6.5).

Leaving the ganglion, the facial nerve runs through the facial canal in the temporal bone. It lies in close proximity to the aditus of the tympanic antrum where it gives off a branch to the stapedius muscle (which limits the

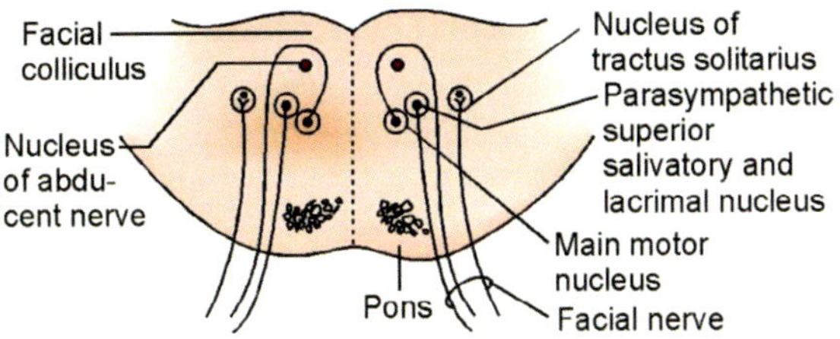

Fig. 6.5: Facial nerve nucleus

movement of the ear drum and ossicles in response to loud noise). It is next joined by the chorda tympani about 6 mm above the stylomastoid foramen. In this part of its course in the facial canal it is enclosed by a bony tube and thus susceptible to trauma and oedema.

After leaving the stylomastoid foramen, the facial nerve passes anteriorly through the substance of the parotid gland and is divides into a number of branches to all the musculature of the face (Fig. 6.6).

Test

Motor

It is helpful to observe the child's face and facial expression. In case of unilateral facial paralysis, the facial furrows are obliterated on the affected side with accumulation of saliva and widening of palpebral fissure. The eyeball rolls up under the upper eyelid rather than the upper lid moving down on the eyeball and blinking may be less forceful on the affected side.

Facial palsy can be confused with the 'congenital cry facies' of the absence of depressor anguli oris. In this case, only the lower half of the face below the angle of the mouth is involved. Bilateral facial weakness may be part of the Guillain-Barre syndrome, some myopathies and the Moebius syndrome.

The following are the tests are done to evaluate the motor function of the 7th cranial nerve.

1. Have the child close the eyes as tightly as possible. Say "can you scrunch (shut) your eyes very tight and don't let me open them". Normally, the upper lid will descend with some movement of the eyeball upward. The

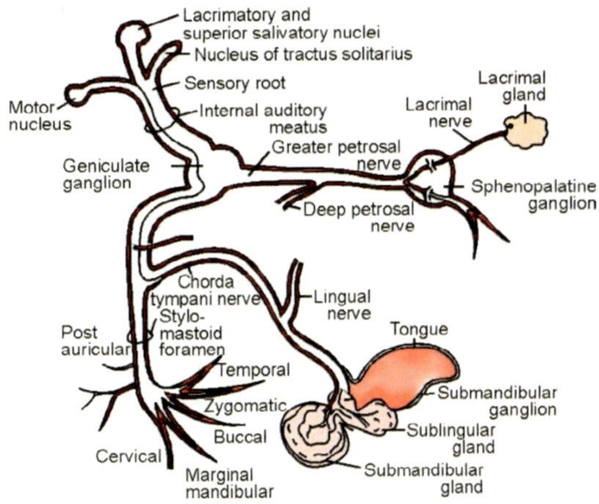

Fig. 6.6: Distribution of facial nerve

eyelashes are generally buried (to some extent) in the eyelids. Note that the child also lifts the corners of his mouth upwards.

In facial paralysis, the eyeball rolls upward during attempted forced eye closure (Bell's phenomenon). The eyelashes are not buried in the closure. The angle of the mouth either does not move at all or moves much less than on the affected side.

2. Ask the child to whistle, if he can understand.
3. Ask him to blow out one cheek. Tap with the finger on the inflated cheek—if air can be made to escape from the mouth, that is the weaker side.
4. Ask the child to smile or show his teeth. An easier way out is to say, "pull a tiger face" and show him how it is done. The angle of the mouth is drawn to the healthy side.
5. If possible, ask the child to frown, the action of which tests the action of the corrugator supercilli muscles.

Sensory

The facial nerve carries the fibres for taste sensation from the anterior two-third of the tongue. Have the child put out the tongue as far as possible and use the following solutions—5 percent glucose (sweet) 3 percent sodium chloride (salty), 1 percent citric acid (sour) and

0.1 percent quinine hydrochloride (bitter). The child should not draw his tongue in but indicate with finger clues or point to cards with the names of the tastes written on them. Taste is lost in lesions of the 7th nerve along its course from the internal auditory meatus to the place where the chorda tympani branches off.

Autonomic

In recent lesions of the facial nerve, increased lacrimation and salivation are common.

Reflexes

The 'glabellar reflex' and 'snout reflex' indicate a regression to infantile status or a frontal lobe lesion. To elicit the glabellar reflex, tap gently and repeatedly over the root of the nose. Normal response is brisk closure of the eyes after the first two or three stimuli. Persistent response (without extinction) with closure of the eyes is abnormal. Puckering of the lips in responses to a tap over the upper lid is called the 'snout reflex.' This is not elicited in normal individuals and is a frontal release sign.

The Chvostek sign is not a reflex but a sign that indicates hypocalcaemia. Ask the child to open the mouth slightly. Tap gently on the facial nerve in front of the ears—there should be abrupt closure of the mouth. In normal individuals, you will elicit only a flicker of movement.

Pathology

Lesions of the facial nerve may be supranuclear (upper motor neuron, UMN), nuclear (lesion in the nucleus) or infranuclear (lower motor neuron, LMN). The supranuclear facial palsy (UMN lesions) chiefly affects the lower part of the face. This is because the muscles of the upper part of the face are bilaterally innervated. A unilateral lesion, therefore, will cause only partial paralysis of the upper part of the face, including eye closure, on one side. Movements of the mouth (lower part of the face) on that side will appear much more severely affected. One school of thought believes that there is little UMN innervation of the facial nerve nucleus. Hence, UMN lesions will not affect the upper half.

The nerves carrying taste sensation run alongside the facial nerve for some part of the LMN course. Therefore, you will appreciate that UMN lesions of the facial nerve do not affect taste. Further in UMN lesions, facial weakness may disappear on volition but is accentuated on emotion. Facial reflexes, elicited by lightly tapping the facial muscles around the mouth are increased.

In infranuclear (LMN palsies) lesions, both the upper and lower parts of the face are involved. The lesion may be in the nucleus or the facial nerve itself. A lesion inside the facial canal (unless it is toward the outer end) involves the fibres of the chorda tympani and therefore causes loss of taste sensation in the anterior two thirds of the tongue. If the stapedius is paralysed, a sound on the side of the facial palsy may seem unusually loud (hyperacusis). A persistent LMN lesion will cause atrophy of the facial muscles. LMN weakness is accentuated on volition and disappears on emotion. Tapping over the supraorbital region may produce ipsilateral blinking (McCarthy reflex).

It may be difficult at times to be certain of facial nerve paralysis. Bilateral facial palsy may be present but usually one of the sides is comparatively stronger. Minimal facial paralysis may also be missed unless specifically looked for. When asked to shut his eyes tightly, the child's eyelashes should normally be buried in. If they are not, you may consider a partial lesion. However, you should remember that this is only possible in the older child who is capable of responding to your command. Another sign of minimal facial palsy is excessive watering and loss of prominence of the nasolabial furrow.

VESTIBULO-COCHLEAR NERVE

Anatomy

There are two components of this nerve—one supplying the cochlea and serving auditory functions and the other supplying the semicircular canals and serving functions of equilibrium. Auditory fibres reach the vestibular nuclei in the pons and medulla. Secondary pathways arise from these locations and terminate in the inferior colliculi and medial geniculate bodies and at the cortical centre for hearing in the temporal lobe.

Test for the Auditory Nerve

In neonates and infants, hearing tests are difficult to perform. There may be clues that point to the problem. A normal newborn will pause briefly during sucking on ringing a bell. After several stimuli the pauses will cease as habituation occurs. The neurologically abnormal infant will not habituate. It is best, however, to test for hearing by auditory evoked potentials or otoacoustic emissions at this age. In the older child with hearing impairment, inappropriate speech and temper tantrums are common. Suspect nerve deafness if there is failure to respond to normal sounds (turns the television on very loud), excessive response to visual stimuli, delayed speech and monotonous voice with normal motor development.

Infant

The best method to check hearing in the infant around 8-9 months of age is the "distraction test". Sit the baby on his/her mother's lap, facing the distracter. The setting ideally should be a sound proof room with no extraneous noise. The distracter has a table in front of the child with a toy to distract the child's attention. The toy should not too attractive and should not make a noise of its own. You should be behind the child and one side at a time. You are required to produce a series of sounds of varying frequencies and intensities. You can either use a device called a "warbler" or tune your own voice to high, mid and low frequencies (pitch or shrillness) and adjust the loudness (intensity) accordingly. Some people use a high frequency rattle to produce the high pitch noises. Whatever be the method, make sure that you are out of the child's visual field as this might give him/her unnecessary clues.

Start the test with the distracter getting the child's attention. At one point the distracter should stop and hide the toy. You are required to produce the sounds at this stage. Watch for the child's expression. A clear pass is when the child clearly turns to the source of sound. For the other side, the distracter has to start all over again and you have to go to the other side. Doing a distraction test needs patience—for the child as well as for the examiners. Very often the child will not cooperate and lose attention. Get some toys to play with the child and work hard to achieve a result. Some children with viral upper respiratory infections may score below par. A middle ear effusion may occur transiently secondary to a viral infection. A hand held meter to assess tympanic compliance, if you have one, shows a damped trace. It is best to repeat the hearing test in a short while to make sure that the discrepancy is not real.

The hearing test is scored on an "audiogram." This is a graph with varying frequencies (kHz) and intensities (decibels). There can be patterns of conductive loss or sensorineural hearing impairment or both.

Toddler

It is quite difficult to do a distraction test on a toddler, as he/she will not easily conform to the rules. A modified distraction may be a way forward. Get the child to play with the distracter while you produce the sounds. A useful toy is "men in a boat." When the child hears the sound, he/she puts the man in the boat. For the older child ask specifically "put the man in the boat when you hear something."

Older Child

A child above the age of five will tolerate the use of headphones. Headphones mask external sounds and you can use pure tone (instead of warbles tones as before). A pure tone audiometry can then be performed using the same principles as the "men in the boat" test. For the school going child put a stick in the child's hand and ask him to tap on the chair as soon as he hears anything.

Rinne's Test

This can only be done on the co-operative child to assess air and bone conductions. Place a vibrating tuning fork near the ear. If the child hears it, put the base of tuning fork on the mastoid process. If it can be heard again, compare to see which sound is heard louder and longer. Normally air conduction is louder and heard longer. In middle ear disease, bone conduction is louder and heard for longer periods. Rinne's test has now largely been replaced by audiometry, which is more accurate (Fig. 6.7).

Weber's Test

Put a vibrating tuning fork on the centre of the forehead and ask the child to comment on which side he/she hears better. In conductive deafness, Weber's test is lateralized to the deafer side. In sensorineural deafness, the reverse occurs. This test, like the one before, is subject to significant subjective variation. It is better to do tympanometry and audiometry where there is suspicion about hearing (Fig. 6.8).

Vestibular Function

Children find it difficult to express vertigo. Benign paroxysmal vertigo may present as unexplained crying, vomiting with change of posture, imbalance and nystagmus. The child may want to bury his face and not open the eyes. You can test for vertigo by changing the position of the head in the semi-reclining or horizontal position. This test is positive for disease in the semicircular canal that is situated low down.

The caloric test is a more objective method but requires the child's full cooperation. It is unwise to attempt this in the younger child as he/she may start to panic. Make sure at the beginning that there is no perforation of the tympanic membrane and that the external meatus is clear. The child is kept in a semi-reclining position (30° with pillows) and held steady. Inject 10 ml of cold water (30°C) slowly over 30 seconds directed at the tympanic membrane and observe the eyes for nystagmus. Normally this should produce slow deviation of the eyes toward the side of injection with the rapid phase of nystagmus away from the side of injection. Warm water (44°C) produces the opposite effect. The above responses may be remembered by the acronym 'COWS.' That is cold–away and warm–same. This response is lost in vestibular damage. Peripheral lesions tend to cause a diminished response on the side (auditory canal paresis), although a directional preponderance (where nystagmus in one direction is more prominent than the other) may also be observed. The latter finding is most likely to occur with central disorders, especially in the brainstem.

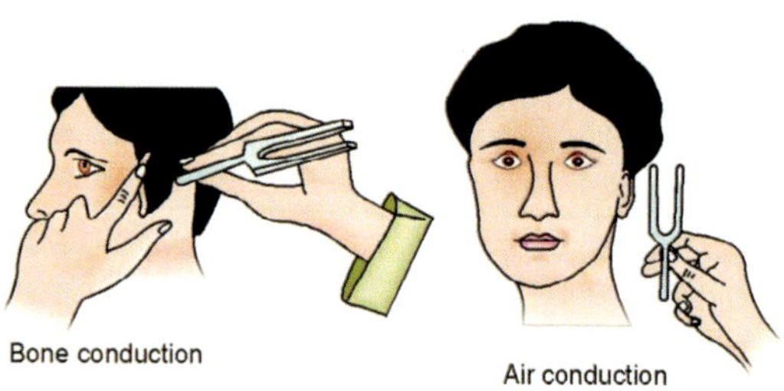

Fig. 6.7: Rinne's test

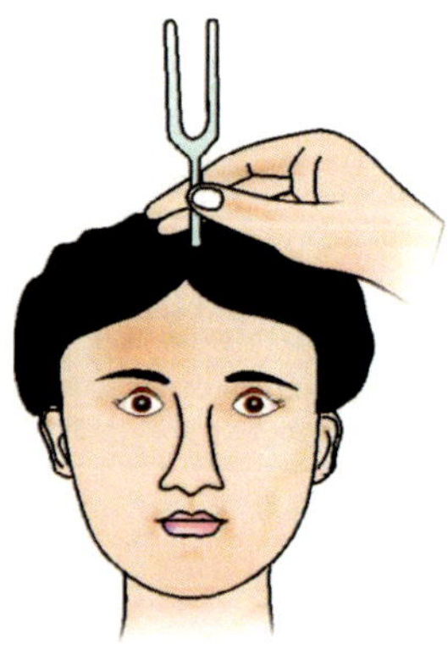

Fig. 6.8: Weber's test

GLOSSOPHARYNGEAL, VAGUS AND ACCESSORY CRANIAL NERVES

Anatomy

The 9th, 10th and 11th cranial nerves are situated in the floor of the 4th ventricle, above downward, in succession. They emerge by several roots along the lateral aspect of the medulla. The spinal part of the accessory nerve emerges from the lateral column of the cord, passes up through the foramen magnum to join its medullary part and emerges with it through the jugular foramen. After emerging, the medullary part joins the vagus nerve while the spinal part supplies the sternomastoid and upper part of the trapezius muscle.

The glossopharyngeal nerve is sensory. It carries sensation from the posterior third of the tongue and the mucous membrane of the pharynx. It supplies motor fibres to the middle pharyngeal sphincter and the stylopharyngeus muscle. It also carries taste fibres from the posterior third of the tongue.

The vagus is motor for the soft palate (with the exception of the tensor palati), pharynx and larynx. It is sensory and motor for the respiratory tract, the heart and, by the parasympathetic ganglia, most of the abdominal viscera. The vagal fibres to the soft palate, pharynx and larynx originate in the nucleus ambiguous and traverse through the accessory nerve. The visceromotor and cardio-inhibitory fibres are derived from the dorsal nucleus of the vagus in the floor of the fourth ventricle.

Test for the 9th and 10th Nerves

It may not always be practical to distinguish between lesions of the 9th and 10th cranial nerves. The only clue to ipsilateral paralysis of the 9th nerve may be a slight flattening of the arch of the palate on the affected side at rest. In general the following should alert you to the possibility of 9th and/or 10th nerve problems (Table 6.8).

Table 6.8: Defects of 9th and 10th cranial nerve

1. Stridor in the absence of mechanical obstruction suggests recurrent laryngeal nerve paralysis (10th cranial nerve)
2. Hoarseness of voice, aphonia (10th cranial nerve)
3. Loss of swallowing reflex and dysphagia (to fluids in LMN lesions; to solids in UMN lesions)
4. Nasal regurgitation when swallowing liquids
5. Ineffective cough, 'bovine cough,' slurred speech - features of recurrent pharyngeal paralysis
6. Inability to pronounce words such as 'Egg' (sounds as 'Eng') and words ending with a 'K' sound

Palatal Paralysis

To examine the soft palate, place the child facing a light source. Instruct him/her to open mouth wide and introduce a tongue depressor. The position of the uvula at rest is variable, even in health. You should watch the movement of the palate during phonation. Ask him/her to say 'Aah' (loud and clear) and observe whether both sides of the palate arch upwards. In unilateral paralysis, the palate on that side will be immobile and the median raphe will be pulled towards the healthy side. In bilateral paralysis, the whole palate is immobile.

Gag Reflex

The afferent of the pathway is the 9th nerve while the efferent is the 10th. While testing for the palate, touch the base of the tongue, soft palate or the pharyngeal wall with your tongue depressor. You could use a swab stick instead. The normal response is elevation of the pharynx and retraction of the tongue. When there is no reflex, ask the child if the pharyngeal stimulus was felt. Presence or absence of sensation will differentiate interruptions of the afferent or efferent limb of the reflex arc.

11th Cranial Nerve

The 11th cranial nerve (or the cranial part of the spinal accessory) is purely motor in function, contributing to the innervation of the larynx and pharynx, as well as the sternomastoid and trapezius muscles.

Test for the 11th Cranial Nerve

Ask the child to shrug his/her shoulders, first on his own and then against resistance. This tests the upper part of the trapezius muscle. To test the lower part of trapezius, have the patient prone with arms adducted to 90° and rotated laterally. Ask him to adduct the scapula against resistance. The movement should take place between the scapula and the thorax. Next test the sternomastoid by asking the child to rotate the head to one side when resistance is applied against this movement at the chin. This tests the muscle of the opposite side. To test muscles of both sides at the same sitting, have the child bend his chin down while you apply resistance to this movement.

Torticollis implies rotation of the chin in a direction opposite to that of the direction of rotation of the occiput. Torticollis and head tilting are seen in athetoid cerebral palsy, hiatus hernia, rheumatoid arthritis with cervical spine involvement, cervical lymphadenopathy, retropharyngeal abscess, mastoid abscess, paralytic torticollis and as compensatory mechanisms in diplopia. Gastro-oesophageal reflex is occasionally associated with intermittent torticollis (Sandifer's syndrome).

HYPOGLOSSAL NERVE

This is a pure motor nerve and arises from a nucleus in the lower part of the floor of the fourth ventricle, close to the midline. It emerges from the brain stem between the anterior pyramid and the olive.

Test

Look at the normal position of the tongue in the floor of the mouth, with the mouth slightly open. If the tongue is in the midline, ask the child to put out the tongue as far as possible. If there is any paralysis, the tongue is pushed to the paralysed side, because of the mechanical positioning and peculiarities of the origins and insertions of the muscles of the tongue. This deviation to the weaker side may be difficult to interpret in the presence of facial weakness. Therefore, in such situations it is better to compare the position of the tongue in relation to the tip of the nose.

Fibrillation is noticed when the tongue lies relaxed in the mouth. These are worm like movements, associated with spinal muscular atrophy and are seen on the under surface of the tongue. Test for the power of the muscles of the tongue. Look for signs of wasting. Ask the child to move the tongue from side to side and protrude it into each cheek in turn, while you press against the tongue from the outside. You are looking for asymmetry, wasting and reduced power.

Motor System

Examination of the motor system entails the following: muscle mass, abnormal movements, tone, power, reflexes, gait and coordination. However it may be cumbersome to perform the examination in the strict order. It is, therefore, simpler to have a "system" of examination that covers all the aspects. We shall discuss about the individual points in greater detail. For now, you could have a system that is as follows (Table 6.9).

Talk to the child and put him/her at ease. There may be vital clues to be obtained—a child with Friedreich ataxia will have characteristic cerebellar speech. Look for such clues that will help you fit the pieces of the jigsaw puzzle. Make a note of anything that catches your eye and try and correlate these with your findings.

Expose the lower limbs to get a good view of the shape and symmetry on both sides. There may be scars (from muscle biopsy), wasting or pseudohypertrophy. If the child is on the bed, make him sit up. Be careful not to walk a child

Table 6.9: Scheme of motor examination of lower limbs

- Inspection of lower limbs
- Sitting up
- Swinging leg side by side
- Standing
- Standing eye closed
- Walking
- Walking on instep, outer edge of the feet, toes and heels
- Running
- Gower test

who has paraplegia. Then ask him to swing his legs to the side of the bed and stand up slowly. Be patient – the child may have Charcot-Marie-Tooth disease with lower limb wasting; he needs an effort to stand up. When the child is up on both feet, you can use the opportunity to test for ataxia—the Romberg test. Ask him to put two feet together and then close his eyes. A child with cerebellar ataxia will sway even with his eyes open. In contrast in sensory ataxia the child will be stable with eyes open (he uses visual sense to compensate for loss of sensation from his feet) but not when they close.

When you are certain that the child can be steady on his feet, make him walk and assess his gait. Allow him to walk up to the door and turn back. Use different techniques to bring out minimal weakness—walking on the instep, outer edge of the feet, toes and heels. Watch for signs of minimal asymmetry and weakness. Does the child swing his hands? Does he bend more on one side? Ask him to run—this is a good way of assessing gait if you do not have time to do the above manoeuvres. In a clinic situation, a quick way of estimating power and function is to make the child hop on each leg (provided he is of the age to do so).

Now play a game with the child—the modified Gower test. Sit down on the floor and ask the child to do the same. Now tell him "let's see who can get up faster." This tests the proximal muscle strength—you are observing if he demonstrates the Gower sign. The child who has Duchenne dystrophy will "climb up," holding on to his knees and thighs.

You can next go on to examine the tone, power and reflexes. Talk to the child when you are checking tone. This keeps the child's attention distracted and does not affect the tone of the muscles. Examine tone by moving the joints passively and feel the resistance against your movement. Examine pronation-supination, flexion-extension of the wrists and forearm. Do similar flexion-extension at the knees and elbows. Roll the knees from side to side for resistance.

Examine power in the different muscle groups of the upper and lower limbs. For convenience, divide the muscles as flexors and extensors, abductors and adductors. Ask the child to do the movement on his own and then against resistance. Grade the power (Table 6.12).

Explain to the child that you are about to use a patellar hammer and that it does not hurt. Examine the different reflexes, superficial and deep, and note aberrance, if any. You can then go on to examine the cerebellar signs – upper and lower limb coordination.

Let us now discuss about the individual components in more depth.

Muscle Mass

Wasting of muscles is usually caused by lower motor neuron type lesions. Inspection gives us an idea of asymmetry. Corroborate this with limb circumference measurements on two sides (at identical sites). Wasted muscles are not only smaller, but also softer and flabbier on contraction. When muscle wasting is accompanied by fibrosis, they become shortened. They then develop contractures—it may be difficult to stretch them passively to a normal degree.

Wasting may be proximal (myopathies) or distal (peripheral neuritis). Generalized wasting is not only seen in neurological conditions – cachexia and malnutrition may confuse the picture. Hypertrophy occurs with excessive use (athletic training) and can be a possibility in a child with good physique. On the other hand, pseudohypertrophy is more local and due to pathological changes in the muscles themselves—the calves, buttocks and infraspinati are involved. There is fat deposition in the muscles that are rendered ineffective. The muscles appear rounded and the feel is firm and rather woody.

Involuntary Movements

Observe for the following movements. Some of them can be exacerbated by volitional activities (Table 6.10).

Table 6.10: Some involuntary movements
• Tics
• Fasciculation
• Chorea
• Myoclonus
• Athetosis
• Dystonia
• Myokymia
• Asterixis
• Tetany

i. Tic—Purposeless, repetitive movements, that usually affect the ocular, facial and upper limb muscles. They disappear in sleep and do not interfere with the child's day-to-day activities. Tics can be a problem with the Tourette syndrome.

ii. Fasciculation-This is due to twitching of groups of muscle fibres. It occurs in slow dysfunction of anterior horn cells as in Werdnig–Hoffman disease. Besides skeletal muscles, the tongue is also a good place to observe for such movements (no submucus coat) where it is termed fibrillation.

iii. Chorea—The term means a 'dance' and is defined as semi purposive, non-repetitive movements affecting the face, limbs or trunk. The movements are often very brief and difficult to discern. Ordinary voluntary movements such as walking or picking up a cup and may be embellished with smooth, rapid extra little flourish of movement. Sydenham chorea can be a result of rheumatic fever, still a common condition. To diagnose this, ask the child to stretch out his arms above his head. The arms and palms turn outward to give a "pronator" sign. If you ask the child to stretch his arms in front, you may see a spooning of the extended hand by flexion of the wrist and extension of the fingers ("choreic hand"). They are increased by agitation or nervousness.

Unilateral chorea may occur with deeply placed lesions in one hemisphere such as the subthalamic nucleus of Luys. They may appear as violent, flinging movements of one of the limbs (hemiballismus). They are sometimes to be associated with tuberculous meningitis.

More commonly the movement of chorea is associated with athetosis and is therefore termed choreo-athetoid. Typical examples are dystonic cerebral palsy, tuberculous meningitis, glutaric aciduria and paroxysmal kinesogenic choreoathetosis. The last mentioned disease is rare but has a typical manifestation. The child with this condition acts and behaves normally but will tell you that he/she finds irresistible episodes of abnormal movements which get better on their own. Have the child lie down on the couch and instruct him to start running at a signal. You will see a dramatic representation of the movement. The child will get up, run a few steps and fall to the ground and show frank choreoathetoid movements.

iv. Myoclonus—Rapid, irregular jerking movement of a group of muscles in a limb or even of the whole body constitutes myoclonus. A sudden start when surprised or bodily jerks when falling asleep (or waking) are examples of benign myoclonus. Myoclonus can be part of major generalised epilepsy. Myoclonus also occurs in association with lesions of brain stem nucleii and reticular formation.

v. Athetosis—Slow writhing movements, more pronounced in distal muscles, brought on by voluntary activity and emotional stimuli.

vi. Dystonia—This is an abnormally maintained posture, resulting in strange positions and torsion spasms. It disappears in sleep. This commonly occurs with the conditions with choreoathetosis. Other causes are Wilson disease, drugs (phenothiazines, metoclopramide, chloroquin) and dopa-responsive dystonia.

vii. Myokymia—Persistent twitching, often rhythmical affecting the periorbital muscles. This is often a benign response to fatigue.

viii. Asterixis—An irregular, abrupt, brief loss of posture evident in the outstretched hand. It occurs in decompensated hepatic failure (hepatic flap), viraemia, poisoning with hypnotic drugs and respiratory failure.

ix. Tetany—This characteristic posture is due to hypocalcaemia or alkalosis. The fingers and thumbs are held stiffly adducted and the hand is partially flexed at the meta-carpophalangeal joints; the toes may be similarly affected (carpopedal spasm). You can inflate a sphygmomanometer cuff and hold the pressure above the systolic for 2 to 3 minutes with a similar result (Trousseau sign). Light tapping in the region of exit of the facial nerve from skull (about 3-5 cm below and in front of the ear), results in twitching of facial muscles with each tap (Chvostek sign).

Power

A quick and preliminary assessment of muscle power is by watching the child lie, sit, stand, walk, dress or undress. These movements involve proximal and distal strength and coordination to a certain degree and thus observing such routine behaviour can provide us with important clues. It is good practice to comment on the functional ability of the child. This acquires great importance in the child with severe physical disability. Testing the muscle power in such a child has little practical implication. Activities of daily living are more useful to judge the independence of the child. Ascertain from the history if he can dress or undress, eat and drink and care for himself independently.

Test

There are two principles to testing groups of muscles—active movements without resistance and then against resistance. Try and test as many groups of muscles as possible (Figs 6.9A to C). They are given in Table 6.11.

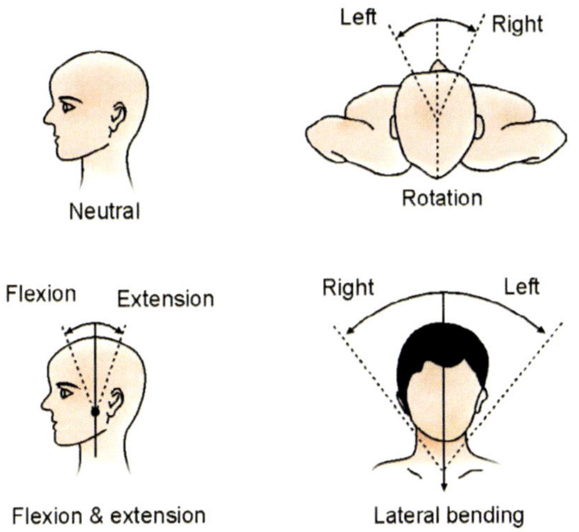

Fig. 6.9A: Movements of the neck

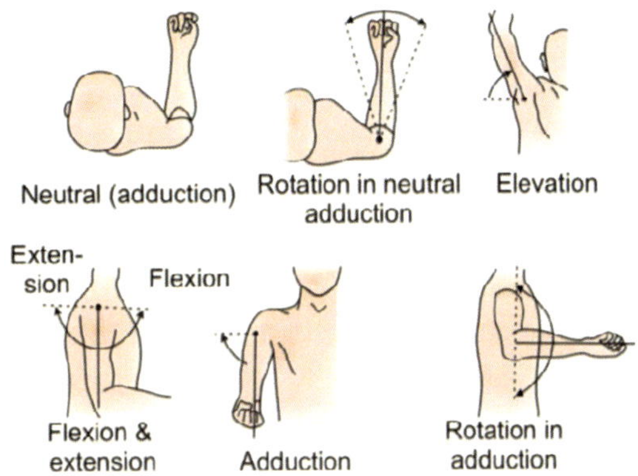

Fig. 6.9B: Movements of the shoulder

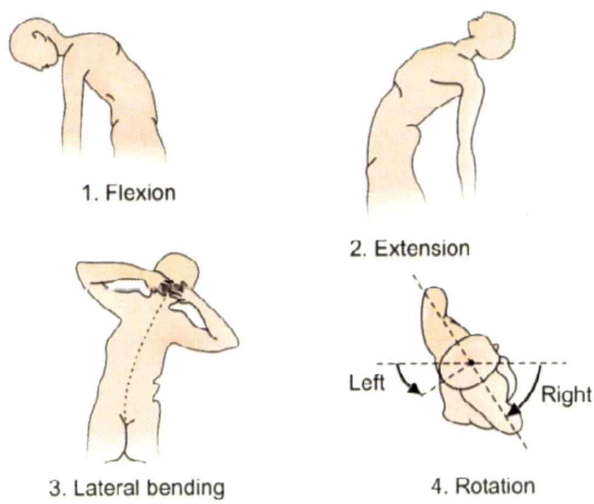

Fig. 6.9C: Movement of the lumbar and dorsal spine

Table 6.11: Movement of different joints

- *Neck:* Flexion, extension, sideways rotation
- Shoulder: abduction, adduction, flexion, extension
- *Elbow:* Flexion, extension
- *Wrist:* Flexion and extension of the wrist, pronation and supination of the forearm
- *Fingers:* Abduction, adduction of the fingers, opposition of thumb and little finger, hand grip
- *Trunk muscles:* Flexion, extension, lateral flexion
- *Hips:* flexion, extension, abduction, adduction
- *Knees:* Flexion, extension
- *Ankle:* dorsiflexion and plantar flexion, inversion and eversion
- *Toes:* Flexion, extension

When testing for power, it helps to have a uniform command to give to the child for each step. For example say to the child "lift your leg in to the air and hold in there, don not let me push it down." Or say "push my hands away," or "pull your legs towards your bottom." For testing power at the shoulder girdle say "fold your arms like the wings of an aeroplane – do not let me push it down." As you examine more and more children you will start developing a system of your own. Practise the commands so that the examination looks slick and you miss little of vital importance. At the end, grade muscle power as per the grading recommended by the medical research council (MRC) (Table 6.12).

The tests of individual muscles are given below:

Upper limb

1. Abductor pollicis brevis–Ask the patient to abduct the thumb in a plane at right angles to the palmar aspect of the index finger. The muscle in the thenar eminence can be seen and felt to contract.
2. Opponens pollicis–Ask the child to touch the tip of the little finger with the point of the thumb. Oppose the movement with your thumb or index finger.
3. First dorsal intraosseous–Ask the patient to abduct the index finger against your resistance.

Table 6.12: Grading of muscle power

0 -	Complete paralysis
1 -	A flicker of contraction only
2 -	Power detectable only when gravity is excluded by appropriate postural adjustment
3 -	The limb can be held against the force of gravity but not against the examiner's resistance.
4 -	There is some weakness, usually described as poor, fair or moderate strength (4-, 4, 4+)
5 -	Normal power is present

4. Interossei and lumbricals—The lumbricals flex the metacarpophalangeal joints and extend the distal interphalangeal joints. The interossei adduct and abduct the fingers. Instruct the child to button his shirt to test the lumbricals. To test the interossei, spread out the fingers and try to appose them (and vice versa).
5. Flexors of the fingers—Allow the child to squeeze your index and middle fingers. This tests for strength of grip, and also tests other associated muscles.
6. Flexors and extensors of the wrist—Ask the child to make a fist and try to forcibly flex or extend the wrist.
7. Brachioradialis—Place the arm midway between the prone and supine position and ask the child to bend up the forearm while opposing the movement by grasping the hand. The muscle will stand out prominently in the upper part.
8. Biceps—Ask the child to bend up the forearm against resistance, with forearm in full supination.
9. Triceps—Ask the patient to straighten out the forearm against resistance.
10. Supraspinatus, deltoid—Instruct the child to lift his arm straight out at right angles to the side. The first 30° of movement are by the supraspinatus, and the remaining 60° by the deltoid. This movement may be resisted to gauge the power.
11. Infraspinatus—Keep the forearm at a right angle and then ask the child to tuck the elbow into the side. With the elbow held

against the side, ask him to rotate the forearm like a lever, during which the muscle may be seen and felt to contract.

12. Pectorals—Ask the patient to stretch the arms out in front and then to clap their hands together. You can resist the movements by separating the hands.
13. Serratus anterior—Have the child push (with the hands) against a wall. A weakness of the serratus anterior may take the shape of a 'winged' scapula.
14. Latissimus dorsi—The process is similar to that of testing the pectorals except that the child has to clap behind his back.

Lower Limb

1. Intrinsic muscles of the foot—These are difficult to test and a paralysis of the above muscles may be inferred from the foot deformity. For example, in familial peripheral neuropathies, a hollow wasted foot deformity 'pes cavus' is characteristic. Note also that normal children, especially avid swimmers, also have hollow arches. Tendon reflexes will help in the differentiation.
2. Dorsiflexors and plantar flexors—Test by elevation or depression of the foot against resistance.
3. Flexors and extensors of knee—Bend the knees and ask the child to push his feet pull toward himself (flexion) as you resist. Then ask him to push your hand away (extension) against your resistance.
4. Extensors of the hip—With the knee extended, ask the child to lift the leg off the bed. Push down while the child tries to hold in the same position.
5. Flexors of the hip—As above, but now ask the child to push down on the bed while you try to keep the leg elevated.
6. Adductors of the thigh—Abduct the limb and then ask the patient to bring it back to the midline against resistance.
7. Abductors of the thigh—Keep the legs together in the midline and try to separate against resistance.
8. Rotators of the thigh—Ask the patient to rotate the limb outside or inside against resistance.

Sometimes it becomes difficult to decide whether weakness is real or feigned. Functional weaknesses can piggy back real weakness. It may be helpful to assess the child's functional ability in these circumstances. A child who can dress himself and yet shows motor weakness in his upper limb (with normal muscle bulk and reflexes) is likely to have functional paresis. Another test (Hoover sign) is applicable to h emiplegics in older children. With the child lying on his back, place your hands beneath the heels on the bed. Ask the child to lift one leg and then another. In case or true hemiplegia, when the patient attempts to lift the paralysed leg off the bed, you will feel a counter pressure on the non-paralysed heel. In 'hysterical' hemiplegics, the child is not making any effort at all to raise his leg and so you will feel no pressure on your hands.

Tone

Muscle tone is the state of tension or partial contracture of a muscle at rest. It may be thought of as the readiness, steadiness and awareness of a muscle waiting to contract. Tone can be normal, hypotonia or hypertonia. Normal tone is difficult to describe and requires experience to define. Hypotonia occurs in sleep, use of certain drugs, lower motor neuron lesions, neurogenic shock and cerebellar disease. You will come across the 'floppy' infant with differentials of spinal muscular atrophy, congenital myopathies and congenital myotonic dystrophy. In these conditions, note that the child is weak as well as being 'floppy.' The 'floppy' but strong child can have hypotonic cerebral palsy or Down syndrome. Sudden and episodic hypotonia signifies akinetic attacks or syncope. Lesions of either corticospinal or extrapyramidal pathways cause hypertonia. Upper motor neuron lesions of the corticospinal tract give rise to 'spasticity.' The limb involved shows a 'clasp knife' character when flexed or extended fairly rapidly. Note that the resistance to stretch increases during the initial phase and then suddenly gives way, just like opening a penknife.

Spasticity due to cerebral or brain stem lesions result in typical postures. The upper limbs are flexed and the lower limbs extended and feet in plantar flexion (think of a quadruped that has predominance of forefoot flexors and hind foot extensors). This distribution is most evident in the erect posture and may be reversed if the patient is lying head down, hinting that it may as a result of labyrinthine or vestibular activity.

Hypertonia resulting from extrapyramidal disturbance is 'rigidity.' The resistance to passive movement in this disorder is described as 'cog-wheel' (like a lever rubbing on the teeth of a cogwheel). The resistance is intermittent and jerky. Rigidity can also be of the 'lead-pipe' type, where the resistance is present throughout the range of movement. Extrapyramidal signs are present with dystonic cerebral palsy, metabolic disturbances, tuberculous meningitis, hypoxic ishaemia and Wilson disease.

Test

Tone is measured passively and therefore patient effort has to be minimized. Talk to the child about his friends, his school and his hobbies. Divert attention whilst you are moving the various joints passively. If this does not help, ask the child to let his muscles go floppy. The tone of a particular group of muscles is felt while performing the opposite function—that is the tone of the biceps is felt while extending the elbow.

Reflexes

For practical purposes, these are of two types – deep tendon reflexes and superficial reflexes. The so called developmental reflexes will be described at the end of the chapter. We shall describe the tendon reflexes first. Tendon reflexes or jerks test for the entire path of a spinal reflex. This includes the afferent impulses from the sensory endings of the muscle spindles in the stretched muscle, the nerve pathways and synapses leading up to and through the spinal cord and the efferent motor response. There is also the influence of the corticospinal tract above the anterior horn cells of the nerve roots being tested—the so-called upper motor neurons. Depending on the pathology, reflexes can be hyper-reflexia (upper motor neuron lesions) or hypo-reflexia (lower motor neuron lesions) (Table 6.13).

Use a patellar hammer to elicit tendon reflexes. The head should be well padded with rubber, so that you do not hurt the child. Explain the procedure, as otherwise this can lead to apprehension. As you strike the tendon, there is brief contraction of the stretched muscle. Look for this contraction in the muscle belly. The movement of the relevant joint is secondary.

In the event of absence of reflexes, there are two possibilities. The reflexes may be truly absent, or else there is difficulty in trying to elicit them. Differentiate the two by using reinforcement (Jendrassik's maneuver). Instruct the child to clench his teeth tightly or to hook one hand with the other, and pull apart. This should make a reflex prominent (if truly present).

Hyporeflexia may be as a result of lesion in the reflex arc in afferent or efferent limbs. Examples are poliomyelitis, peripheral neuropathies and primary muscle disease. *Hyperreflexia* occurs with upper motor neuron lesions at levels above the anterior horn cells. It is proposed that the higher control over the muscle spindles responsible for the reflex is lost. If symmetrical and generalised, it does not always indicate neurological pathology. There may be elements of anxiety, hyperthyroidism or drug toxicity if there are generalised brisk reflexes.

Table 6.13: Deep tendon reflexes can be graded as follows:

0	Absent
1	Present (as a normal ankle jerk)
2	Brisk (as a normal knee jerk)
3	Very brisk
4	Clonus

Table 6.14: Root value reflexes

- Biceps—C_5, C_6
- Tricpes—C_6, C_7
- Supinator—C_5, C_6
- Knee—L_2, L_3, L_4
- Ankle—S_1
- Plantar—S_1, S_2
- Abdominal—T_8 - T_{12}

The following are the reflexes you will be expected to examine (Table 6.14).

Knee jerk: The quadriceps contract when the patellar tendon is tapped. The second, third and fourth lumbar spinal roots are involved. You can put the child in the sitting (with legs dangling from the side of the bed) or supine position. In the supine state, bend the knees and pass a hand underneath the knee to be tested. Tap the patellar tendon midway between its origin and insertion. This should be followed by a contraction of the quadriceps and brief extension of the knee. Knee jerks are normally brisk. In unusually hyper-reflexic states (UMN lesions), you will find a progression reception area of the knee jerk. You may well see that tapping and even touching other distant areas (like the shin) will lead to a brisk response. This type of response is particularly common in pyramidal cerebral palsy and hypoxic ischaemic encephalopathy (Fig. 6.10A).

Ankle jerk: The segments concerned are the first and second sacral. Place the foot in such a way that it lies everted on the bed. Dorsiflex the foot slightly and tap on the Achilles tendon with your hammer. There should be contraction of the calf muscles and plantar flexion of the foot. (Fig. 6.10B).

Triceps jerk: This reflex depends upon the sixth and seventh cervical segments. Flex the elbow and rest the forearm across the chest. If the child is sitting, you could rest the weight of the forearm on your hand. Feel the triceps tendon above the olecranon process of the humerus and tap on it gently. There should be contraction of the belly of the triceps muscle. The triceps jerk is important to ascertain the level of lesion in problems of the cervical spine. Unusually brisk triceps reflexes may mean a spinal lesion above the level of the sixth cervical segment. Conversely, the absence of a triceps reflex may herald ascending spinal paralysis and possible diaphragmatic involvement (Fig. 6.10C).

Biceps jerk: The fifth and sixth cervical segments are concerned in this reflex. Flex the elbow at a right angle in the semi prone position. Place your thumb or index finger on the biceps tendon and tap with the hammer. The result is a contraction of the biceps and flexion of the elbow. The biceps jerk is useful like the triceps in delineating the level of a cervical spinal cord lesion (Fig. 6.10D).

Supinator jerk: Like the biceps jerk, this also is dependent on the fifth and sixth cervical segments. A tap on the styloid process of the radius with forearm in the mid prone position causes supination of the elbow. Lesions of the cervical 5th and 6th spinal segments are often associated with hyperexcitability of the anterior horn cells below the C_5/C_6 level. This gives rises to brisk flexion of the fingers, even though the elbow supination is lacking. This phenomenon is known as 'inversion' of the supinator reflex. You may not find the supinator reflex to be great practical use in your day-to-day practice and it can be threatening to the child because of the pain. However if cervical lesions are on your agenda, then do check this, by all means (Fig. 6.10E).

Jaw jerk This test for the fifth cranial nerve the jerk is sometimes absent in health and is increased in upper motor neuron lesions above the trigeminal nerve nucleus. Open the patient's mouth lightly, not too wide. Put a finger horizontally on the chin and tap on your finger. There results a muscle contraction closing the jaw. Cortical lesions can give rise to a brisk jaw jerk (Fig. 6.10F).

Clonus: Clonus is the regular oscillation of contraction and relaxation on sustained stretch of a muscle group. Sustained clonus (usually more than 6 oscillations) is evidence of an upper motor neuron lesion. Unsustained clonus may

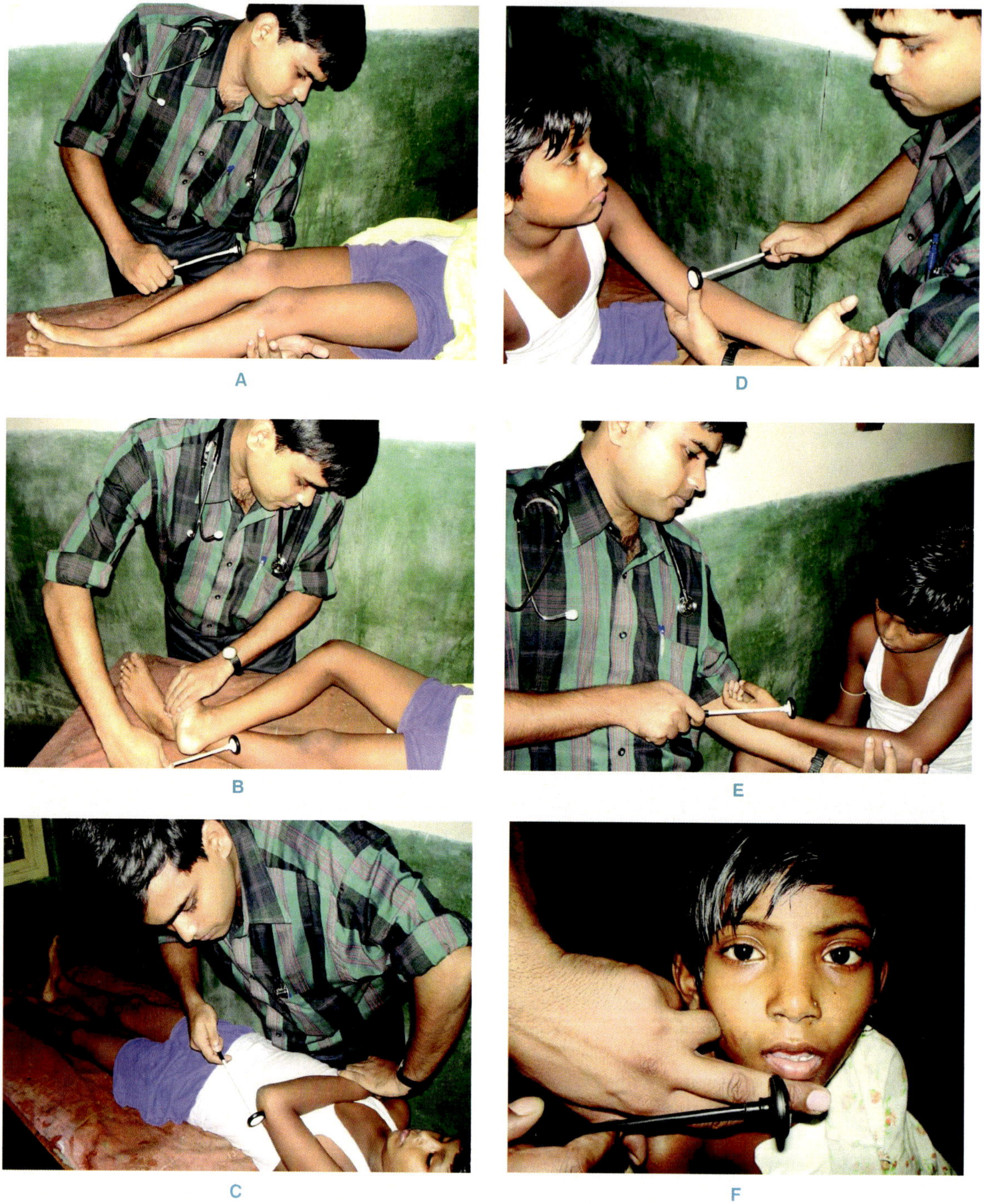

Figs 6.10A to F: Jerks. (A) Knee jerk; (B) Ankle jerk; (C) Triceps jerk; (D) Biceps jerk; (E) Supinator jerk; (F) Jaw jerk

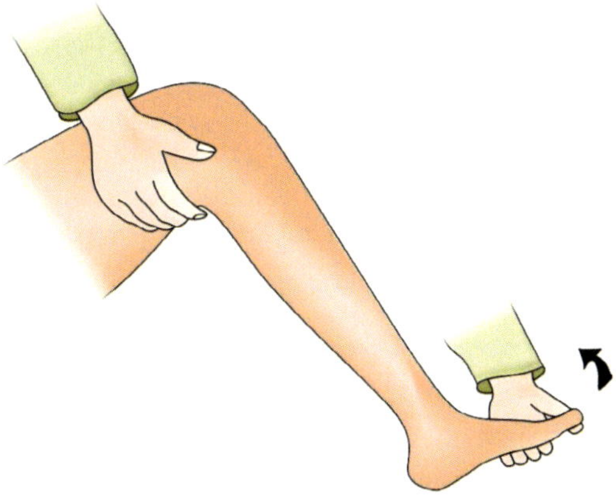

Fig. 6.11: Ankle clonus

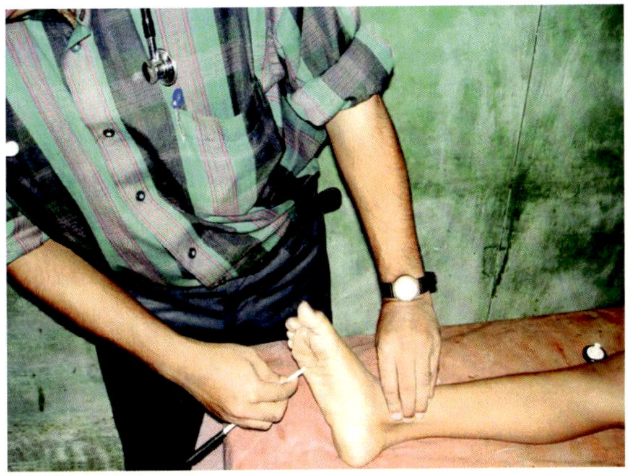

Fig. 6.12: Plantar reflex

occur in anxious persons. The places to look for clonus are the ankle and the knee (Fig. 6.11).

To test for ankle clonus, bend the child's knee slightly with your hand as support beneath it. Hold the forefoot with the other hand and dorsiflex in a quick movement. Keep the foot in dorsiflexion without putting too much pressure to achieve this. There is a brief reflex contraction of the calf muscles that then relax; continued stretch causes a regular oscillation called clonus.

To test for patellar clonus, put the patient in the supine position with knees extended. Pull a portion of skin proximal to the upper part of the patella, upward. Then quickly push downward toward the feet (and also a degree towards the bed). You will notice the patella to move up and down in patellar clonus.

Let us now come to the superficial reflexes. They are elicited by sensory stimulation of the skin and are not carried by afferents of the muscle spindles. The plantar reflex is clinically the most important, and has great relevance in distinguishing upper and lower motor neuron lesions.

Plantar reflex (Babinski response): Stroke the outer edge of the sole of the foot from the heel gently towards the little toe and then medially across the metatarsus (without touching the ball of the little toe). Minimal stimulus should cause contraction of the tensor fascia lata, accompanied by a slight contraction of the adductors of the thigh and sartorius. With a slightly stronger stimulus, there is flexion of the outer four toes. This flexion increases with the strength of the stimulus and leads to dorsiflexion and inversion of the ankle (Fig. 6.12).

In upper motor neuron lesions there is extension of the big toe instead of flexion. This response is however normal in infants under a year of age. In a child with upgoing plantars, the first response is extension of the great toe followed by spreading out and extension of the other toes. This is better elicited by stroking the more outer edges of the foot. A more medial stimulus evokes flexion of the toes as part of the 'grasp response' and can be quite misleading. In major corticospinal lesions, the area of receptivity enlarges, spreading inward and over the sole of the foot and then spreads upward along the leg to the knee or higher. The following stimuli may then elicit a Babinski response:

Oppenheim sign—Squeeze the calf or press along the inner border of the tibia.

Gordon reflex—Pinch the calcaneus tendon.

Gonda's method—Flex and twist any toe.

Bing's method—Stroke the big toe along the lateral side.

Flexor spasms (Sherrington's nociceptive flexion withdrawal response) - Sometimes while testing for the plantar reflex, the whole limb is suddenly drawn up into flexion and the great toe extended. This occurs particularly in spinal cord disease and in some patients with bilateral UMN lesions at a higher level.

Plantar equivalent (Hoffmann sign): Hold the child's hand is held at the level of the wrist. Grasp the tip of the middle finger with your thumb and index finger. Flex the distal interphalangeal joint and let go suddenly, so as to snap the tip back to its normal position. There should be no movement of the thumb. In an abnormal response the thumb flexes and adducts. The other fingers may also flex in a more widespread lesion.

You would normally test for plantar reflex in children (with sensitive skin) with your thumbnail. Quite often in children who go barefoot, you may find it difficult to get a response. Use the end of a key (make sure that it not too sharp) and go to the outer aspect of the foot for a try. The skin of the feet can be thick and keratinised to impair response. If you use too much of a pressure, the child may 'withdraw' by showing a flexor response of his knees with a false up going of the plantars. Equally you may be at a loss to be absolutely certain if the plantars are up or down. In such cases, it is best to call the response 'equivocal'. Use corroborative evidence to judge if the patient has an upper or lower motor neuron lesion.

Always test both sides and look for asymmetry. Up going plantars on one side may be indicative of spinal cord lesions on the opposite side. This may not hold true for those higher up. Cortical lesions can occur with a crossed plantar response. Further the reflex may be in evolution (of appearance or disappearance) and this may be reflected in the absence on one side and the presence on the other.

Abdominal reflex: This tests for the reflexes from the different quadrants of the abdomen. You elicit a muscle contraction by stimulating the skin in that particular quadrant. You should not attempt to do this in the younger child as he/she will be frightened by it. Lie him/her down and have the tummy uncovered. Use a light stimulus (key, wooden stick) and pass across the abdominal skin from the outer aspect towards the midline. The usual response is a ripple of contraction of the underlying muscle. The level of the umbilicus is the thoracic tenth segment. As you stroke above and below this line, you test for two cord segments superior and inferior to the T_{10} segment (Fig. 6.13).

In UMN lesions above the spinal level, the abdominal reflex is absent. In thoracic cord lesions, absence of this reflex indicates segmental involvement of the cord below that level. In cerebral palsy this reflex is preserved till late.

Anocutaneous reflexes: The perianal skin should ideally be stimulated by a sharpish object. The normal response is a contraction of the external anal sphincter with resultant in-drawing of the anal opening. A loss of this reflex indicates lesion at the levels of the sacral segments S_2, S_3 or S_4. These lesions can be of importance with lesions like spina bifida and cauda equina. You could at this juncture corroborate the sensation in the perianal area by using the cold metal end of your patellar hammer.

Palmomental reflex: Normally, tapping the thenar eminence or the hand should not result in movements of the face. A bilateral frontal lobe lesion results in contraction of the mentalis and orbicularis oris muscles on the ipsilateral side.

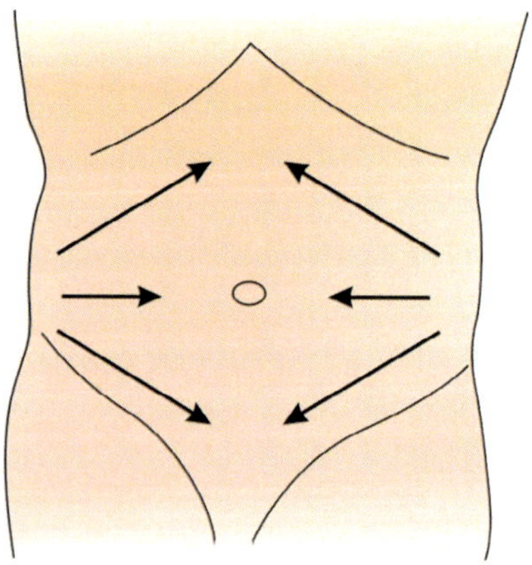

Fig. 6.13: Superficial abdominal reflexes

Cremasteric reflex: This is mediated through the 1st and 2nd lumbar segments. Stroking the skin of the upper and inner part of the thigh from above downward (or pressing the sartorius in the lower third of the Hunter's canal) results in upwards movement of the testicle. Children can be put off by this reflex – so don't venture to do this unless you suspect spinal cord lesions at the level of L_1 or L_2.

Coordination

Coordination of a group of muscles involves recruitment, interaction and cooperation among the individual muscles (and also the cerebellum). Ataxia results from imperfect coordination and is defined as an abnormality of the rate or extent of movement of muscles or muscle groups. The following are important in defining coordination:

1. Afferent impulses from muscle and joint receptors.
2. *Cerebellar function*—The cerebellum develops predominantly in the postnatal period and full cerebellar activity may not be evident until 9 to 10 years of age. You will not be able to say with certainty if a child who cannot walk in tandem (heel to toe gait) at the age of five has cerebellar dysfunction. The same applies for hopping on one foot before the age of seven. These signs (soft neurological signs) ought to be taken with the full picture in view, and you should not lay too much on them alone.
3. *State of tone and power of the muscles*—Children with paresis find it difficult to coordinate. Make allowances also for the child with hypertonicity leading to contractures.
4. *Vision*—This in itself is not directly connected with maintenance of coordination but sight is important to control and direct the movements that constitute the motor act. When there is loss of joint or position sense, the child uses his/her eyes as a compensatory mechanism.

Test for Coordination

Upper Limbs

- *Finger-nose test*—Ask the patient to touch the nose with one forefinger and then with another. Alternatively have him touch your finger (kept at a distance) and then his nose in a sequence. Instruct him to do so quickly. In cerebellar ataxia, the errors of movement occur at right angles to the direction of movement (Fig. 6.14).

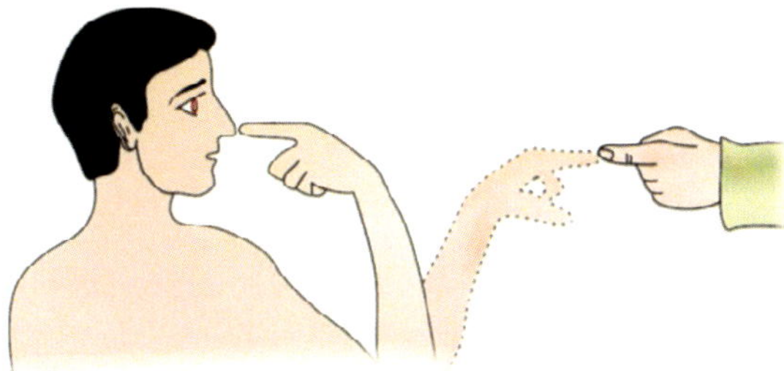

Fig. 6.14: Finger-nose test

- *Dysdiadochokinesia*—Alternate supination and pronation of the forearm as rapidly as possible. In cerebellar incoordination, movements are clumsy and awkward (Fig. 6.15).

Minor degrees of ataxia can be evidenced by noticing clumsiness of movements like buttoning up, tying shoelaces or dropping objects from the hand. Dyspraxia is a term used for minor degrees of motor incoordination and is often present in children born prematurely.

Lower Limbs

- *Tandem gait*—Show the child how to walk along a straight line with the heel of one foot touching the toes of the other. It is a sensitive test for lower limb incoordination. Making

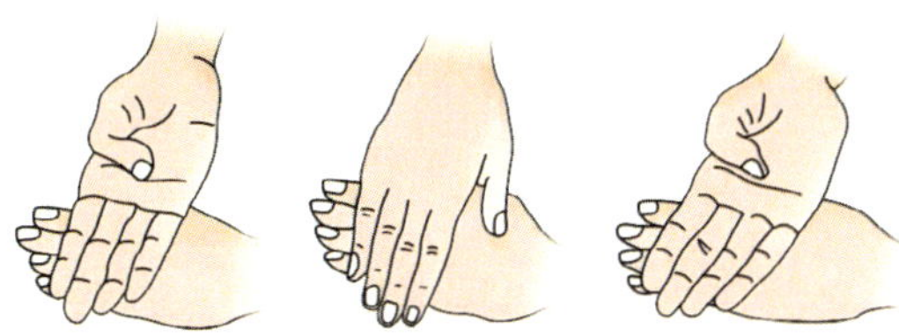

Fig. 6.15: Dysdiadochokinesia

a child walk can actually bring out other useful information. Not only will it test for ataxia and cerebellar function, but it may also amplify minor degrees of limb weakness. Children with minimal hemiplegia will be find it hard to do the test and may flex the elbows as an associated movement (Fog sign).

- *Heel-knee test*—Show the child how to lift one leg high in the air, to place the heel of this leg on the opposite knee and then slide the heel down the skin towards the ankle. Instruct him/her to do this on his/her own and rapidly. The child with lower limb coordination problems will clearly find it impossible to do the test without help (Fig. 6.16).

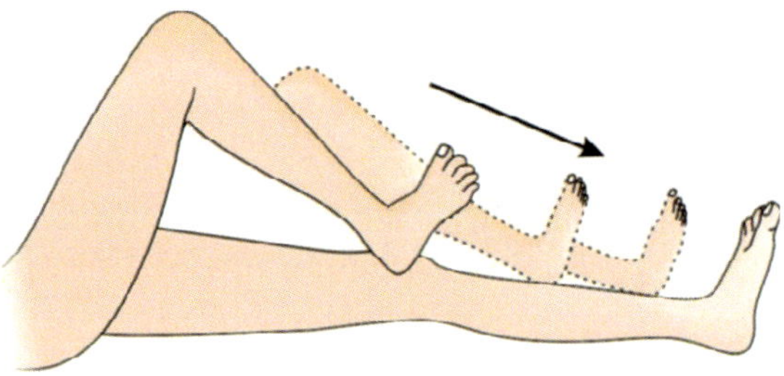

Fig. 6.16: Heel-knee test

- Romberg sign—It is a test for sensory ataxia and not cerebellar ataxia. We however use the principles of this test to detect both when we make the child stand up to examine the motor system. If a child cannot stand with his eyes open (and feet close together), then he has sensory ataxia. Closing his eyes will exaggerate the unsteadiness. With cerebellar lesions, the child can be steady with his eyes open but not when they are closed (Fig. 6.17).

Gait

Understanding gait is central to any effort to examine the motor system. Gait tells us about the aspects mentioned before—tone, power, coordination, and much more. If you have a careful eye, gait will guide you the source of the problem. For example a child with an asymmetric gait make you worry about hemiplegia. Ataxic gait should make you suspicious of Friedreich ataxia.

Gait itself is a cycle and consists of events occurring between heel strike on one side and the subsequent heel strike on the same side. In each cycle, the lower limb goes through 2 phases —stance and swing. The stance phase occurs between heel strike and toe-off, while the swing

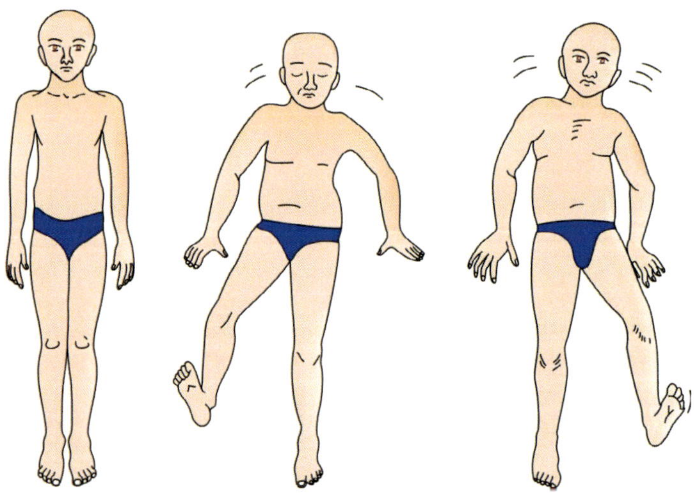

Fig. 6.17: Romberg's test

phase is between toe-off and heel strike. To test gait, have the child walk a few steps forward (ask the mother at a distance to call her child, who walks up to her) and observe for the following:

a. Can the child walk at all?
b. Is help needed?
c. Does the child walk in a straight line or waver to one side?
d. Look at the ankle, knee, hip and spine?
e. Look also at the movement of the hands for the period of the gait.

Here are some examples that you may come across.

Trendelenburg gait – In the stance phase, lateral trunk bending toward the side bearing weight suggests abductor weakness (gluteus medius and minimus) of that side (Fig. 6.18).

Posterior trunk bending: Gluteus maximus paralysis.

Waddling gait: This is comparable to that of a duck. The body is usually tilted backwards with an increase in lumbar lordosis. The feet are planted wide apart; the body sways from side to side. As each step is taken, the heel and toe are almost brought down simultaneously. This disorder suggests proximal muscle weakness as in myopathies and muscular dystrophies. The causes of waddling gait are given in Table 6.15.

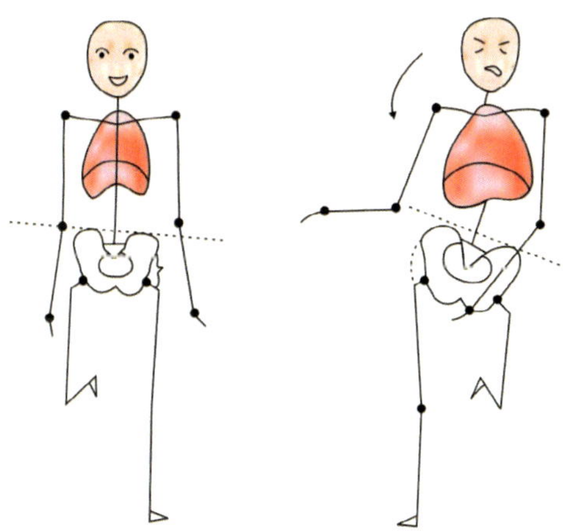

Fig. 6.18: Trendelenburg's sign

Table 6.15: Causes of waddling gait

- Bilateral dislocation of hips
- Duchenne muscular dystrophy
- Polymyositis
- Bilateral slipped epiphysis
- Bilateral coxa vara
- Glycogen storage disease - acid maltase deficiency
- Achondroplasia
- Morquio disease
- Progressive diaphyseal dysplasia
- Myelodysplasia
- Exostrophy of bladder - separation of the pelvic bones

Ataxic gait: Walking with a wide-based gait in staggering unsteady fashion: Guillain-Barre syndrome, posterior fossa tumours, Friedreich ataxia, and phenytoin toxicity.

In-toeing gait: Associated with metatarsus varus, tibial torsion, femoral neck anteversion, pronated feet.

Limping gait: Trauma, fractures, thigh contusions, improper fitting shoes, periostitis, Perthes' disease, arthritis, slipped femoral epiphysis, transient synovitis of hip, leukaemia, osteosarcoma, leg length discrepancy, peripheral neuropathy, spinal cord tumour, muscular dystrophy, cerebral palsy, appendicitis.

Toe-walking (equinus gait): Normal up to 3 years of age, and is often as a result of habit. More serious causes need evaluation: cerebral palsy, dislocation of hip, Duchenne muscular dystrophy, contracture of Achilles tendon, glycogen storage disease (acid-maltase deficiency), intraspinal tumours, filum terminale tumours. Check if there are abnormalities in the anatomy of the foot. Examination of the power and reflexes will give you clues as to the exact aetiology.

Sensation

It is often very difficult to examine the sensory system in children partly because they cannot cooperate and also because they are easily distracted or fatigued. It may be necessary to test on more than one occasion to avoid confusion. The following forms of sensation can be tested (Table 6.16).

Test

It is better to start testing for touch and position sense and later use a pin (if at all) when you have gained the child's confidence. Apply the sensory stimulus first to an area of impaired sensation and then to the area of normal sensation (the patient readily notes the change). Explain clearly to the child the procedure and instruct him/her to close the eyes. Whilst applying your stimulus, make sure that you test bilaterally. Ignore small differences as they may seem to upset the broader picture. Use some dummy tests (no stimulus applied) to test if the child's responses are genuine.

Light touch: Use a wisp of cotton wool (or the tip of the index finger) and touch over a certain area. Ask the child to indicate if he/she felt anything. Compare with other areas and the opposite side if that felt any more or less than normal. Areas of diminished sensation should be marked out. Use a map for the dermatomes of the skin. Instead of testing sensation on all areas represented by a certain dermatome, it is easier to test a certain predetermined part e.g. the tip of the thumb tests for C_6, the tip of the middle finger for C_7 and that of the little finger for C_8. Device a way to test all the dermatomes - be selective but not exhaustive (Figs 6.12A and B).

The ability to discriminate between 2 points is tested by the use of blunt dividers. Ask the child whether one or both points can be felt. Normally 2 mm of separation of points can be recognized as 2 separate stimuli on the finger-tips. The separation is slightly wider on the pulps of the toes. This test is useful in cases of posterior column disease or parietal cortical lesions.

Table 6.16: Sensory system examination

1. Tactile sensibility—light touch, pressure, tactile localization, discrimination
2. Position sense—appreciation of passive movement
3. Recognition of size, shape, weight and form of objects
4. Vibration
5. Pain
6. Temperature

Position sense: This is essentially a posterior column sensation. Explain to the patient that you will move part of a finger (or toe, or elbow) up or down and that he must respond by telling you which way it had been moved.

Movement sense: The appreciation of movement is closely related to the sense of position. With the patient's eyes closed, gradually move a digit or limb into a new position and ask him to respond as soon as the movement is perceived (Fig. 6.19).

Recognition of size, shape, weight and form: In the older child, have the eyes closed and place in his palm familiar objects such as coins, a pencil, and a marble. Ask him to identify the objects or to describe their form. Loss of this faculty (astereognosis) occurs in parietal lesions.

Vibration sense: Place the foot of a vibrating tuning fork (frequency 128 Hz) on a bony prominence (e.g. the patella) and ask the child to comment on the feeling. He/she will generally describe it as a buzzing feeling. Perception of the cessation of vibration is a more sensitive marker than perception of the presence. Put the base of the tuning fork on a

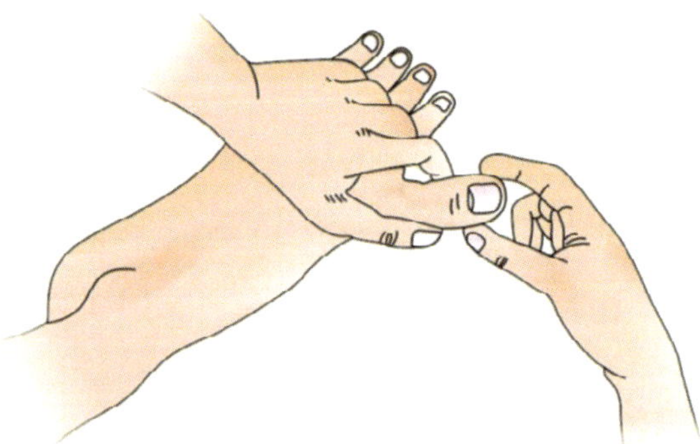

Fig. 6.19: Testing for joint sense

bony prominence and ask the child to close his/her eyes. Ask him/her when the buzzing stops. Repeat the tests from distal to proximal joints, bilaterally. Testing for vibration sense may have significance in posterior column lesions as in Friedreich ataxia (Fig. 6.20).

Pain: Pain can be either superficial (skin, subcutaneous tissue) or deep (muscles, bones). For superficial pain a pin (the tip should be reasonably blunt) can be used. For deep pain, press the calf muscle or press over a bony surface. Do not test for pain unnecessarily – you will appear intimidating in your examination (Figs 6.21A and B).

Temperature: You can test this with two test tubes – one containing warm and the other cold water. Ask the child to comment on the sensation perceived. In syringomyelia, temperature sense is lost so that the child may get a burn without feeling it.

Other disturbances of sensation: Sensory inattention/sensory extinction/sensory neglect – have the child close his eyes and stimulate homologous points on opposite sides of the body by touch or pinprick. Ask the child to indicate which side or sides are touched. In sensory inattention, the stimulus on the pathological side is not felt, though on separate testing, no difference can be elicited. Sensory inattention occurs chiefly with parietal lobe lesions.

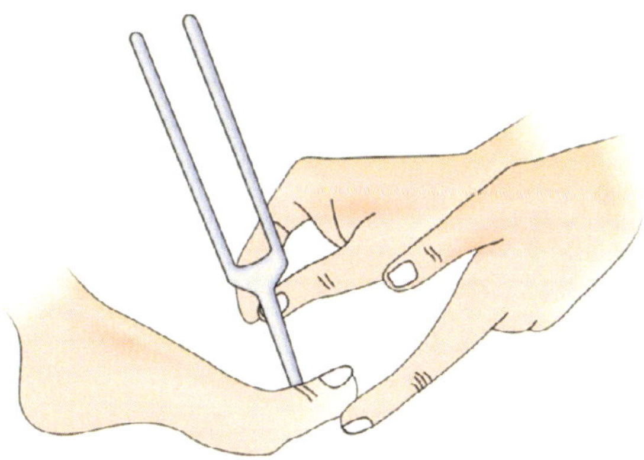

Fig. 6.20: Testing for vibration sense

Spatial summation: In other types of parietal lobe lesions, the child will perceive a stimulus only if an area of skin larger than a certain critical area is stimulated.

Temporal summation: Here rapidly repeated stimuli applied to the same point are perceived but not the application of a single stimulus.

Agnosia: This is a term to denote a condition arising out of higher perceptual defects. The child loses perception of part of his/her body e.g., finger agnosia.

Apraxia: The patient fails on constructional tests like copying a map, a complex diagram or a human face. Constructional apraxia occurs in right parietal lesions, and is an early marker of hepatic encephalopathy.

Neurodevelopmental Examination—Developmental Reflexes

Please see **Neonatal examination** (Chapter 9).

Autonomic Function (Table 6.17)

These consist of sympathetic and parasympathetic systems with a small degree of voluntary control. They are concerned with modulating the functions of the cardiovascular system, gastrointestinal system, temperature regulation, pupillary and respiratory reflex control mechanisms.

Table 6.17: Autonomic function
1. Heart rate
2. Pupillary reflex
3. Micturition, defaecation – history of abnormality
4. Blood pressure – hypotension, transient rise
5. Sweating
6. Deglutition
7. Deep breath test
8. Orthostatic hypertension

The following are tested:

Deep breath test: Do this in the older child. With the patient flat on the back, count the pulse rate during maximal deep breaths. In normal

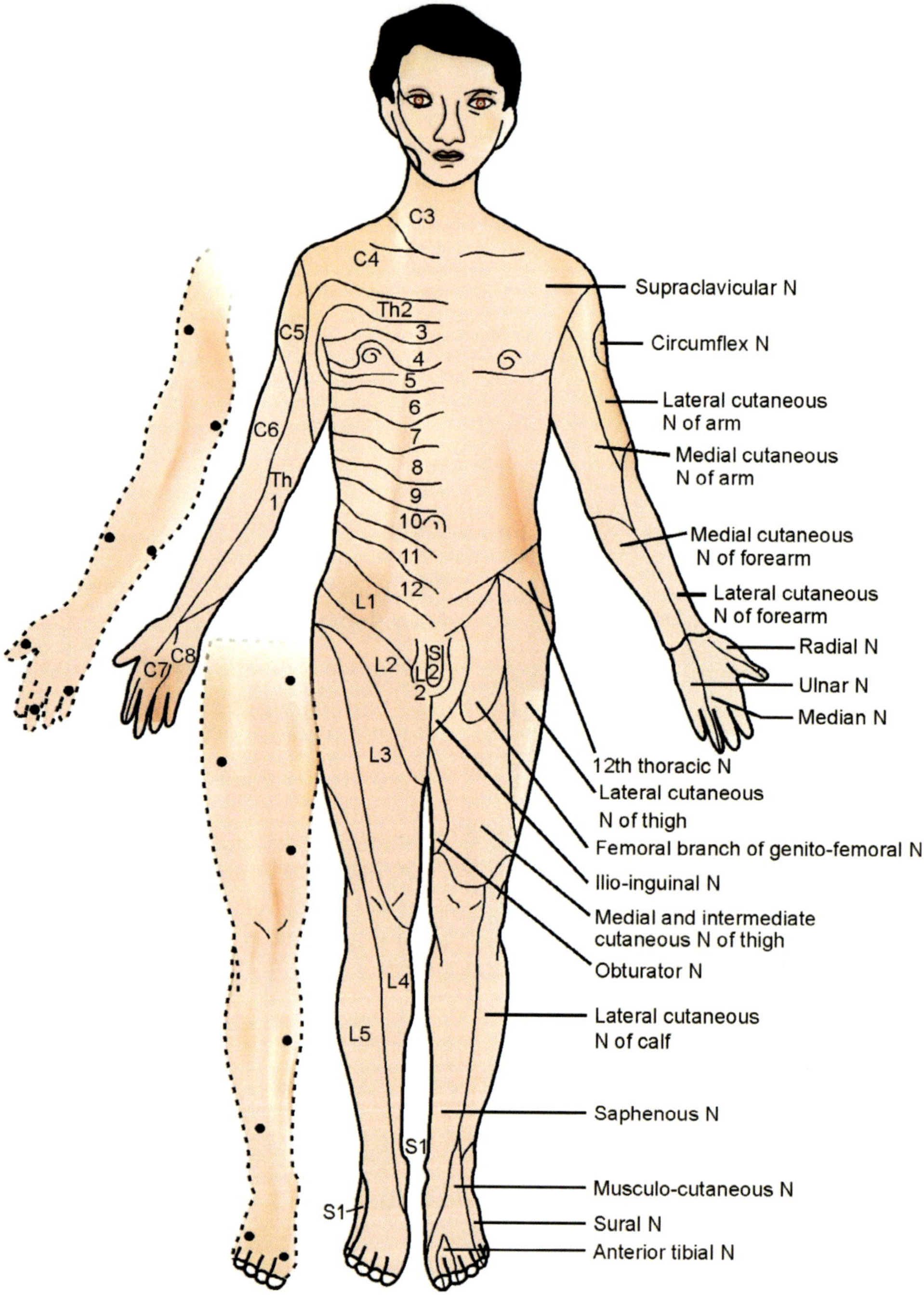

Fig. 6.21A: Sensory nerve distribution in front

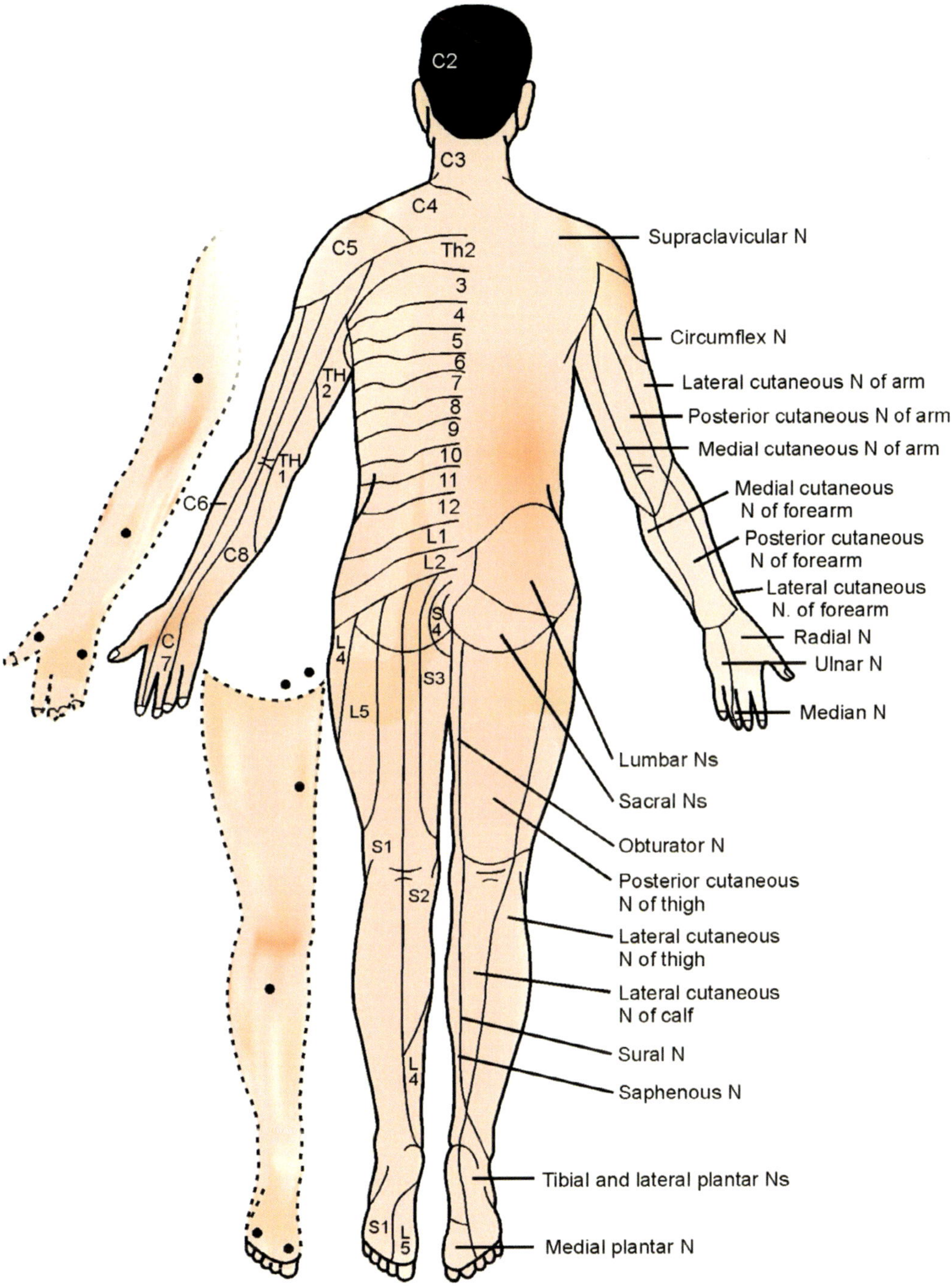

Fig. 6.21B: Sensory nerve distribution at back

subjects, the pulse rate should fall by more than 15 beats per minute. In autonomic dysfunction, the pulse rate slows by less than 10 per minute.

Orthostatic hypotension: Check resting blood pressure with the child initially lying down, then in the sitting and finally in the standing position. Note the blood pressure at one minute and three minutes after standing. A systolic blood pressure drop of more than 10 mm Hg indicates autonomic disturbance.

Autonomic dysfunction: can occur as part of a bigger problem. Head injury and brain tumours can present with such a picture. So also can spinal lesions like poliomyelitis or the Guillain-Barre syndrome. You should know that some conditions are termed as autonomic neuropathies—familial dysautonomia, Hirschsprung disease and reflex sympathetic dystrophy.

7 EXAMINATION OF THE ENDOCRINOLOGICAL AND METABOLIC SYSTEMS

The examination of the system is not a separate entity, rather it incorporates parts from the general survey and from each of the 4 major clinical systems—gastrointestinal, neurological, cardiovascular and respiratory. It is therefore essential to perform accurately the clinical examination in the above system to form an opinion of the endocrinological status of the child.

HISTORY

- Poor weight gain, failure to suck, lethargy, convulsion without evidence of septicaemia in the infant—metabolic dysfunction (urea cycle defects, aminoacidopathies, organic acidaemias, galactosaemia)
- Abnormal body odour-Maples-syrup urine disease, isovaleric acidaemia
- Vomiting refusal to feed, dehydration and skin manifestations—multiple carboxylase deficiency
- Seizures, enlarging head circumference—Canavan disease, Alexander disease, Tay-Sachs disease
- Hypopigmentation, seizures, mental retardaton—Phenyketonuria
- Jaundice, irritability, vomiting - Galactosaemia, Tyrosinosis Type I
- Tall stature, thin long hands and fingers, refractory errors—Marfan syndrome homocystinuria
- Abnormal startle response—Tay-Sachs disease
- Strabismus, Trismus, Dorsiflexion of head-infantile Gaucher disease
- Pain in the extremities, skin eruption around umbilicus - Fabry disease
- Joint pain with swelling - Farber disease, Mucolipidosis
- Family history of early myocardial infarction, pancreatitis - Lipid disorders (familial combined hyperlipidaemi, lipase deficiency)
- Abdominal pain, skin changes, psychiatric manifestations - Porphyrias
- Polyuria, Polydipsia - Insulin dependent diabetes mellitus (IDDM), Hyperparathyroidism, Compulsive water drinking, Diabetes inspidus
- Tremor, palpitation, neck swelling - thyrotoxicosis
- Deteriorating scholastic performance, failure to grow, excessively 'sleepy' - Juvenile hypothyroidism
- Obesity, hirsuitism - Cushing's syndrome, Polycystic ovarian disease
- Ambiguous genitalia - Congenital adrenal hyperplasia, Maternal progestogen use, Maternal tumours, Defects of testosterone biosynthesis, Camptomelic dwarfism, Mixed gondal dysgenesis, Androgen insensitivity syndromes
- Precocious puberty (Table 7.1).

INSPECTION

Short stature—Measure accurately (see anthropometry on page 140) (Table 7.2) for length, upper segment, lower segment, span - height ratio.

- Disproportionate short stature (abnormal span - height and upper: lower body ratios)

Table 7.1: Common causes of precocious puberty

- Hypothalamic hamartomas
- Post trauma, encephalitis
- Congenital adrenal hyperplasia
- McCune Albright syndrome
- Adrenal tumours
- Ovarian tumours
- Exogenous oestrogen/androgen

Table 7.2: Common causes of short stature

Proportionate short stature	*Disproportionate short stature*
Constitutional delay of growth Hypothyroidism Malnutrition Hypopituitarism IUGR baby Systemic illness	Rickets Skeletal dysplasia Untreated congenital hypothyroidism

- rickets, skeletal dysplasia, untreated congenital hypothyroidism

- Goitre—EU/Hypo/Hyperthyroid
- Needle marks - IDDM
- Moon facies, buffalo hump, central obesity—Cushing syndrome
- Male hypogonadism—Noonan, Kallmann's syndromes, XX, XYY males, X-linked congenital adrenal hyperplasia, Post-radiation
- Pigmentation, vitiligo—Addison's disease
- Frontal bossing, small triangular facies, hemihypertrophy—Russell-Silver syndrome
- Tall stature—Cerebral gigantism, Sotos syndrome, Klinefelter's syndrome, Marshall and Weaver syndromes, XYY males, XXX female, Marfan's syndrome
- Abnormal facies, hypertelorism, cleft palate— DiGeorge syndrome
- Doll facies—Glycogen storage disease type 1, Hypopituitarism, Pseudoparathyroidism
- Xanthelasma—Hyperlipidemia
- Late puberty (Table 7.3)
- Proximal muscle weakness (Table 7.4)
- 'Mongoloid' appearance, high forehead, hypoplastic supraorbital ridges - Zellweger's syndrome.

Table 7.3: Common causes of delayed puberty

- Constitutional delay of growth and puberty
- Gonadotropin deficiency
- Space occupying lesion of the brain
- Primary gonadal dysgenesis
- Kallmann's syndrome
- Systemic illness
- Proximal muscle weakness

Table 7.4: Common causes of proximal muscle weakness

- Cushing syndrome
- Glycogen storage disease
- Hypokalaemic periodic paralysis
- Kocher-Debré-Sémélaigne syndrome

- Coarse features—Hypothyroidism, Mucopolysaccharidoses, mucolipidoses, GMI gangliosidosis
- 'Rosary' at costochondral Junction—Rickets, scurvy, chondrodystrophy.

Examination

Hypertension

- Cushing's syndrome
- Hyperparathyroidism
- Phaeochromocytoma.

Hyperventilation

- Organic acidaemias
- Diabetic ketoacidosis
- Salicylate poisoning
- Glycogen storage disease type 1
- Subacute necrotizing encephalopathy
- Carnitine deficiency
- Tachycardia—Thyrotoxicosis, diabetic ketosis, hypoglycaemia, Addison's disease
- Warm flushed extremities—Thyrotoxicosis, hypoglycaemia.

Ejection Systolic Murmur

- Williams syndrome (supravalvular aortic stenosis)

- Noonan syndrome (Pulmonary stenosis)
- DiGeorge syndrome (conotruncal defects)
- Thyrotoxicosis.

Retinitis Pigmentosa

Table 7.5: Important causes of retinitis pigmentosa

- Refsum syndrome
- Laurence-Moon-Bardet-Biedl syndrome
- Hunter-Hurler syndrome
- Zellweger's syndrome

Peripheral neuropathy
- IDDM
- Metachromatic leukodystrophy

Cherry Red Macula

Table 7.6: Causes of cherry red spot in macula

- Tay-Sachs disease
- Sandhoff's disease
- GMI Gangliosidosis
- Mucolipidosis
- Sialidosis

Hypotonia
- Canavan disease
- Tay-Sachs disease

Spasticity/Rigidity

- Late onset GMI gangliosidosis
- Niemann-Pick disease
- Neurogenic cretin
- Metachromatic leukodystrophy
- Wilson disease
- Delayed tendon reflex—Hypothyroidism
- Visual field defect—Cranipharyngioma
- Hepatomegaly - Glycogen storage diseae types I, VI, IX, X.

Hepatosplenomegaly

- Glycogen storage disease types II, IV
- Gaucher disease
- GMI gangliosidosis
- Rickets
- Mucopolysaccharidoses
- Mucolipidosis.

8 HAEMATOLOGY - ONCOLOGY

Most components of examination of this system have been discussed in the individual systems. Start by asking the relevant questions. Do a thorough general survey, with special emphasis on pallor, lymph node examination, bleeding manifestations and swellings of any part of the body. Look for central lines and old scars. Look for the tell tale signs of drug side-effects – alopecia, gum hyperplasia, obesity. Always bear in mind that the child with a cancer may be in unbearable pain. Be sensitive to this and respect the parents' feelings. This chapter provides a brief round up of the salient features you would expect to see in a child with a malignancy or haematological disorder.

HISTORY

- Exercise intolerance–anaemia, leukaemia, solid cell tumour
- Respiratory distress–mediastinal mass, blood loss, gram-negative sepsis, *Pneumocystis carinii* infection
- Weight loss–malignancies, poor nutrition, post chemotherapy
- Weight gain–steroid use in leukaemia/lymphoma regimes, postoperative craniopharyngiomas
- Fever–pancytopaenia, leukaemia, febrile neutropaenia, bacterial, viral and fungal infections
- Rash–leukaemia, immune thrombocytopaenia, herpes zoster, viral rash, HIV
- Jaundice–glucose-6-phosphate dehydrogenase deficiency (G6PD) from drugs (quinine, primaquine, sulphamethoxazole), naphthalene balls, graft versus host disease
- Diarrhoea–post chemotherapy, gastroenteritis, cryptosporidiosis
- Constipation–vincristine, mass effect
- Blood in stool–hookworm induced iron deficiency anaemia, bleeding disorder
- Sore mouth–mucositis (dactinomycin, anthracyclines), infectious mononucleosis, herpetic gingivostomatitis
- Joint swelling–Haemophilia A or B, leukaemia, osteosarcoma, Ewing's sarcoma, synovial sarcoma, sickle cell disease
- Bleeding from umbilical cord–Factor XIII deficiency
- Epistaxis–von Willebrand disease, acute leukemia, juvenile angiofibroma, rhabdomyosarcoma
- Red urine–G6PD deficiency, Paroxysmal Nocturnal haemoglobinuria, haemorrhagic cystitis (cyclophosphamide, ifosfamide)
- Poor urine output–dehydration, tumour lysis syndrome, renal failure (nephrotoxic agents).

Examination

- Pallor–anaemia, sepsis
- Cyanosis–methaemoglobinaemia, sulphaemoglobinaemia
- Swelling–superior vena cava syndrome, local mass effects, inflammation, venous thrombosis
- Jaundice–haemolytic anaemias (Thalassaemia major, autoimmune haemolytic anaemia, G6PD deficiency)

- Bleeding into skin/mucous membranes – Idiopathic thrombocytopaenic purpura (ITP), acute leukaemias, disseminated intravascular coagulation, scurvy, meningococcaemia
- Erythema–radiation effects, red man syndrome (vincristine), allergic reaction, vasomotor response
- Eczema like rash–graft versus host disease, radiation
- Vesicles–varicella, herpes zoster, extravasation injury
- Hyperpigmentation–Fanconi anaemia, dyskeratosis congenita, Leishmaniasis, post chemotherapy pigmentation of skin, radiation scars
- Bony tenderness–acute leukaemia, bone marrow infiltration by lymphoma, scurvy, extramedullary haematopoiesis
- Proptosis–retinoblastoma, rhabdomyosarcoma, cavernous sinus thrombosis, neuroblastoma, osteopetrosis
- Hepatomegaly–neuroblastoma, haemolytic anaemia, hepatoblastoma, leukaemia, lymphoma, metastasis to liver
- Lymphadenopathy–leukaemia, lymphoma, autoimmune diseases, infectious mononucleosis, cat scratch disease
- Patch over tonsils–acute leukaemia, infectious mononucleosis, agranulocytosis
- Splenomegaly–leukaemia, lymphoma, haemolytic anaemias, congenital hypoplastic anaemia, osteopetrosis (Fig. 8.1)

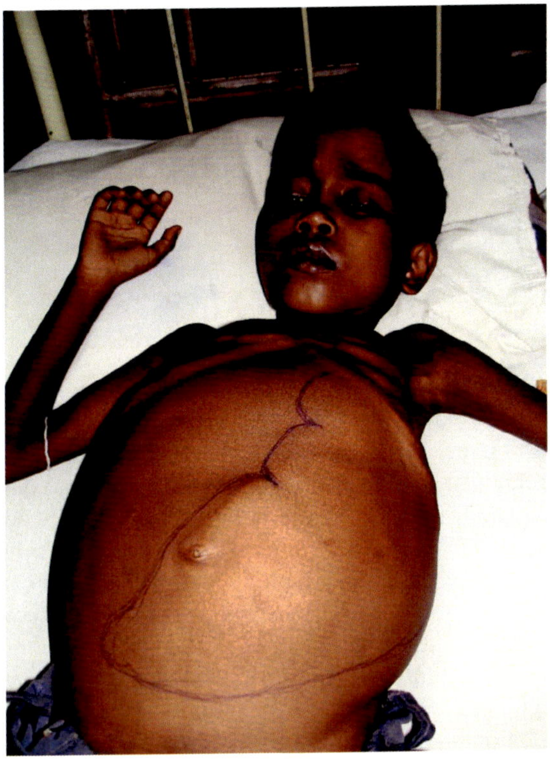

Fig. 8.1: Huge splenomegaly

- Abdominal mass–Wilm's tumour, neuroblastoma, lymphoma, ovarian cyst, rhabdomyosarcoma
- Neurological dysfunction–brain tumours, neuroblastoma, raised intracranial tension, haemophilia, leukaemia, vincristine.

9 NEONATAL EXAMINATION

Examining the neonate is different from the child, but not necessarily more difficult. This chapter deals with the standard format of examination, but you will find that you have to refer to the other systems for more clues. A lot of the examination hinges on whether the baby is "unwell." Children in this age are very susceptible to infection and therefore do think of sepsis as a prime suspect. Newborns respond well to treatment, but only if instituted early on. A baby with frank septicaemia in disseminated intravascular coagulation is extremely difficult to salvage. Therefore, it is of paramount importance to look for early signs. With experience, you will develop a 'nose' for suspecting problems, even when the baby seems to be feeding and growing normally.

In your day to day practice, you will come across two broad types of babies - the apparently healthy baby on the postnatal ward who needs a first day examination or a discharge check and the ill child in intensive care needing careful nursing support and monitoring. Although tedious and time consuming, you should aim to get as much experience as possible in examining normal neonates. You will then be able to contrast the normal from the subtly abnormal. It is helpful to have a 'scheme' of examination for each. Here is a typical checklist for the newborn in the postnatal ward (Table 9.1).

You will come across a range of conditions on the intensive care unit—prematurity, respiratory distress syndrome, necrotising enterocolitis, perinatal asphyxia, intestinal obstruction, duct dependent complex cardiac malformations, convulsions, etc. The child may be ventilated on breathing on his/herself. The level of care required will depend on the severity of the illness. Your examination should take these factors into consideration. It is best to have a problem list and address the issues in each. This enables you to cover all the problems from a diagnostic and management point of view (Table 9.2).

It is beyond the scope of the book to detail all aspects of neonatal care. We shall be limited to the basic 'clinical' examination of the newborn. The general system of examination is

Table 9.1: Checklist for the newborn

- Date and time of examination
- Age of the baby
- Gestational age – dates, ultrasound examination, any abnormalities
- Birth weight, length, and head circumference and current anthropometry
- Method of feeding
- Colour, perfusion, general well being
- Scalp, hair, head shape
- Anterior fontanelle, posterior fontanelle
- Eyes – appearance, red reflex (ophthalmoscopy)
- Face, nose, ears, neck
- Mouth – any clefts, other abnormalities
- Chest – respiration, chest wall, type of breathing
- Cardiovascular – femoral pulse, heart rate, rhythm, murmurs
- Abdomen – appearance, organomegaly, feed tolerance, meconium, urine, anal orifice, umbilicus, genitalia, hernial sites
- Extremities – digits, symmetry, movement
- Hips
- Behaviour, reflexes, 'handling'

Table 9.2: Problem list

- Date and time of examination
- Age of the child in days
- Gestation of the baby, corrected gestation for age
- Birth weight, current weight, head circumference, rate of weight gain, growth chart
- List set of problems – most important first
- Overall progress in the last 24 hours
- Ventilation – type, parameters, blood gases, surfactant, chest movement, breath sounds, work of breathing, chest X-ray, drains, oxygenation index
- Cardiovascular system – heart rate, blood pressure, inotropes, heart sounds, regularity, murmurs, femoral pulse
- GI system – feed tolerance, aspirates, abdominal distension, tenderness, umbilicus, organomegaly, genitalia, urine, stool, bowel sounds
- Neurology – 'handling', fontanelles, reflexes, behaviour, cranial ultrasound examination, retinopathy of prematurity screen, audiology screen
- Skin – colour, ulcers, breakdown, maturity
- Infection – organism, sensitivities, antibiotics, blood markers
- Fluids – intake and output
- Medication – drugs, doses, day of treatment, side effects
- Lines – peripheral, central, arterial catheters
- Investigation – glycaemia, blood counts, biochemistry, jaundice
- Parents – awareness, involvement, breast feeding
- Vaccination status
- Home conditions, social environment

not too different from the older child. The principles of examination are the same with some modifications and adaptations. Some aspects like neurology have a slightly different approach— we shall make note of these changes.

HISTORY

Start at the antenatal period and the events of pregnancy and labour. Detail the obstetric history on the following aspects:

i. *Previous obstetric history:* Ask for the maternal age, consanguinity, abortions, still birth, marital status, parity, diabetes mellitus, syphilis, malnutrition, immunisation status, birth weight, gestational age, perinatal complications. Is there a history of early neonatal deaths? These can be from conditions like early septicaemia, congenital adrenal hyperplasia, genetic defects, transposition of great arteries and hypoplastic left heart syndrome. It is important that you remain vigilant of the possibility of recurrence of the previous problem in the current pregnancy. Also note the Rh and blood group of the mother.

ii. *Pre-pregnancy health state:* Diabetes mellitus, smoking, hypertension, tuberculosis and anticonvulsant use are associated with adverse outcomes in the baby.

iii. *Antenatal history:* Ask about illnesses suggestive of the intrauterine infections—toxoplasma, cytomegalovirus and rubella (fever, rash, cervical lymphadenopathy). Ask about the use of medication during the duration of pregnancy. Drugs like valproic acid, alcohol, diethylstilbestrol, phenytoin, oestrogen-progesterone combinations are liable to cause congenital malformations. Platelet disorders arise from thiazides, quinine and salicylates. Seizures may result from drug withdrawal syndromes and accidental injection of local anaesthetic into the fetal scalp. Deafness may be due to quinine, streptomycin or chloroquin. Enquire about maternal Grave's disease as antibodies may cross the placenta and cause neonatal thyrotoxicosis.

Ask the mother about the quality of foetal movements, if she had fever and whether there was meconium-stained liquor at birth. Get information on the antenatal ultrasound scans to assess the well being of the foetus. Was there any comment about a congenital anomaly like hydrocephalus, cleft palate, diaphragmatic hernia or major cardiac anatomic malformation? "Soft" signs on antenatal scans like that of a dilated pelvi-calyceal system or left ventricular "pea" (associated with Down syndrome) need to have follow-up in the post-natal period.

Ask for rupture of membranes and whether the baby was preterm. Check whether there was prolonged rupture of the membranes, instrumentation, emergency caesarean section and the use of anaesthetic agents (spinal or general). Was there foetal distress before delivery? Were antenatal steroids prescribed in anticipation of a premature delivery? Is there a hint that the mother had chorioamnionitis?

iv. *Events at delivery:* Note whether baby cried at birth or suffered hypoxia. Check the notes for details of resuscitation. Note the details of the Apgar score (at 1, 5, 10 and 20 minutes) – does it support a possibility of perinatal asphyxia? The score is given in Table 9.3.

Table 9.3: Apgar score

Sign	*0*	*1*	*2*
Heart rate	Absent	Below 100	Over 100
Respiratory effort	Absent	Slow, irregular	Good, crying
Muscle tone	Limp	Some flexion of extremities	Active motion
Response to catheter in nostril	Response	Grimace	Cough or sneeze
Colour	Blue, pale	Body pink, extremities blue	Completely pink

The score is useful to assess hypoxia but you should not rely fully on this as false positives and false negatives can occur. A low Apgar score (less than 3 at 20 minutes) is associated with a poor outcome but higher scores do not necessarily indicate normal outcomes. Judge the score in the context of the events at delivery. A child may have low Apgar scores, but have a perfectly normal outcome. Conversely, a baby who suffered intrauterine anoxia and has low Apgar scores is likely to have some neurological dysfunction. Events with poor outcomes are prolonged resuscitation and the use of epinephrine at delivery.

It is best to document in detail the baby at birth, at one minute, five minutes, ten minutes and if necessary, at twenty and thirty minutes. Your descriptions should cover the headings of respiration, heart rate, perfusion, colour, tone and movements. Write down resuscitation procedures—cardiac compressions, what volume of fluid bolus given, whether ventilated and if epinephrine was used. What were the oxygen saturations? Collate results including blood gas (acidosis) and blood counts (antepartum haemorrhage, septicaemia). This will build up a composite picture of the exact condition of the baby at birth.

v. *Neonatal progress:* Determine if the baby was roomed in or transferred to the intensive care unit. Was the baby ventilated? Did the baby need intensive monitoring? Was the child fitting and put on anticonvulsants? What were the events in the first few days of life? It is important to ask about neonatal care—ventilation, cardiovascular status, bowel movements, neurological progress, jaundice, glycaemic status, resuscitation, feeding and growth. Summarise your information and associate this with your examination findings.

Examination

i. *Anthropometry:* Measure the weight, length, chest and head circumferences (Table 9.4). The head circumference is preferably measured a day after birth but which time caput succadaneum will have subsided. By this time there will also be less overriding of the cranial bones from moulding at birth. Record the weight on a growth chart at the appropriate gestation. Subsequent weight records should be corrected for prematurity. For example if the child was born at 28 weeks of gestation, then you should allow for 12 weeks of correction every time you plot his/her weight or height (till the age of 2 years). Babies over 38 weeks of gestation need not have this correction.

Table 9.4: Anthropometry to be done in all newborns

- Weight
- Length
- Head circumference
- Chest circumference

Categorise the baby as large for date, appropriate for date or small for date. A large for gestational age (LGA) baby is one whose birth weight is more than the 90th centile for age (large parental build, infant of diabetic mother, transposition of great arteries, Marshall, Sotos', Weaver-Bottom syndromes). An intrauterine growth retardation (IUGR) baby is one whose birth weight is less than the 10th centile for age (malnutrition, intrauterine infections, smoking, genetic defects, multiple pregnancies, hypertension, long standing diabetes, heart disease, working mothers). The terms IUGR and small for gestational age (SGA) are often used interchangeably. Strictly speaking, a baby less than the 10th centile in weight (or length) should be classified as SGA. An IUGR baby has decreasing growth velocity in the uterine period but may not be less the 10th centile at birth, and therefore not SGA. For example, a baby growing normally along the 90th centile may drop to the 25th centile over a period of 2 weeks when he/she stopped growing in utero. Technically this child is not SGA but is clearly a case of IUGR.

Measuring the occipito-frontal circumference helps you determine if the IUGR neonate has "symmetric" or "asymmetric" growth retardation. Those children on the lower centiles for weight, length and head circumference are "symmetric" IUGRs. Genetic causes are predominant in such children and their catch up is generally less than expected. On the other hand poor placental nutrition in the late stages of pregnancy is the chief cause of "asymmetric" IUGR.

It is useful to determine the infant's length and the target centile based on the midparental heights. Children born IUGR demonstrate a catch-up height (and weight) gain over the first few years. Documentation of catch up is important – IUGR babies who are otherwise well but do not exhibit adequate catch up to the target centiles need consideration of growth hormone treatment at 4 years of age.

It is now well established that infants born IUGR are more likely to develop cardiovascular complications, type 2 diabetes mellitus and the insulin resistance (metabolic) syndrome in later life if given energy dense calorie intake in the postnatal period. You may therefore want to outline the calorie and fat intake after birth as also the pattern of weight gain.

ii. *Assessment of gestation:* Check the dates of the mother's last menstrual cycle. This should give you an expected date of delivery that you can use to calculate the gestation of the child. Ultrasound examination for gestational age is in some ways a more reliable indicator. It is helpful to note the two readings if both are available. You can also assess the gestational age by clinical examination. The Dubowitz, Ballard and other scoring systems utilise the assessment of certain external features and neuromuscular maturity. When ultrasound assessment of gestation is available, such scores are more of academic interest. However, one should know the principles and application of such a scoring system for use in the event of a conflict between the scan age and gestational age calculated from the last menstrual period (Figs 9.1A and B).

Knowing the gestational age is crucial in very premature babies. Infants less than 23 completed weeks of gestation are below the limits of viability. Babies more than 26 weeks of gestation have a particularly good chance of survival and to be free of neurodisability. The chances of the baby needing surfactant at or below the 28th week are high. Gestation becomes relatively less important as the baby becomes more mature than 33-34 weeks of gestation.

Physical maturity	Score						
	-1	*0*	*1*	*2*	*3*	*4*	*5*
Skin	Sticky friable, transparent	Gelatinous red, translucent	Smooth, pink, visible veins	Superficial peeling and/or rash, few veins	Cracking, pale areas, rare veins	Parchment like deep cracking, no vessels	Leathery, cracked, wrinkled
Lanugo	None	Sparse	Abundant	Thinning	Bald areas	Mostly bald	
Plantar surface	Heel-toe 40-50 mm : 1 < 40 mm : 2	< 50 mm, no crease	Faint red mark	Anterior transverse crease only	Creases on anterior 2/3rd	Creases over entire sole	
Breast	Imperceptible	Barely perceptible	Flat areola, no bud	Stripped areola, 1-2 mm bud	Raised areola, 3-4 mm bud	Full areola, 5-10 mm bud	
Eyes/ears	Lids fused loosely (-1) tightly (-2)	Lids open, pinna flat, stays folded	Slightly curved pinna; soft, slow recoil	Well-curved pinna, soft but ready recoil	Formed and firm, instant recoil	Thick cartilage, ear stiff	
Genitals male	Scrotum flat, smooth	Scrotum empty, faint rugae	Testes in upper canal, rare rugae	Testes descending, few rugae	Testes down, good ragae	Testes pendulous, deep rugae	
Genitals female	Clitoris prominent, labia flat	Prominent clitoris, small labia minora	Prominent clitoris, enlarging labia minora	Majora and minora equally prominent	Majora large, minora small	Majora cover clitoris and minora	

Fig. 9.1A: Assessment of gestational age by new Ballard score

Neuromuscular maturity

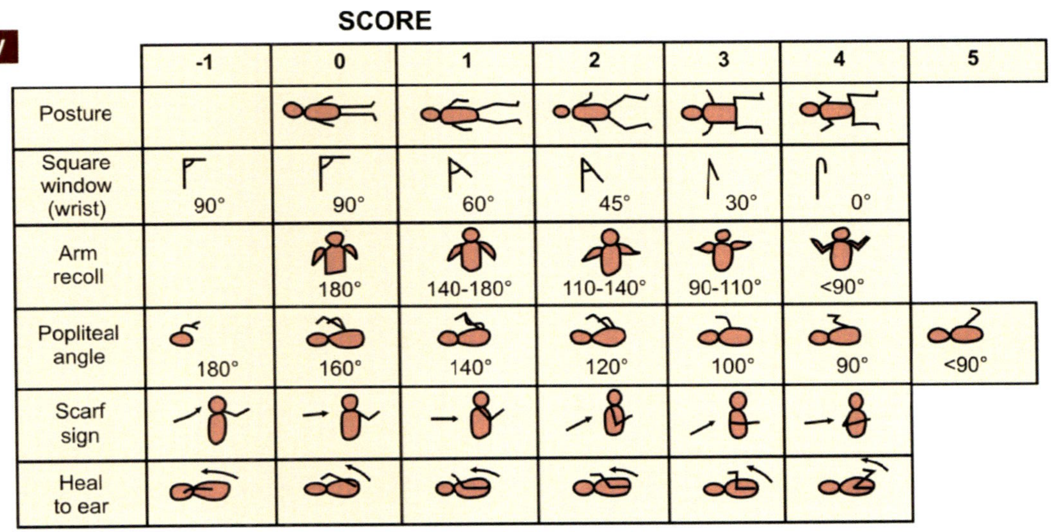

Adapted from Ballard JL, Khoury JC, Wedig K, Eilers- Walsmae BL, Lipp R. New Ballard Score, expanded to include extremely premature infants. **J. Pediatr 1991** : 417-423

Maturity Rating	
Score	**Weeks**
-10	20
-5	22
0	24
5	26
10	28
15	30
20	32
25	34
30	36
35	38
40	40
45	42
50	44

Fig. 9.1B: Assessment of gestational age by new Ballard score

iii. *Systemic examination:*

a. *Signs of acute illness*

The signs of infection may be very subtle. The baby may just be feeding marginally slowly. The nurses may have noticed him/her to be quieter than usual. He/she may not be waking up at the right time looking for food. If any suspicion, it is best to insert a cannula, check the baby's bloods, obtain a blood culture and start antibiotics. You should have a low threshold to treating sepsis. If sepsis is advanced you will find that the baby is less responsive to pain (like a venous cannula), lethargic and has a poor cry. There may be tachypnoea, jaundice, apnoeas and bradycardias. Check the temperature – the baby may have hypothermia (core temperature less than 35.5°C). In severe cases you will come across convulsions, an increased bleeding tendency and skin thickening (sclerema).

The signs of infection are rather non-specific and therefore often difficult to differentiate from other conditions. Look for signs of respiratory distress (tachypnoea, grunting, recession), pallor and cyanosis for clues relating to cardiorespiratory problems. Is there abdominal distension suggesting ileus or intestinal obstruction? Have there been convulsions suggestive of intraventricular bleeds, meningitis or metabolic disturbance?

Neonatal units have a low threshold for treating infections and you should commence antibiotics pending the results of the sample for culture. You should keep a record of how the child improves when treated. Hypoplastic left heart syndrome and some of the metabolic syndromes masquerade as septicaemia. Be prepared to think laterally about these conditions if the baby deteriorates inspite of treatment.

b. Recognition of major malformations - anencephaly, hydrocephalus, myelomeningocele, extrophy of bladder, cleft lip and palate, imperforate anus, Amelia.

c. General survey–This is done in the same way as for children, except for some modifications. Make additional notes to record the activity of the neonate. Does the baby appear to be unusually quiet? Is there abnormal movement of the limbs and mouth? Does the baby pacify with breast-feeding? Does he/she appear to be irritable despite your best efforts? Tone is another important marker of the neurological state of the infant. It is best to assess tone when the baby is in 'Brazelton' stage 3 or 4. Brazelton described different 'states' in the neonate, which are given in Table 9.5.

Table 9.5: Stages of Brazelton's neurological state

State 1	Deep sleep, regular breathing, no movements
State 2	Light sleep, irregular breathing, rapid eye movements (eyes closed)
State 3	Drowsy, eyes open or closed, some activity – smooth
State 4	Alert, minimal motor activity, mildly fussing
State 5	Eyes open, considerable motor activity
State 6	Crying

Hypertonia (or hypotonia) signifies brain injury. This may be due to hypoxic insult, intraventricular haemorrhage, hypoglycaemia, hypocalcaemia, mitochondrial defects, meningitis or metabolic dysfunction.

d. Regional examination: Examine the different regions of the body, much like that outlined in general survey for older children. Some aspects are unique to newborns and need to be addressed differently. Asymmetry of the skull and overlapping of cranial bones at the sutures are present shortly after birth. 'Caput succedaneum' overlies the presenting part of the head as a soft, nonfluctuant oedematous swelling of the scalp, the edge of which is ill defined. 'Cephalohaematoma' is characterised by fluctuant swelling with clearly defined edges that do not cross suture lines (except multiple cephalohaematomas or subgaleal haematoma). Examine the scalp, fontanelles, head size, ears, eyes, face, nose, mouth and pharynx.

Come down to the neck and search for swellings, fistula, neck size, intertrigo or pustular melanosis. Next examine the chest starting from the clavicle (fracture in shoulder dystocia) downward. Examine for asymmetry, movement, accessory nipples, apex beat and heart sounds. Examine the limbs for deformity, fractures, and movement. Palpate the abdomen for lumps and organomegaly. Note if there is distension (intestinal obstruction, necrotising enterocolitis) or tenderness. The liver is normally palpable 3 cm below the costal arch. The spleen tip and lower pole of left kidney may just be palpable. Examine the genitalia, look for hernial sites (common in preterm infants) and listen to bowel sounds.

Turn the baby prone to examine the back. Look for spinal defects (spina bifida) at sites marked by a hollow in the lumbosacral region. Check anal sphincter tone and reaction. Check the skin in all regions for erythema toxicum, pustules, bullae, melanocytic naevi, capillary haemangioma and Mongolian spots.

e. Cardiovascular system: Count heart rate, assess rhythm disturbances, check situs, femoral pulses, blood pressure, murmurs, cyanosis, heart failure.
f. Respiratory system: Observe for signs of distress (tachypnoea, grunting, chest retraction), desaturation (drops in oximetry readings), chest transillumination and adventitious sounds.
g. Gastrointestinal system: Look for vomiting, stools, feeding, sucking, swallowing, abdominal distension, umbilicus, periumbilical cellulitis, ambiguous genitalia, perineal defects, hernia.
h. **Neurodevelopmental examination – developmental reflexes**

It is postulated that the child goes through a process of developmental maturation of the nervous system. The child acquires and loses certain reflexes (primitive reflexes) en route to the fully functioning neurological state. Multiple centres in the brain and spinal cord are responsible for posture and balance. They help the child progress to the characteristic human form of bipedal walking. Normally at birth, spinal cord reflexes are present and disappear within one or two weeks. Brain stem reflexes start appearing at about the second week of life and should disappear by the 6th month. Midbrain reflexes start appearing at about the 4th month but become suppressed by cortical influences after two years of age.

It is often useful to have a practice of the normal neurodevelopmental state in an infant. There are some postures and reflexes that are normal for a certain age and not for others. Persistence of reflexes beyond the normal time for disappearance should make you worry about brain damage in utero or in early life, as in cerebral palsy. Conversely the absence of reflexes can imply states of hypotonia, sensory dysfunction or motor paralysis.

Test

It is good practice to comment on the attitude of the child before rushing in to examine the child. If you stand back and look you may pick up vital clues. For example, the hypotonic infant may be lying placidly on his back without making any movements. The spastic child with limb contractures may find it difficult to lie flat on a bed. Note the position of the limbs whilst at rest and in motion. The hemiplegic child will display an asymmetry of one side. A good neurodevelopmental examination will also take into account the child's responses to you and the environmental stimuli. The child with nystagmus and looking 'past' you has visual cortical impairment. Do not ignore the padded bed and the wheel chair. They speak volumes of the child's inability to sit up or stand erect.

In the younger child (less than six months) you can do the **'180 degree examination.'** The infant must be lying on a flat surface to start with. Note the posture of the child and the way that he/she lies on the bed. Is the face turned to one side with arm and leg extended on that side (the asymmetric tonic neck reflex)? Is there abnormal posturing as in chorea or athetosis? Next, draw the child into the sitting position, by pulling on his/her arms. Note the degree of head control or head lag. When the child has been brought to the sitting position, note if there is head and trunk control. Can the child sit unsupported? Next, hold up the child to check weight bearing. This may bring out lower limb scissoring (spastic diplegia) or help detect lower limb hypotonia (neuromuscular disorders). Now, hold the child in the ventral suspension (if the weight permits) and describe the position of the head, trunk and limbs. A hypotonic child may demonstrate a 'C' curve over your hand. Conversely, the child with cerebral palsy may have an exaggerated extensor posture. Finally lay the child prone. Put the child's hands on either side of the shoulders with palms apposed to the bed and elbows slightly flexed. Note the ability of the child to raise the head and trunk when prone.

You can now check the primitive reflexes (Figs 9.2A to I). These reflexes are important when trying to ascertain the neurodevelopmental age of the child. Their persistence or absence (allowing for a spectrum of normality) can tell you at what age the child functions. You do not have to be exhaustive in testing the primitive reflexes, but it is worthwhile to know a few, along with their chronology. A suggested order is given below, but it is best to leave the Moro and parachute reflexes till the very end as it may upset the child.

1. Sucking and rooting: Birth to 4 months, until 6 months when asleep
2. Palmar grasp: Birth until 3 months
3. Flexor withdrawal: Keep the child in the supine position with head in the midline and legs in extension. Pinch the sole of the foot – there should be slow response of the foot with uncontrolled flexion of the knee. Persistence of this reflex beyond 2 months is abnormal. Do not confuse this reflex with the brisk avoidance response seen in older children.
4. Extensor thrust: One foot should be flexed in the supine position. Pinch the sole of the flexed leg. There should be slow extension (without attempting to kick the stimulus away) in children up to 2 months of age.
5. Placing, stepping: Birth until 6 weeks – hold up the infant and place the plantar aspect of the feet on a firm surface (stepping) when the feet are lifted up. Touching the dorsum with an object also evokes a similar response.
6. Landau reflex: Hold the child in the prone position with your hand under the tummy. The child should normally extend the head, trunk and hips. Next flex the head and neck—the response is flexion of the trunk and hips. The first stage is from 4 months of age and the second stage is from 9 months onwards. The reflex should be gone by 2 years.
7. Asymmetric tonic neck reflex (ATNR): With the child in the supine position, rotate the head to one side. A 'fencing' posture results. There is extension of the ipsilateral upper and lower limbs and contralateral flexion. This reflex is said to be present normally between 2 and 6 months of age. Persistence beyond the age of 6 months may be indicative of upper motor neuron lesions.

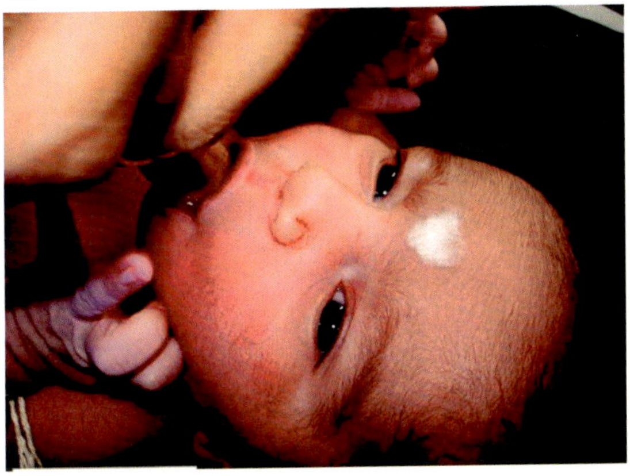

Fig. 9.2A: Sucking reflex

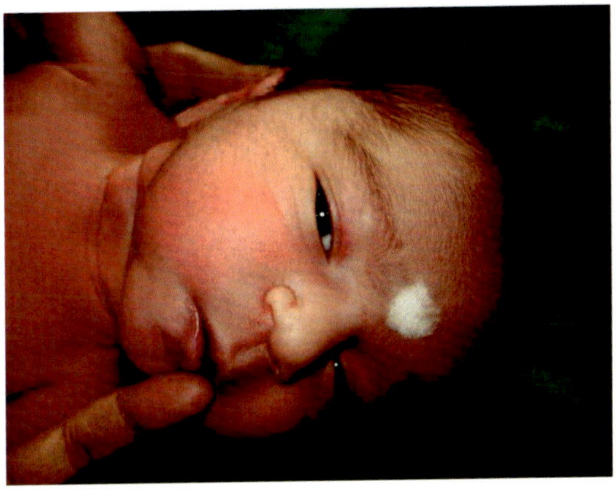

Fig. 9.2B: Rooting reflex

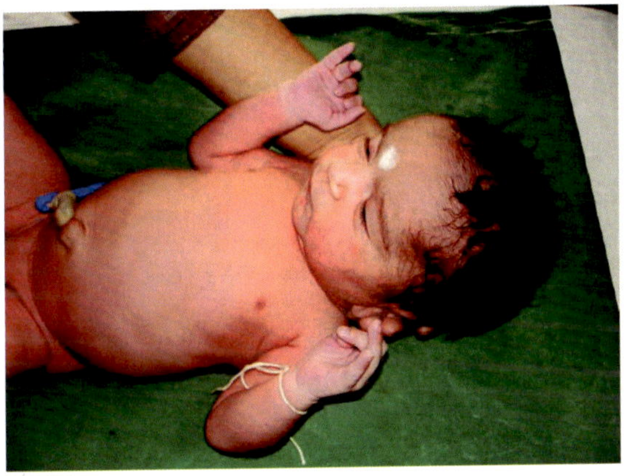

Fig. 9.2C: Moro reflex (viewed from side)

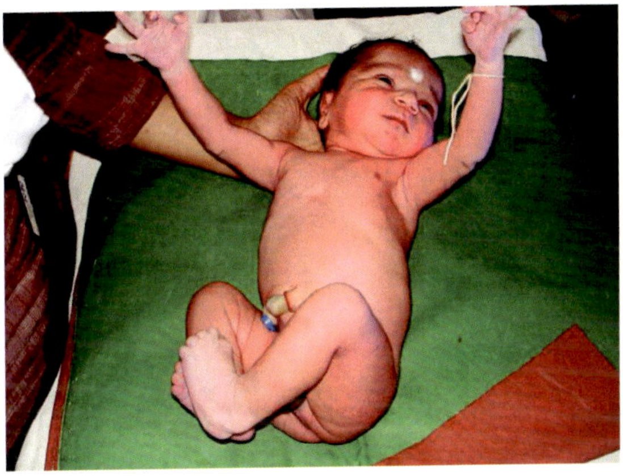

Fig. 9.2D: Moro reflex (viewed from foot end)

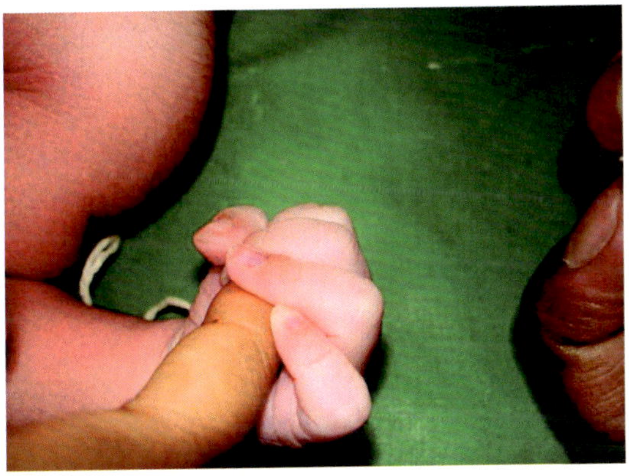

Fig. 9.2E: Palmar grasp

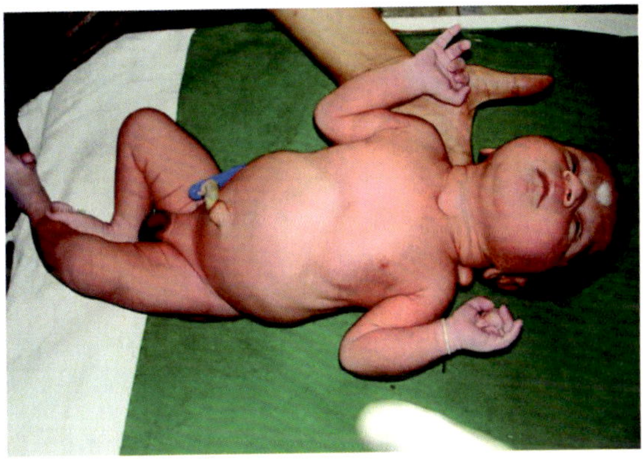

Fig. 9.2F: Symmetric tonic neck reflex

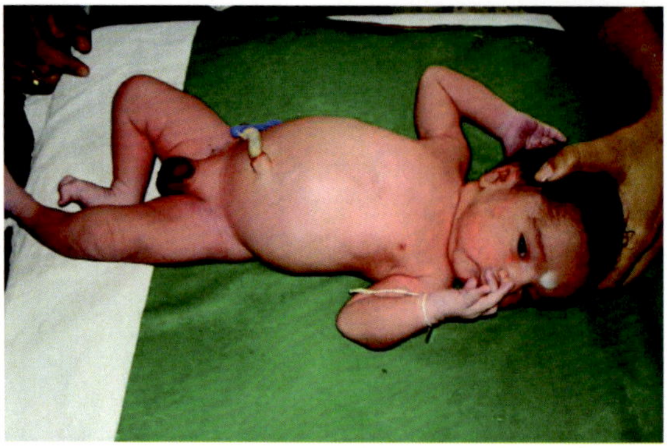

Fig. 9.2G: ATNR

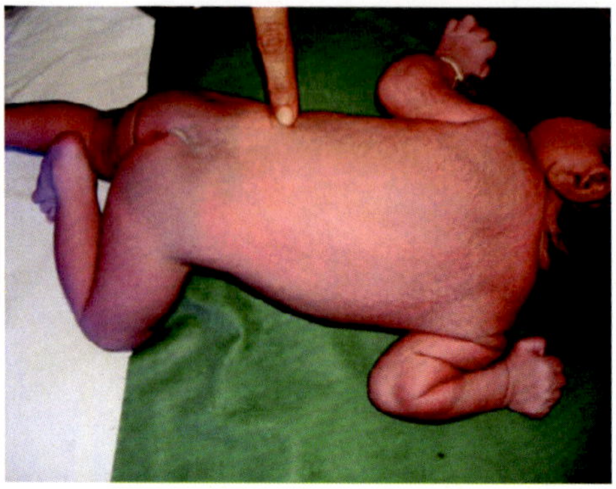

Fig. 9.2H: Gallant reflex

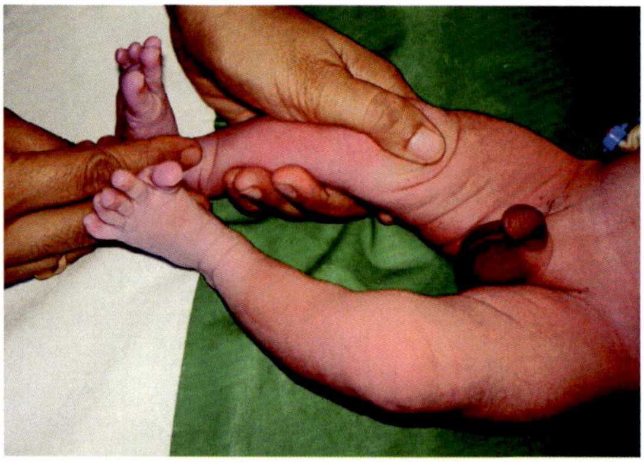

Fig. 9.2I: Crossed extensor reflex

Figs 9.2A to I: Neonatal reflexes

8. Symmetric tonic neck reflex: Support the child prone on your thigh whilst you are seated on a chair. Flex the neck downward – the arms should flex and the legs should extend. Conversely when the neck is extended, the reverse happens. The response should normally disappear after 6 months of age.
9. Positive supporting reaction: Pick up the child by holding under the axillae and bounce his feet several times. When the feet now touch the floor gently, there should be increased extensor tone in the legs, suggestive of bearing weight. This reaction is present at birth and disappears by 3 months. It later reappears at 6 months in preparation for the child to walk around the age of a year. Increased plantar flexion and adductor tone is abnormal (after 4 months) and suggestive of lower limb spasticity.
10. Negative supporting reaction: Try the same maneuver as above, but this time, hoist him up into space. The child has increased flexion tone in the legs with flexion at the knees. This reflex should disappear after 4 months.

11. Neck righting reflex: Rotate the head to one side and you will notice the trunk following suit. This is normally present between 6 months and 2 years.
12. Moro reflex: Birth to 4 Months – support the child in the semi-sitting position and suddenly drop the head and upper part of the body (make sure your hands are beneath to catch the fall). There will be sudden extension of the shoulders quickly followed by flexion at the shoulder and elbow in an embrace like movement. The fingers open during the reflex and also there is change of facial expression (watch for this in hemiplegia).
13. Parachute reflex: Hold the infant in the prone position with your hand under the tummy. Move the child, face downward towards the floor. The child will extend both upper limbs, as if to break the fall. The reflex appears between 6 and 12 months and persists. Absence of parachute reflex is abnormal, as is asymmetry (hemiplegia).

Neurological system: Examine the anterior fontanelle, head circumference, dysmorphic features, and abnormal movements. The position of the child when lying on the bed may provide clues to the underlying diagnosis. For example, the hypotonic neonate lies in a "pithed frog" position. Assess how the baby 'handles.' The child with clavicular fracture may be reluctant to move the arm on that side. Does he/she desaturate or appear fretful whilst being examined? Does he/she not respond, as you would expect for a baby of that gestation? Is there any abnormality on the recent cranial ultrasound examination? Is the baby encephalopathic? This may be difficult to define especially in the context of mechanical ventilation and sedation with morphine. In general, does the baby show any response to stimuli? Is this associated with abnormal movements and altered tone? Babies in stage 1 hypoxic ischaemic encephalopathy have a 'staring' look.

Examine for possible deficits in the cranial nerves. Test vision using a brightly coloured object (red wool). The examiner's face may itself serve the purpose. The neonate fixes the object of interest, in its line of vision. Note that visual acuity at birth is 3/60, at 3 months is 6/60 and 12 months of age is 6/18.

Assess the third nerve by observing the pupillary reflex (present at 28-30 weeks of gestation). The doll's eye movement tests for ocular palsy. Tapping the nasion leads to closure of the eyes (5th and 7th nerves) and evaluates movements of the upper face. The rooting reflex gives information about the lower face. Look for deviation of the angle of the mouth during crying in a facial palsy. Clinical examination of hearing is not reliable. Watch the baby for a startle response, blinking of the eyes and sudden changes in alertness at a noise. A negative response does not automatically mean that the child is deaf, as many other variables modify the auditory response.

Observe for nasal regurgitation and any abnormalities in sucking and swallowing. Asymmetry of the tongue may be due to 12th cranial nerve lesions.

To examine the motor system, start by observing the normal range of spontaneous movements. Does the baby move both arms spontaneously? There may be asymmetry on one side with an Erb's palsy. Look at the posture of the baby (elbows, hips, knees flexed) to have an idea of the tone. In the lower limb, test for the popliteal angle; in the upper limb test the 'scarf' sign. Use grading for post-asphyxial encephalopathy as follows (Table 9.6).

Elicit deep tendon reflexes by tapping gently with a patellar hammer. It is sometimes easier to use the index finger for the knee and ankle reflexes. In states of cerebral insult they appear brisk. Persistence of certain primitive reflexes may be suggestive of neuronal insult. You should be able to demonstrate asymmetry and abnormal response, reflecting on neuromuscular immaturity. Here are some examples:

Asymmetric Moro–Brachial plexus injury
Depressed Moro–Cerebral ischaemia

Table 9.6: Clinical features for grading post-asphyxial encephalopathy

Mild	*Moderate*	*Severe*
Irritability Hyperalert Normal tone	Lethargy Seizures Differential tone:egs > arm, neck extensors > flexors	Coma Prolonged seizures Severe hypotonia
Weak suck Sympathetic dominance	Poor suck, requires tube feeds Parasympathetic dominance	No sucking reflex Coma, requires respiratory support

Incomplete Moro–Preterm less than 35 weeks of gestation
Exaggerated startle–Tay-Sachs disease
Persistent palmar, plantar grasp–Cerebral palsy

Sensory testing, as part of the neurological examination, is of limited value in neonates. Nevertheless one must remember that neonates, no matter how premature, are perfectly capable of feeling pain, but the response is not always consistently reproducible. Pain may be assessed by observing the behavioural response of the baby. The newborn in pain appears irritable and unsettled. He or she may be desaturating more frequently than usual. Assessment of pain is very subjective and cannot be relied upon. Routine testing for pain is, therefore, not recommended. This applies for the other sensory examinations as well. However, in neural tube defects it is important to test the anal reflex as sphincter involvement denotes a poorer prognosis.

i. Hips: Use Barlow's modification of Ortolani's maneuver to identify dislocated and dislocatable hips. Undress the baby and place him/her in the supine position(Figs 9.3A and B). Steady the infant's pelvis between the thumb resting on the symphysis pubis and fingers under the sacrum. Use the other hand to test for dislocation. Alternatively, both hips can be tested at the same time. Take a grip over the flexed hip with the thumb over the femoral triangle and the middle finger behind over the greater trochanter. Try to bring the flexed thigh to the position of mid-abduction. In congenital dislocation of the hip, there is limitation of abduction to that side. In the hip that can be brought to

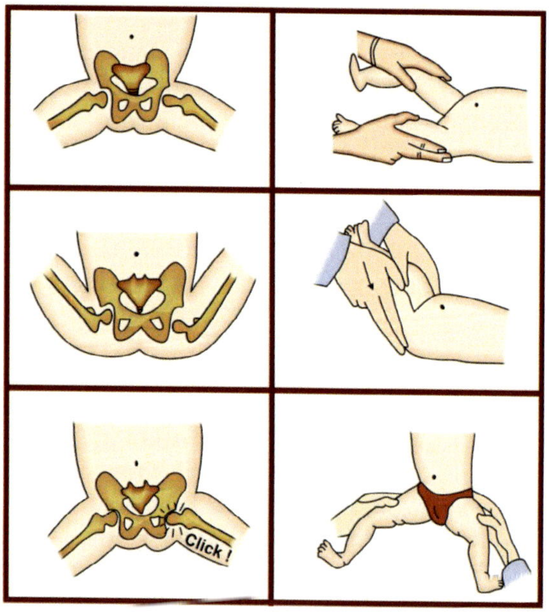

Fig. 9.3A: Barlow's maneuver for examination of hip

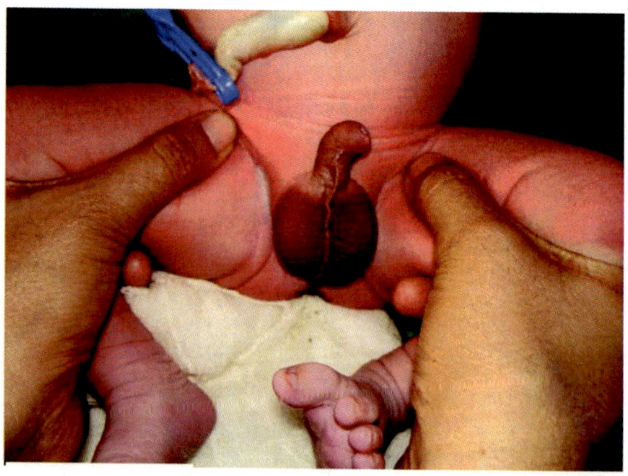

Fig. 9.3B: Ortolani maneuver for examination of hip

mid-abduction, press over the greater trochanter in a forward direction with the middle finger. If a 'clunk' results with movement of the femoral head anteriorly, then obviously the hip was already 'dislocated' before pressure was applied.

If the above section of the test is negative, then proceed to the next step. Press gently with the thumb over the medial aspect of the thigh. If a 'clunk' results with the femoral head moving out of the acetabulum (and going back when the pressure is released), the hip is probably 'unstable.'

Some signs of minor significance:

- Jittery (metronomic movements with equal amplitude, stops when part of limb is held)—Normal newborn, hypoglycaemia, hypocalcaemia
- Pedal oedema—Prematurity, Turner syndrome
- Oedema of eyelids—Chemical irritation by antiseptic
- Acrocyanosis—Normal in newborns
- Harlequin colour change (division of the body from forehead to pubis into red and pale halves)—A transient, harmless condition
- Lanugo hair—Fine, soft, immature hairs over scalp and brow occur in the preterm infant and are replaced by vellus hair in the term infant
- Pustular melanosis—Small benign pustular lesions predominantly in many ethnic communities on the chin, neck, back, extremities, palms and soles, and lasts typically 2-3 days
- Subconjunctival haemorrhage/retinal haemorrhage—Normal variant
- Corneal size—Diameter more than 1 cm suggests congenital glaucoma
- Erythema toxicum—Firm, yellow-white papules or pustules with surrounding erythematous flare (or occasionally only areas of blotchy erythema), sparing palms and soles, with peak incidence on the 2nd day of life in normal newborns
- Salmon patch—small, symmetric, pale, pink, flat lesions of vascular ectasia on glabella, eyelids, upper lip, neck region, prominent on crying and ultimately fading away over a period of time
- Port wine stain (naevus flammeus)—Unilateral, permanent, sharply circumscribed pink to purple lesions in head and neck region due to mature dilated dermal capillaries
- Capillary haemangioma (strawberry naevus)—Bright-red protuberant, compressible, sharply demarcated lesions heralded by an erythematous mark or area of pallor which develops into a area of fine telangiectasia before undergoing expansion.

10 Assessment of Child Behaviour

No assessment of a child is complete without a behavioural and developmental assessment, the development of an infant and child has been outlined in the chapter of history taking, Chapter 1. Different scales are available to quantify the defect (Denver developmental screening test, Baroda scales, Trivandrum development screening chart, etc.) and one may proceed to use these screening tests to assess the behavioural aspect or proceed to more sophisticated scales (Rutter scales).

HISTORY

History is taken of the child's problem and the interplay of the environment in shaping the child's outcome and prognosis. Ask general and informal questions like 'what does he enjoy playing with?', 'Does he play with his friends'?, 'Can he tell a story'? to get an idea of the developmental level. The current level of functioning is assessed under areas of play, language comprehension and expression, gross motor, social skills and behaviour. Do not rely on the parent's interpretations as they may be incorrect (e.g. reply to the question 'can he understand what you tell thy baby?' is 'He understands everything').

Ask the following questions (discreetly) to obtain information about the environment in Table 10.1.

Emotional Development

Erikson divided the emotional development of a child as shown in Table 10.2.

Table 10.1: Questionnaire interaction with environment

- Is this a wanted child?
- Is there marital discord or separation?
- Any parental experimental disruptions?
- Socioeconomic situation pressing?
- Abnormal health in antenatal period?
- Prolonged maternal depression related to pregnancy?
- How she sees herself in mothering?
- How helpful is the father in running the household?
- Does the mother work?
- If so who looks after the child?
- Father out of job?
- Is he ill tempered, alcoholic?
- Any complaints of the child at school?
- What do the parents think is wrong with the child?
- What do they expect to be done by the paediatrician?

Table 10.2: Emotional development

Period of life	*Core problem being mastered*
Infancy	Trust – Mistrust
Toddler	Autonomy – Shame
Preschool	Initiative – Guilt
School	Industry – Inferiority
Adolescence	Identity – Identify diffusion

Behaviour

The core problem in each period of development correlates with the major developmental task set for that period.

Trust-Mistrust: In infancy the child is entirely dependent on the mother. He needs a sense of security and how secure he feels depends on how effective is the security provided by the mother. He needs to develop his sense of trust before he can emotionally venture on his own.

Autonomy-Shame: This equivalent of the Freudian Anal Stage is characterised by his control of bowel and bladder functions, giving the child more independence. The negative feeling at this stage is 'Shame'.

Initiative-Guilt: As the child explores new objects and activities, he also comes into contact with other children. The interaction gives vent to a sense of competition and resulting frustration and guilt feeling.

Industry-Inferiority: In the school years, he has considerable physical and mental energy (industry) he uses his newly acquired skills in all games and physical exercises. However, though he believes he can be 'a jack of all trades' he fails in some and there develops the fear of failure (inferiority) he has to develop a sense of pride in his industry without feeling inferior to his peers.

Identity-Identify diffusion: In adolescence, this is the biggest crisis with the child confused as to his true worth. The parents want him timid and docile, his peers would like him to be aggressive and non-conformatory.

Each age has its own problems. Understanding the core problems for each age period makes it possible for the clinician to guide children and parents appropriately. For example, in a child of 3-6 years age, his problem is initiative versus guilt. At this time a marital discord makes the child feels 'guilty' for the problem and thus he suffers an emotional setback.

If there is a crisis during a period the child may not master the problem and get 'stuck' at that level (emotional developmental delay). The paediatrician should be aware of these problems and carefully observe the baby for:

- Contendedness
- Interaction with mother
- Play with peers
- Activity
- Conversation
- Confidence

A child with autism will not interact socially or verbally with the examiner and hide in a shell of his own, oblivious of the world round him. A child with attention deficit disorder cannot sit still but is always impulsive and jumping at things. A child with a physical handicap has more 'inferior' feelings resulting in poorer performance.

Cognitive Development

It is important to have an idea of the cognition in a child who may be physically normal but parents are worried about unnatural or unseeming behaviour or deteriorating scholastic performance. Like Erikson, Plaget has devised a scheme development of intellectual function as given in Table 10.3.

Table 10.3: Cognitive development stages

Period of Life	*Type*
Infancy	Sensory motor
Toddler	Sensory motor
Preschool	Preoperational
School	Concrete operations
Adolescent	Formal operaitons

Behaviour

Sensor motor stages: In the first few years the child is exposed to a world of different sights, sounds and experiences. Every day he stores new information through his sensory system (explores own body, leaves mother to explore the surrounding) as also he trains his motor system to help him gather the information for his senses.

Preoperational: In this stage of pre-logical ideas, the child is dominated by magical thinking, egocentrism and thinking governed by perception. Magical thinking is the thought of unrealistic causation (e.g. power of wish turning true). Egocentrism is the inability to take another's viewpoint.

Concrete operations: The pre-logical stage give way to the stage where logic and reason exert sway over preconceived ideas.

Formal operations: Upto the above stage the child had to be dependent on someone else's ideas, now he comes of his own and has the capacity to generate abstractions. Though there is no structural change in the brain, cognitive processing has speeded up to include quantitative increases in knowledge, experience and efficiency.

Like the Eriksonian stages, these stages are important to understand the age differences in cognition. A neurological insult to the developing brain may result in cerebral palsy with mental retardation. Repeated convulsions with neuronal cell may cause a child to fare badly in class. Observe the child carefully, talk to him to know his viewpoints, tell him a story and see how he interacts, give him a riddle and see how he can solve it. To assess higher order cognition the following parameters are used:

Concepts – His grasp of understanding the central point.

Problem solving skills – His ability in formulating techniques. To meet a challenge and find out the best solution.

Brainstorming skills – Original ideas to write a topic imaginatively.

Critical thinking – Ability to compare and contrast different views.

Metacognitive abilities – Refers to his capacity to think about thinking (whether the thinking is right or how to correct learning strategy).

Table 10.4: Common age related behavioural disorders

Age	*Disorder*
Infant and Toddler	Feeding problem, 3 months colic, stranger anxiety, breath holding spell, temper tantrum
Preschool	Head banging, body rocking, thumb-sucking, nail biting, masturbation
School	Stuttering, pica, enuresis, encopresis
Adolescence	Juvenile delinquency, homosexuality

Behaviour Problems

A child often presents with behaviour problems which are largely ignored in a bid to establish organic origins for the complaint. Habit disorders, problems of eating, speech, sleep, scholastic deterioration, sexual problems, antisocial activities are quite common in our society and it is primarily the paediatrician's responsibility to be alert to them. A list of common age-related behaviour problems is given in Table 10.4.

11 PSYCHOLOGICAL ASSESSMENT

ASSESSMENT: A DEFINITION

Sundberg and Tyler (1962) defined assessment as the process of bringing together relevant information from a variety of sources, i.e. the systematic collection, organisation and interpretation of information about a person and his/her situations that may be used for predicting his/her behaviour.

WHY ASSESS PSYCHOLOGICAL FACTORS?

In the holistic management of a child, assessment of psychological factors is essential. This is because:

- Illness (chronic as well as acute) have a profound effect on the social, emotional, behavioural and academic functioning of the child.
- Psychological factors (smoking, lack of exercise, substance abuse, treatment non-adherence) can be a major contributor to an illness, in terms of onset, maintenance and treatment (Brown et al, 2002).
- Further psychological factors can interfere with procedures and complicate history-making and symptom assessment.
- In spite of the advancement in the medical field, the inner world of children remains essentially unchanged (Rauch and Jellinek, 2002).

Often paediatricians are considered as the ideal professionals to screen for psychological disorders (Simonian and Tarnowski, 2001). However, studies indicate that psychological problems in paediatric care are under-identified (Costello, et al 1988, Brown, et al 2002). Described below are the barriers to effective assessment.

- *Inadequate training programme:* Training programmes do not provide specific education, knowledge, training and skills to address psychosocial disturbance in patients.
- *Time and financial pressures:* The average visit is less than 15 minutes, barely enough time to assess and manage physical needs. The financial pressures restrict their ability to devote sufficient efforts towards assessment and management of patents psychological functioning (American Academy of Paediatrics, 2002).
- Frequently, incorporation of mental health issues is seen as a *paradigm shift*.
- *Resistance:* Often paediatricians feel that patients would resist addressing psychological issues and thus pediatricians are hesitant in inquiring about the child's behaviour, development and family functioning (Perrin, et al 1999).
- *Nondisclosure on patients/parents part:* Often parents do not report psychological concerns due to stigma attached.

Considering the above-mentioned points, the present chapter is an attempt to provide an overview of psychological assessment with children. The description of detailed clinical conditions and interventions is beyond the scope of the present work.

This chapter outlines the role of psychological assessment under two categories:

1. As part of medical conditions
2. Psychological assessment in general.

AS PART OF MEDICAL CONDITIONS

Each medical condition carries its own unique specific challenges. The stressors examined can be *brief or chronic*. The stressors or psychological concerns commonly faced (and that should be assessed) are highlighted in Table 11.1. The stressors have been classified under three categories, i.e. from the perspective of the *child*, the *parents* and the *treating team*. In cases where the stressor is specific to a given condition, the same have been highlighted in brackets.

Table 11.1: Psychological concerns that need to be assessed

Child	*Parents*	*Treating team*
• Anxiety, Fear • Low mood, feeling sad • Non-adherence/non-compliance • Frequent medical visits/ Hospitalisation • Painful procedures • Physical disability • ↓Physical/exercise endurance (*e.g., cystic fibrosis*) • Fear of death (*e.g., Cancer, HIV*) • Interruption of school and play activities • Monitoring symptoms (*e.g., Glucose levels as in diabetes*) • Adverse effects of medicines • Change in lifestyle, eating habits (*e.g. Cancer, diabetes*) • Appear different from others • Disclosure of diagnosis to peers • Diminished self-esteem • Decline in cognitive functions (*e.g. intelligence, concentration, memory; in epilepsy, cancer*) • Night awakening (*e.g., asthma*) • Social isolation and rejection • Compromised Quality of Life (QOL) • Unpredictable course of illness/ prognosis • Stigma (*e.g., cancer, HIV*) • Intense time consuming medical regimen	• Disruption of family routine and lifestyle (*e.g., absenteeism from work, less time for each other*) • Coping with new anxiety-provoking information • Conflicting information by different team members • Anger/Blame • Uncertainty • Guilt (*e.g., passing defective genes*) • Emotional burst out • Burnt out • Managing mealtime and medicines • Financial strain	• A high stress environment • Long working hours • Conflicts with other team members (nurses, seniors/ juniors) • Sense of helplessness • Burn out

While dealing with chronic illnesses, a developmental approach can be useful. It emphasises how psychosocial challenges and adjustment change from the preschool to school age to adolescence. Psychological assessment is essential to help children cope with chronic medical illness or painful procedures, as per their developmental age.

It is important to keep in mind that children with chronic conditions may not have major psychiatric disturbance but are at an increased risk for psychological adjustment problems (Wallander, Thompson and Alriksoon-Schmidt, 2003).

The following aspects although time consuming, are yet worth exploring:

- What is the hardest aspect of the illness from the child's perspective?
- How does it affect the child's image of him or herself now and how has it changed?
- Does the child have worries about the future?
- How do the illness and treatment impact on peer relations and favourite activities?
- When and how does the child tell others about the illness and why?
- Are there areas of conflicts between the child and the parent or the child and the physician?
- What are the child's perceptions of the parents' worries? (Rauch and Jellinek, 2002).

The author is well aware the sometimes, despite the best intentions the paediatrician is unable to assess these aspects in detail (due to various constraints). A well-trained Paediatric Psychologist (as in West) or a Clinical psychologist (as in India) can effectively assess these aspects and his/her services should be availed to provide holistic care to the child.

In context of medical conditions, pain is one of the most commonly assessed variables. It is challenging to measure pain due to its subjective nature and the important roles played by cognitive and emotional factors. With children the assessment of pain becomes even more difficult because of the following factors:

- Limited vocabulary to describe pain.
- Pain scales require children to discriminate constructs (e.g., intensity and duration) that may be sophisticated for their cognitive development.
- Further, in comparison to adults, children are less accurate in their estimates of pain; more susceptible to situational demands.
- Children are less able to separate pain from emotions such as fear.
- Children have fewer painful experiences with which to compare the current event.

The commonly used assessment measures comprise of:

a. Child Self-report and
b. Observational methods.

Child Self-Report

Visual analogue scale are the most common forms of child pain intensity assessment. These scales involve the graphic representations of pain intensity by marking a point on a line and can be used with children as young as 5-year-old (Dahlquist, 1990). Face Scales are also used which consist of a set of line drawings or photographs of faces that depict pain states (Chambers, Giesbrecht, Craig, Bennett, and Huntsman, 1999). Structured interviews with children and their parents are commonly used to assess the historial and contextual variables contributing to pain experiences (Allen and Matthews, 1998).

Observational Methods

Some researchers argue that behavioural observations are more reliable and valid than self-report measures because they are objective in nature, recording the presence or absence of discrete pain behaviours (Mcgrath, 1987). However, the behavioural observations capture only the overt expression of pain. Once can observe for specific pain behaviours such as limping, grimacing, sighing. It is also important to observe how the parents respond to child's pain (e.g. ignore the pain, over-concerned, minimise the pain by considering it as feigning, a 'drama', too critical/hostile).

To summarise, the choice of specific measure should be determined by the child's developmental level, the setting and whether the assessment is for research or clinical purpose.

PSYCHOLOGICAL ASSESSMENT IN GENERAL

The psychological concerns in children have broadly been classified under two domains: *Internalising and Externalising disorders* (Achenbach and Edelbrock, 1991). The *internalising* disorders are also referred to as disorders of emotions and are characterised by subjective distress in children, feelings of inferiority it, social withdrawal, self-consciousness, shyness, anxiety, crying, hypersensitivity, depression and sadness (Quay, 1979). On the other hand, *Externalising* disorders are marked by conflicts with the environment and include aggressiveness, temper tantrums, lying; which are distressing to others.

The literature on psychological disorders is voluminous. To describe the diagnostic criteria and assessment of each condition would defeat the purpose of the present work. The chapter selectively focuses on the assessment procedures. A detailed account of diagnostic criterion and management of the psychological conditions can be obtained in Walker and Roberts (2001) and Rutter and Taylor.

Psychological Assessment

The psychological assessment is aimed at evaluating the child's psychological and social problems along with his/her limitations and capabilities. It also includes description and analysis of performance of a particular child.

Psychological Assessment: Functions Served

- Provides a picture of current phenomenology
- Helps to build an aetiological hypothesis
- Estimate the potential of the child and
- Provides information on child's assets and limitations.

Assessment for Children: How is it Different from Adult Assessment?

- Unlike adults children rarely come to treatment on their own (Generally, referral is initiated by significant others e.g., parents, teachers).
- Children and youth undergo behavioural, social, emotional and cognitive changes at a rapid pace than adults; and thus their behaviour must be viewed within a developmental context.
- The child assessment involves multiple persons in the child's life, unlike the adult assessment, which involves only the adult client.

The most useful assessment tools for evaluating any child behaviour problem are those that accurately describe the characteristics and impact of the concerned behaviour. For most childhood behaviour problems, a multiple method of assessment is required, which obtains information from at least two different assessment methods.

According to Johnson and Bommarita, the assessment of children traditionally focuses on eight areas (Table 11.2). The commonly used methods for assessment are also describe in the table. It is essential to clarify that the methods are not corresponding to the areas being assessed. These are general methods and each area may be assessed using one or more of the following methods.

Table 11.2: Areas and methods of assessment

Areas of assessment	*Methods of assessment*
• Cognition • Personality • Perception of environment • Self-concept • Environment • Motor skills and brain injury • Physical attributes and • Social behaviour	• Psychological tests • Clinical Interviews (with children and parents) • Direct observation • Standard rating scales

A brief description of the assessment method is illustrated below.

Psychological Tests

Broadly speaking, a test is any systematic and quantified way of describing behaviour (Sergeant and Taylor, 2002). It may be highly standardised as an IQ test, or it may be developed and used for the unique problems of an individual case. The traditional definitions of psychological tests focus on those procedures and instruments that have been standardised through psychometric refinement, have satisfactory reliability and are valid in describing an individual child in relation to the rest of the population. Psychological testing makes mental assessments more reliable and closer to what they seek to measure. A large number of tests have been developed for assessing various functions. It is difficult to enumerate all the tests. Some of the most commonly used tests are depicted in Table 11.3. Details regarding the administration, scoring and interpretation can be obtained from test manuals. In general, to administer tests, one requires specific training that needs to be learnt under expert guidance. Clinical psychologists are trained for this purpose and they can form a part of the team involved in assessing the child. Some of the tests have been adapted specifically for Indian children. The details of the same can be obtained in Kapur (1995).

Clinical Interviews

A. With Parents

Firstly, it is important to ask parents to clearly define the behavior that is of concern. A statement that the child has a "bad attitude" or "never listens" is not enough to address the problem. Parents should be asked to describe the behaviour. Information on the course of problematic behaviour needs to be solicited (e.g., duration; intensity; frequency; do factors such as public setting, hunger, fatigue increase the problematic behaviour). After defining the present problem, an assessment of antecedent and consequences is done. This is important because it helps to establish the conditions under which the child is having difficulty behaving or complying and they also provide targets for interventions. Some of the probable questions to determine Antecedents and Consequences are illustrated in Table 11.4. Characteristics (Family of origin, religious values, knowledge of child development), child characteristics (temperament, handicaps, cognitive level), previous history with professionals (medical,

Table 11.3: Commonly used psychological tests for children

Area	*Commonly used tests*
Cognition	
• Intelligence	Binet's scale Weschlers' Intelligence Scale for Children (WISC) Malin's Intelligence Scale for Indian Children (MISIC) Raven's Colored Progressive Matrices (CPM)
• Specific Learning Disabilities (SLD)	NIMHANS Index of SLD
• Memory	Cattell's Retentivity test Benton's Visual Retention test
Personality	Children's Personality Questionnaire Rosenzweig Picture Frustration test Children's Appreciation test Roscharch Inkblot test Draw A Person test
Perception of environment	Preadolescent Adjustment Inventory
Self-concept	Self Esteem Inventory

Table 11.4: Probable questions to determine antecedents and consequences

Antecedents	*Consequences*
• Where does the behaviour occur and with whom? • What is the child generally doing before exhibiting the problematic behaviour? • How do the parents respond to the child when she exhibits problematic behaviour?	• Is the child praised/rewarded/ignored for positive behaviour/compliance? • Is the child sent for time out, reasoned with, or begged to comply when she refuses to complete a task? • Does the parent complete the task?

school), resources for family support (Relatives, friends, community) and overall stress level.

Some of the other following family factors to be assessed while dealing with parents include:

- The cultural background,
- Socioeconomic status (income, education, living conditions),
- History of family disruption (shifting houses, illness),
- Parental psychopathology (substance abuse, anxiety, depression),
- Marital relationships (separation, divorce, conflicts),
- Parenting characteristics (Family or origin, religious values, knowledge of child development),
- Child characteristics (temperament, handicaps, cognitive level),
- Previous history with professionals (medical, school),
- Resources for family support (Relatives, friends, community) and
- Overall stress level.

B. Child Interviews

An interview with the child can provide valuable information as well as an opportunity to observe his/her behaviour. Most interviews need to include a combination of questions that require a knowledge base (e.g., what she understands about illness and behavioural difficulties), the way the child relates to his parents, sibs and peers and open-ended questions that have no right-wrong answers. The information gathered can provide the clinician with an *understanding of child's perception* of the current problem and his/her *willingness to participate in treatment*. The child interviews also provide the opportunity to evaluate any inconsistency of information provided by the parent versus the child.

A number of structured diagnostic tools have been developed. The most commonly used instruments are: Diagnostic Interview for Children and adolescents-Revised (DICA-R, Herjanic, et al 1975), Diagnostic Interview Schedule for Children (DISC, Costello, et al 1984), Child Assessment Schedule (CAS, Hodges et al, 1981).

Behavioural Observations

Behavioural observation has been an important method of assessing children. The child may be observed under Natural conditions (*Naturalistic observation*) or in a structured situation (*Structured observation*, e.g. school, clinic). During observation, the focus is on verbal as well as non-verbal cues (gestures and behaviour). While observing the child, one can observe for the following:

- General appearance (dress, happy/unhappy, tearful, afraid of being alone with the examiner),
- Motor functions (slow/quick, clumsy, right-left orientation, overactive/under active),
- Speech (talks freely/with hesitations, does not talk, stammering),
- Content of talk and thought (logical flow, expression),
- Mood (happy, depressed, hostile, fearful).

It is also important to observe the interaction between parents, attitude of the parents towards the child and interaction between the parents and child (answer for the child, provide cues, gets angry).

Rating Scales

A number of standardised ratings scales are also used to obtain information from multiple informants, including the parents, teachers and the child. The rating scales provide an indicator of child's conduct and emotional states. Rating scales also provide a way to repeat assessment during and after treatment and after medication changes to monitor progress. Rating scales allow for a child's score to be compared with scores of children of similar ages, providing an important developmental reference for a child's emotional and behavioural functioning. The interpretation of rating scales requires knowledge of the psychometric issues and how the various scales were developed. Some of the commonly used behaviour rating scales are:

a. *Child Behaviour Checklist (CBCL):* As developed by Achenbach (1991) is a commonly used rating scale to assess internalising and externalising problems in children. CBCL is documented to effectively discriminate between normal children and those referred to mental health clinics.
b. *Behaviour Assessment System for Children (BASC):* Has been developed by Reynolds and Kamphaus (1991). It is available in three forms: Parent rating scale, Teacher rating scale and self-report of personality. Scores are reported for behavioural symptoms, externalising and internalising problems, school problems, adaptive skills and atypicality.
c. *Conners Rating Scale:* developed by Conners (1973) is commonly used to assess ADHD with the help of 10 overlapping parent and teacher items.
d. *Developmental Psychopathology Checklist for Children (DPCL):* Has been devised for use with Indian children by Kapur, et al (1994). It consists of 124 items classified under six subsections:
    i. Developmental history,
    ii. Developmental problems,
    iii. Psychopathology,
    iv. Psychosocial factors,
    v. Temperament,
    vi. Social support and asset of the child.

CONCLUSION

While working with children it is important to consider the behavioural/developmental concerns medical/biological, and environmental/psychosocial risk as well as protective factors. It is essential to keep in mind that a bi-directional influence occurs between the infant and the environment. Paediatricians should focus on the patient's discomfort rather than on categorisation of clinical manifestations as either organically or psychologically determined. Psychological factors have a role in the onset, maintenance and treatment of medical illnesses/conditions. Further, psychological difficulties may emerge as a result of the medical condition and all these need to be dealt with in providing holistic care to the pediatric patients. Only on the basis of a thorough assessment can one plan individual and family interventions that are crucial in preventing mental health problems and exacerbating symptoms. To conclude, in order to provide quality care and enhance quality of life, assessment of psychological factors is essential. For this purpose, a well-trained paediatric psychologist needs to be an integral part of the paediatric team.

APPENDICES

GROWTH CHARTS

- CDC
- ALL INDIA (IAP)
- ROAD TO HEALTH CHART
- RAINBOW CHART

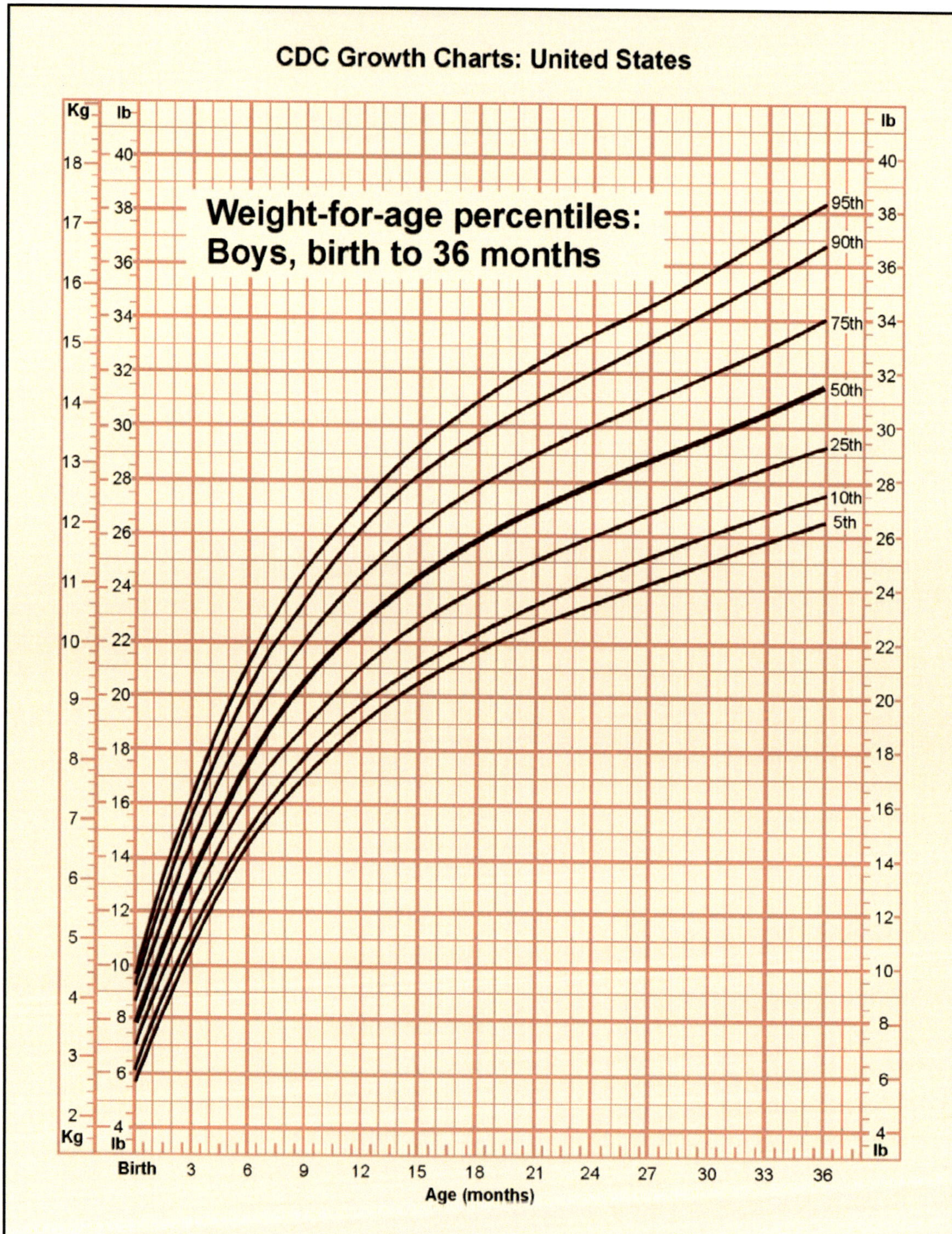
CDC Growth Charts: United States
Weight-for-age percentiles:
Boys, birth to 36 months
95th
90th
75th
50th
25th
10th
5th
Kg
lb
Birth
3
6
9
12
15
18
21
24
27
30
33
36
Age (months)

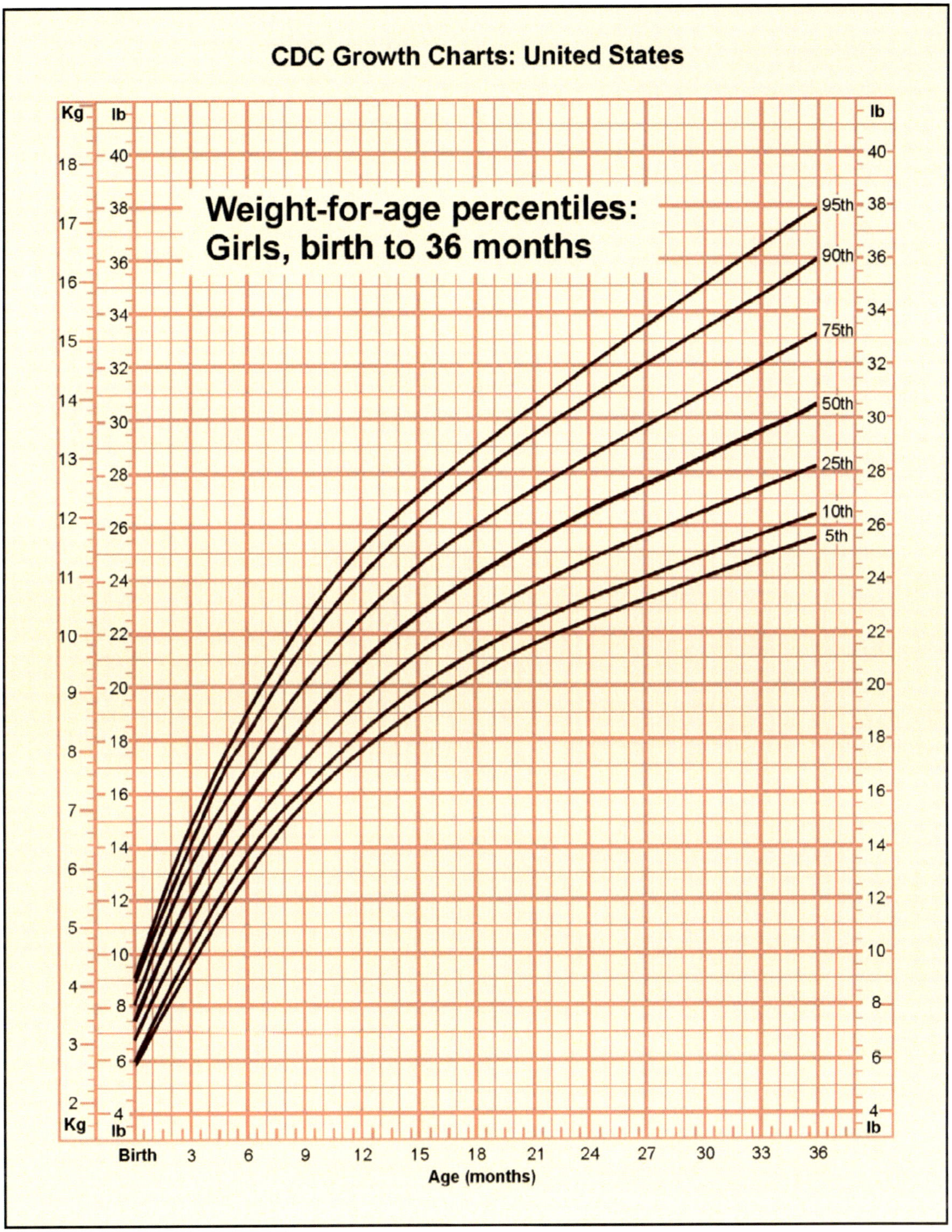

CDC Growth Charts: United States
Weight-for-age percentiles:
Girls, birth to 36 months
Kg
lb
95th
90th
75th
50th
25th
10th
5th
Birth 3 6 9 12 15 18 21 24 27 30 33 36
Age (months)

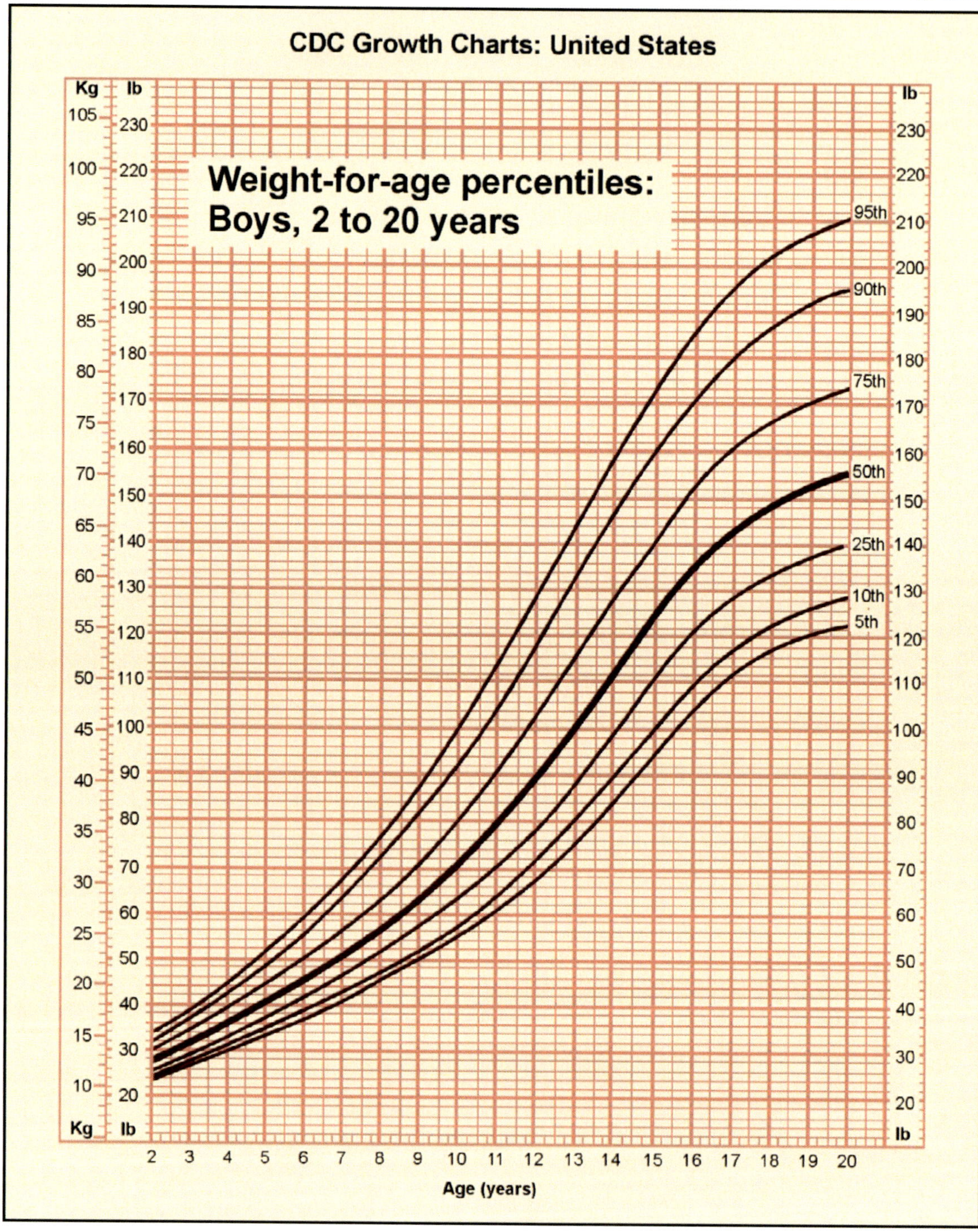
CDC Growth Charts: United States
Weight-for-age percentiles:
Boys, 2 to 20 years
Kg
lb
95th
90th
75th
50th
25th
10th
5th
Age (years)

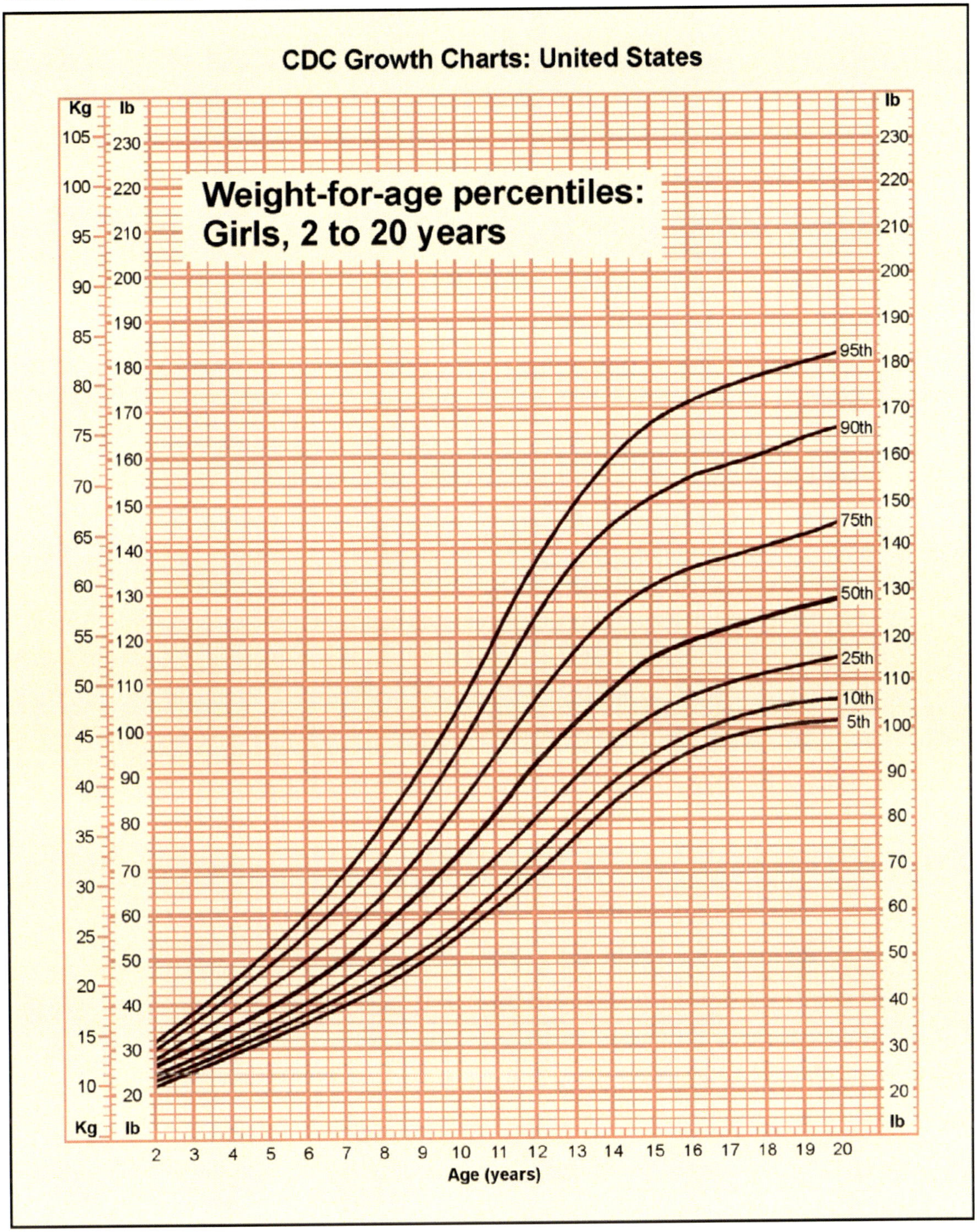
CDC Growth Charts: United States
Weight-for-age percentiles:
Girls, 2 to 20 years
Kg
lb
95th
90th
75th
50th
25th
10th
5th
Age (years)

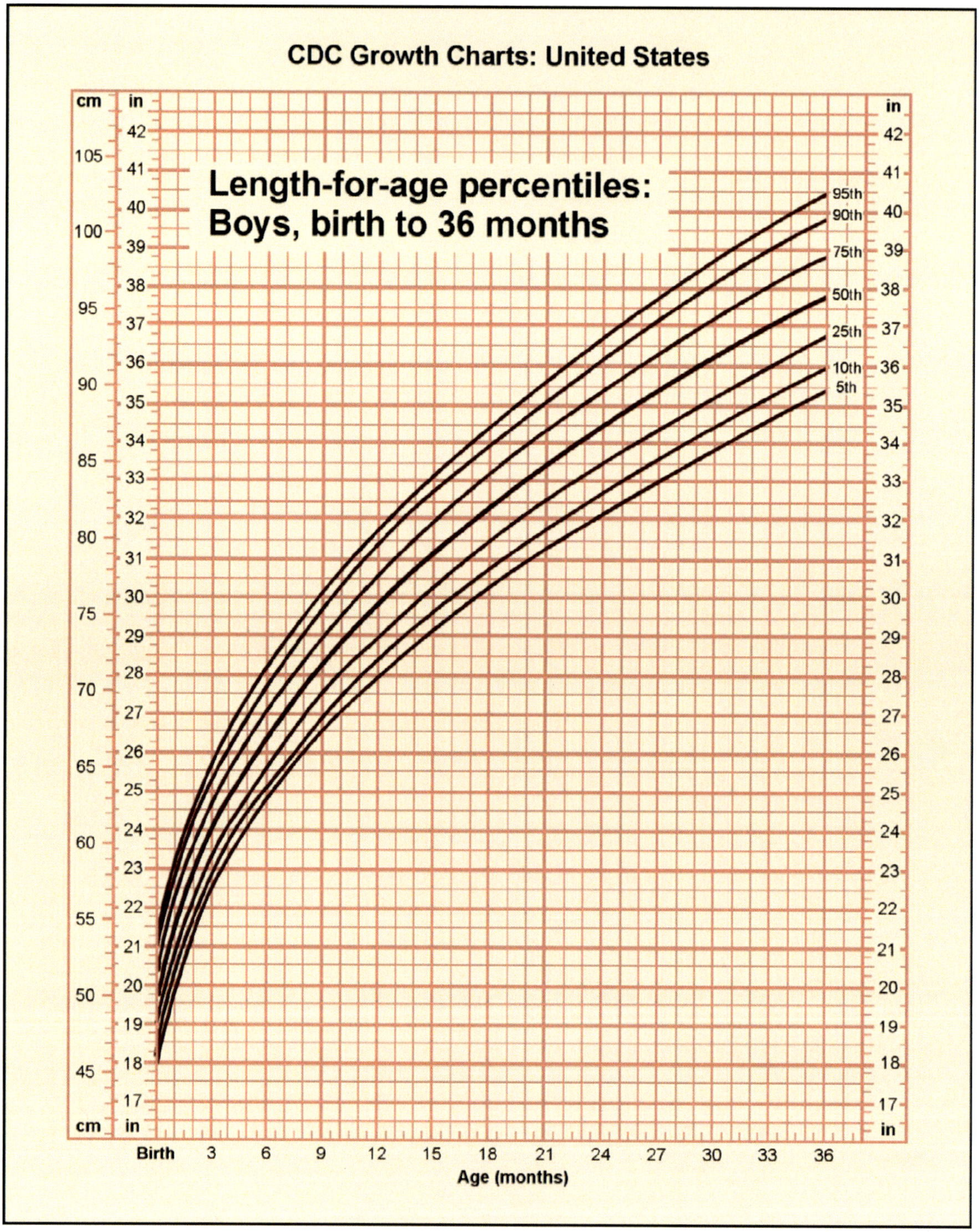
CDC Growth Charts: United States
Length-for-age percentiles:
Boys, birth to 36 months
cm
in
95th
90th
75th
50th
25th
10th
5th
Birth
3
6
9
12
15
18
21
24
27
30
33
36
Age (months)

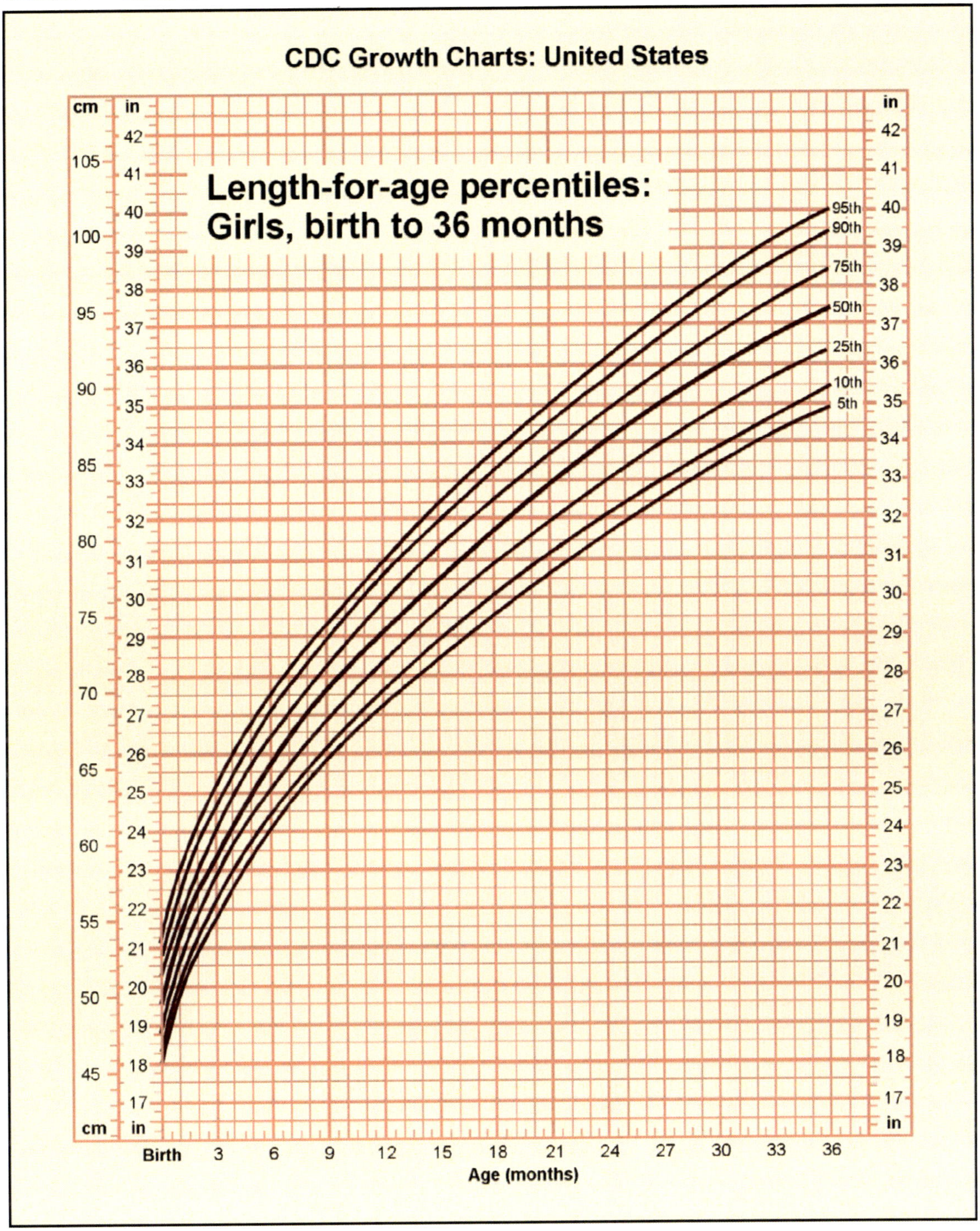
CDC Growth Charts: United States
Length-for-age percentiles:
Girls, birth to 36 months
cm
in
95th
90th
75th
50th
25th
10th
5th
Birth
3
6
9
12
15
18
21
24
27
30
33
36
Age (months)

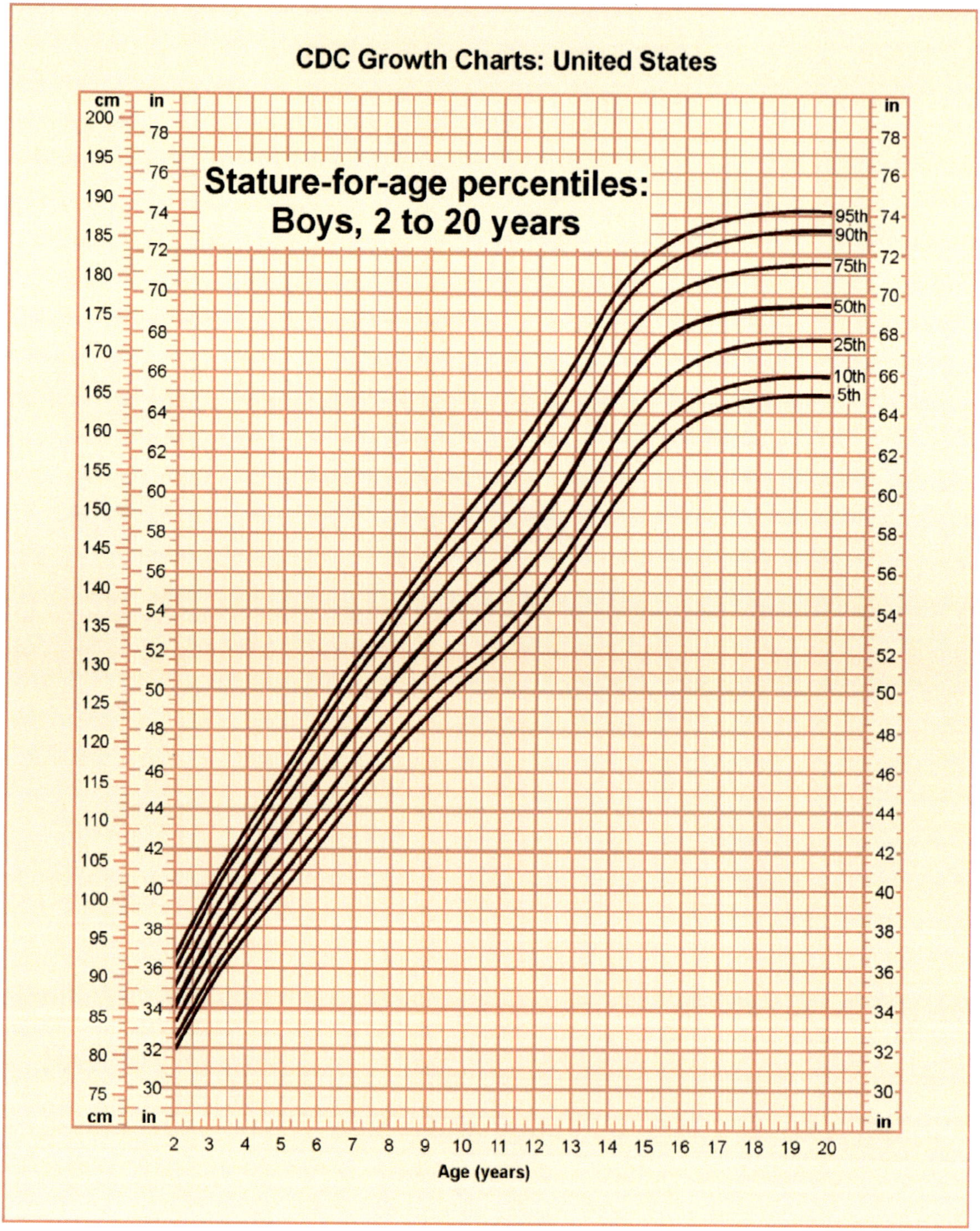
CDC Growth Charts: United States
Stature-for-age percentiles:
Boys, 2 to 20 years
95th
90th
75th
50th
25th
10th
5th
cm
in
Age (years)

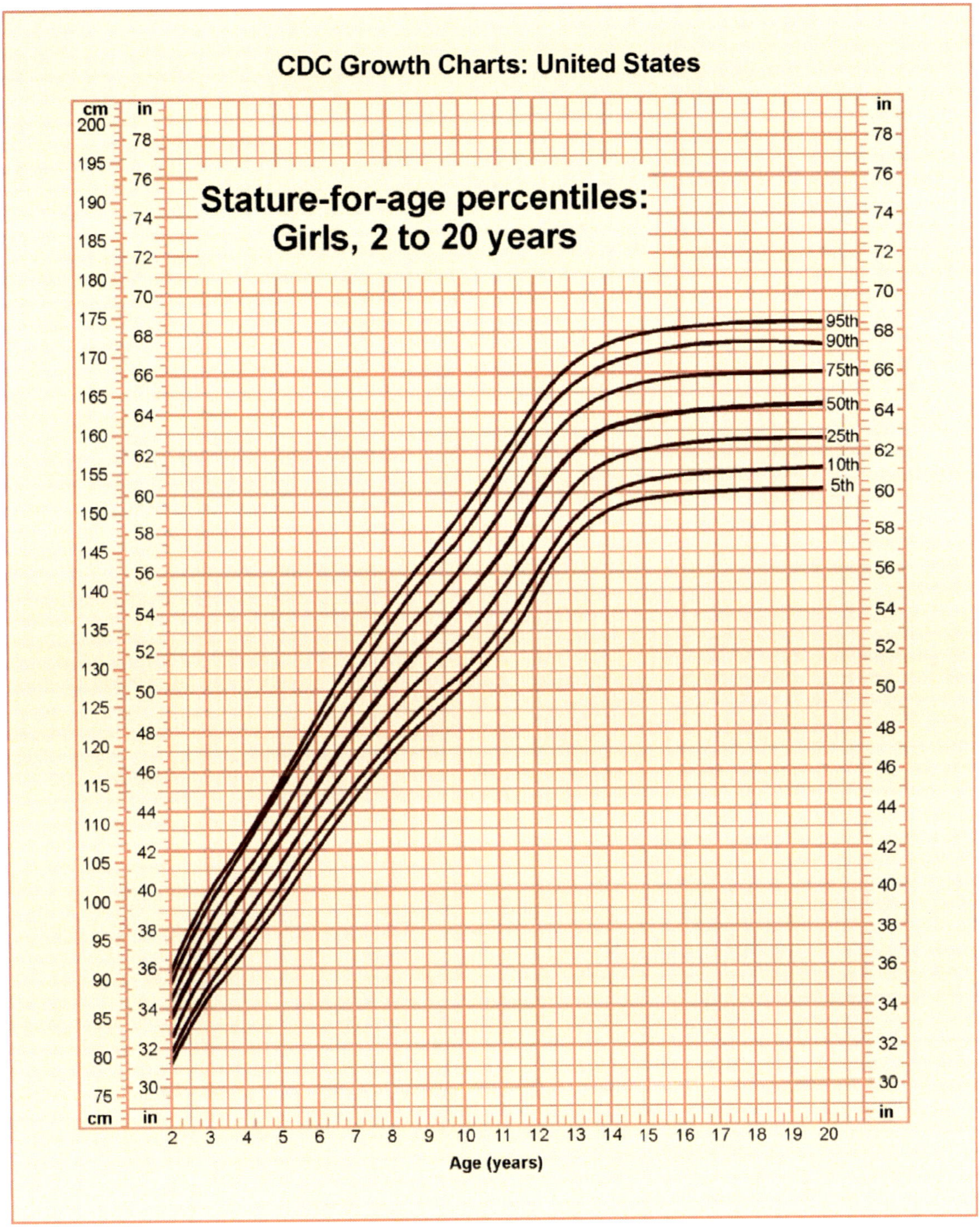
CDC Growth Charts: United States
Stature-for-age percentiles:
Girls, 2 to 20 years
cm
in
95th
90th
75th
50th
25th
10th
5th
Age (years)

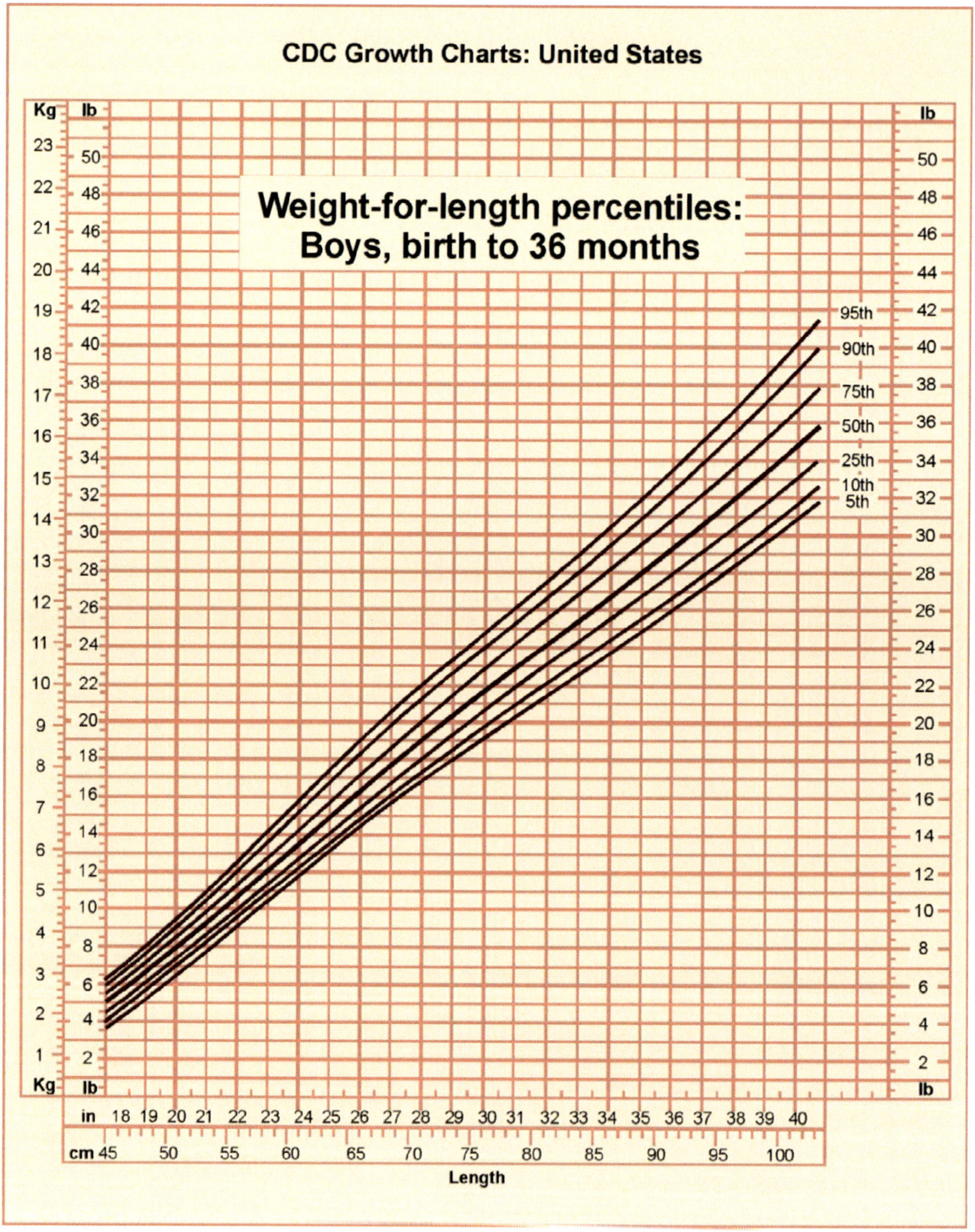
CDC Growth Charts: United States
Weight-for-length percentiles:
Boys, birth to 36 months
95th
90th
75th
50th
25th
10th
5th
Kg
lb
in
cm
Length

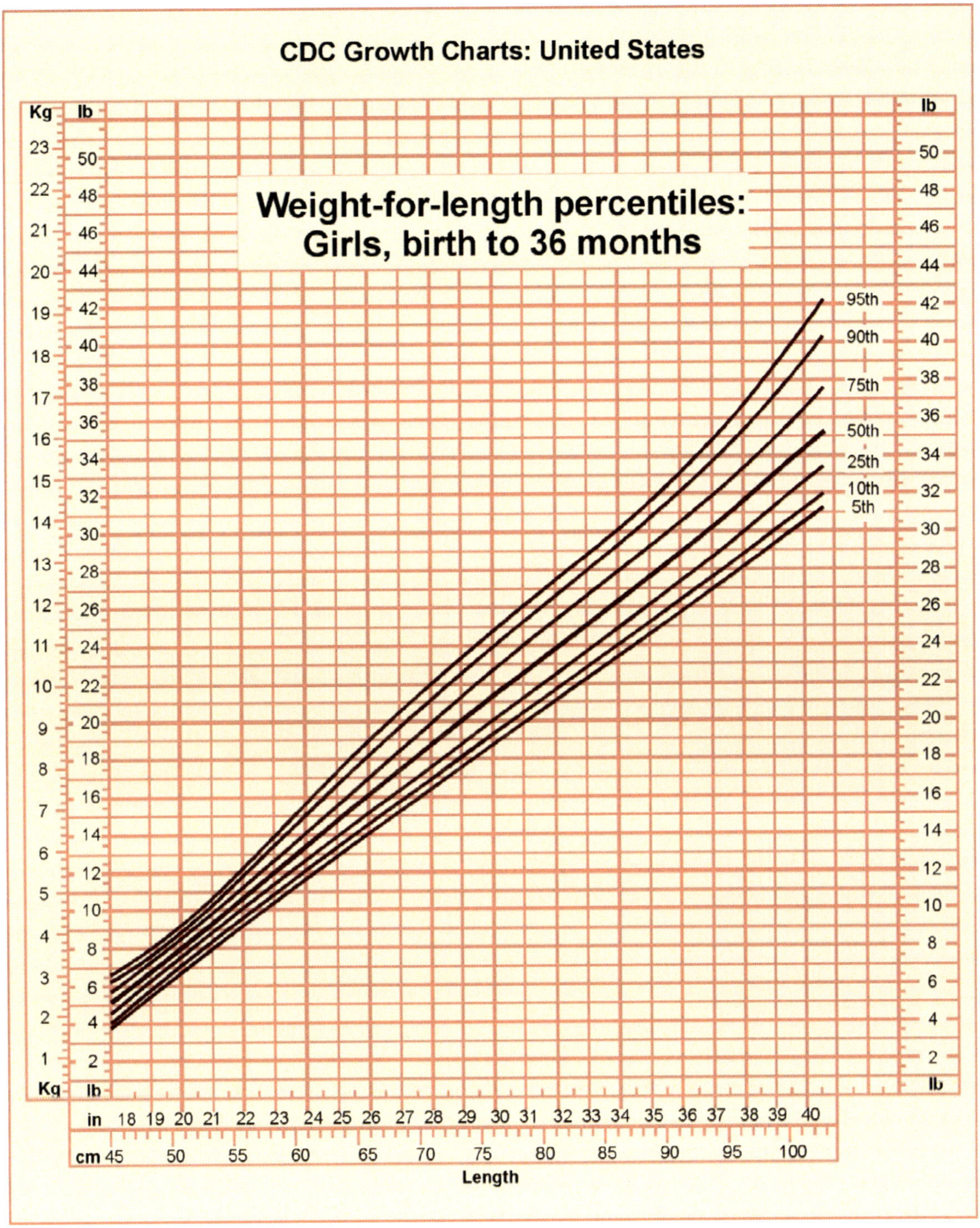
CDC Growth Charts: United States
Weight-for-length percentiles:
Girls, birth to 36 months
Kg
lb
95th
90th
75th
50th
25th
10th
5th
in
cm
Length

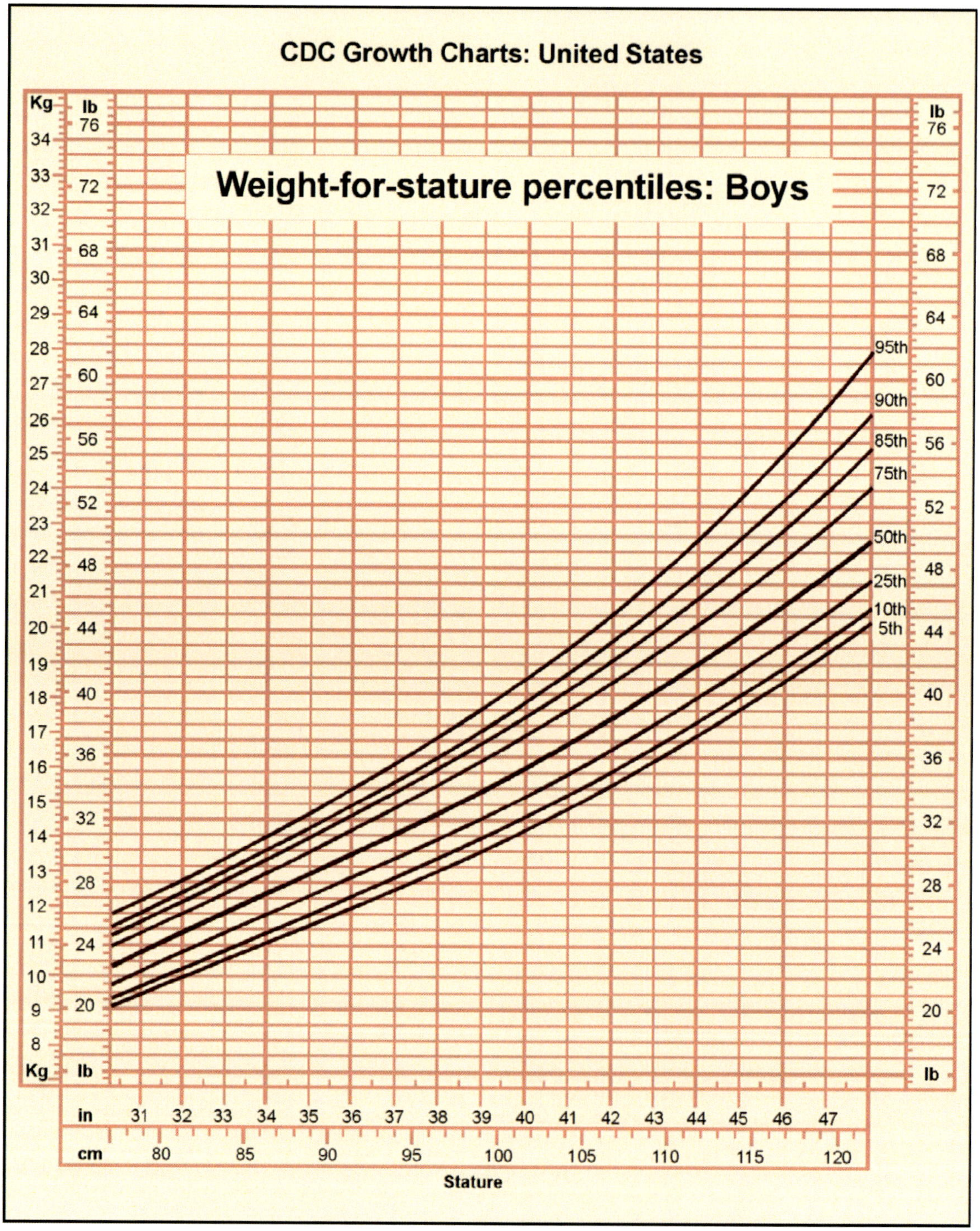
CDC Growth Charts: United States
Weight-for-stature percentiles: Boys
Kg
lb
95th
90th
85th
75th
50th
25th
10th
5th
in
cm
Stature

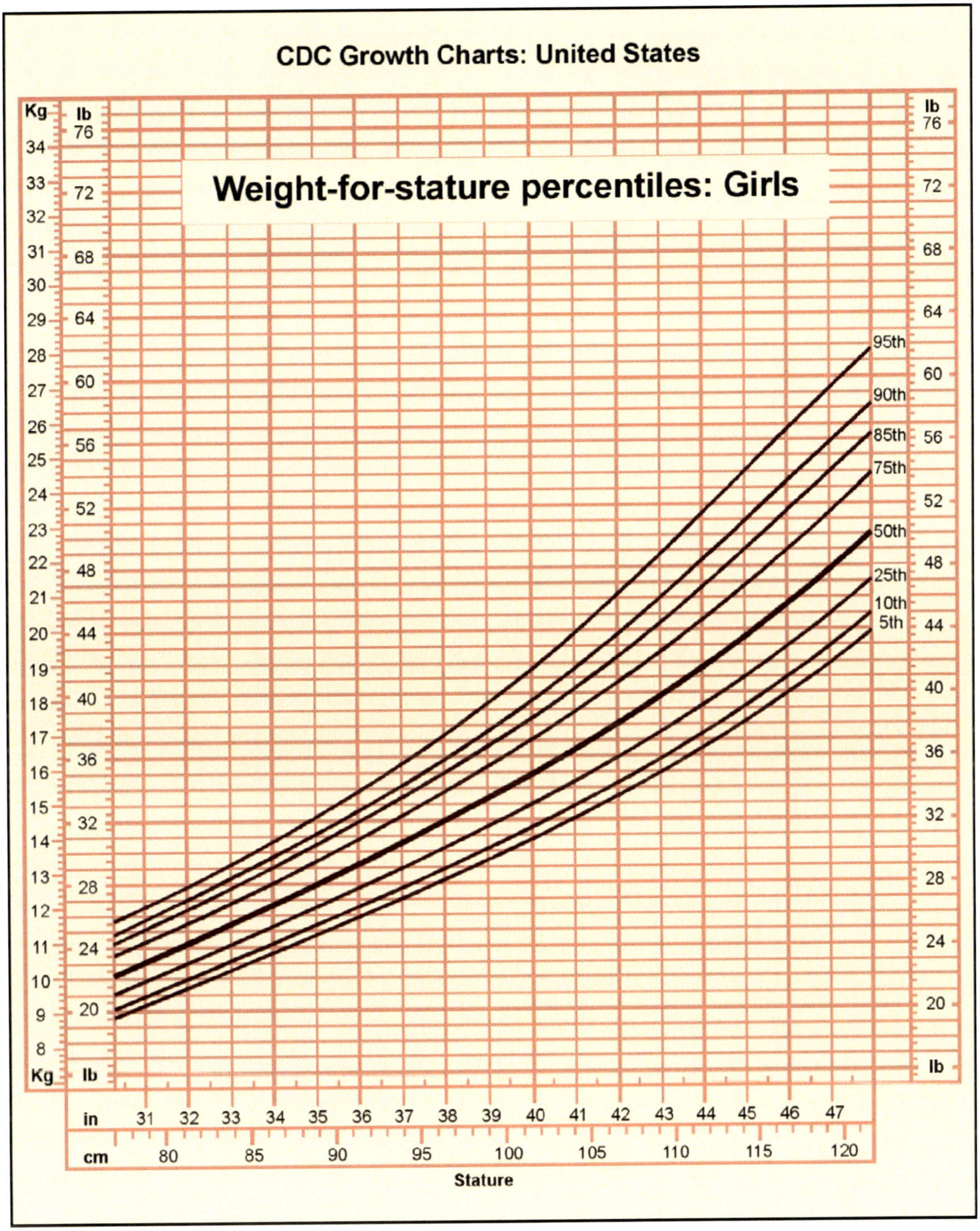
CDC Growth Charts: United States
Weight-for-stature percentiles: Girls
Kg
lb
95th
90th
85th
75th
50th
25th
10th
5th
in
cm
Stature

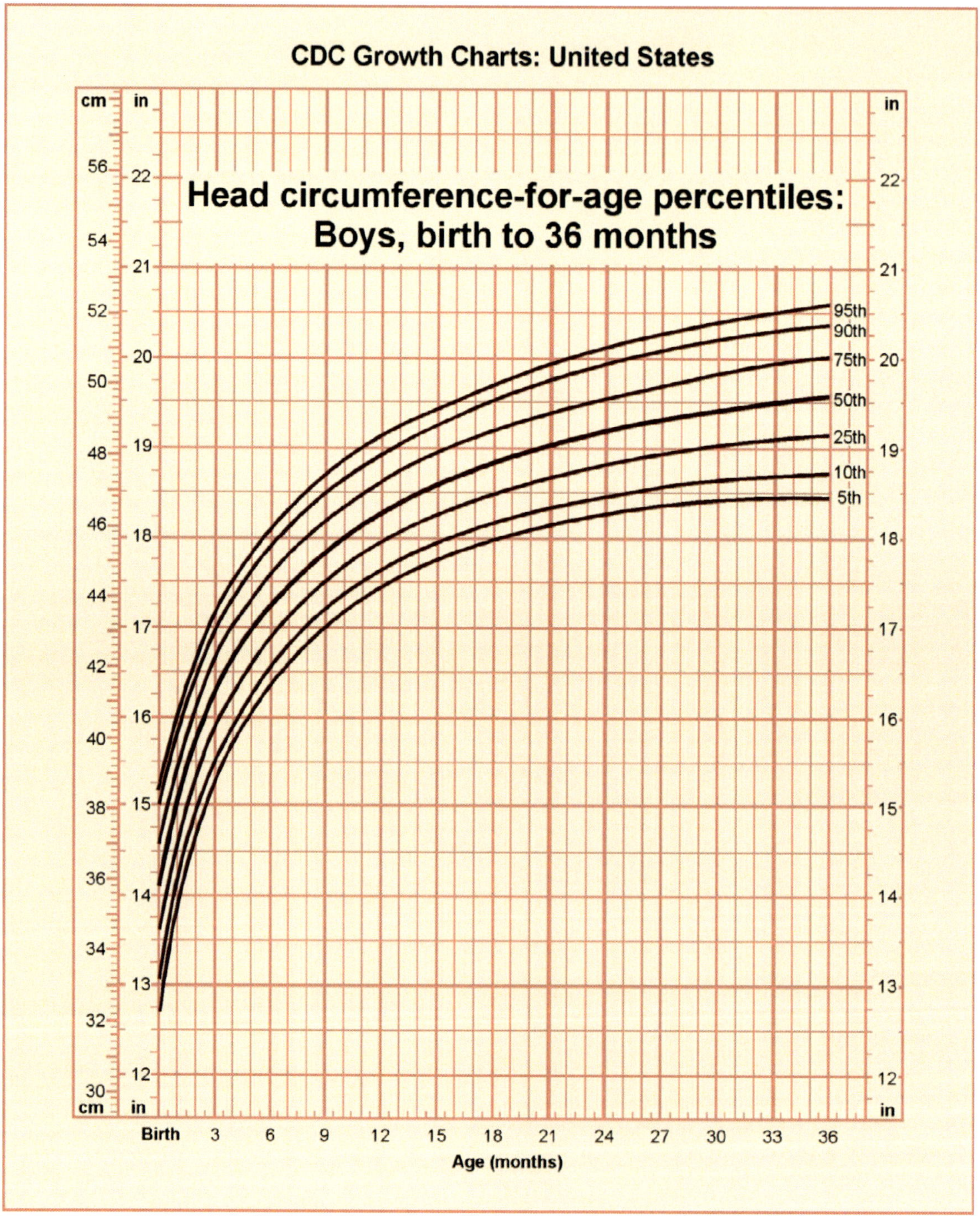
CDC Growth Charts: United States
Head circumference-for-age percentiles:
Boys, birth to 36 months
cm
in
56
54
52
50
48
46
44
42
40
38
36
34
32
30
22
21
20
19
18
17
16
15
14
13
12
95th
90th
75th
50th
25th
10th
5th
Birth
3
6
9
12
15
18
21
24
27
30
33
36
Age (months)

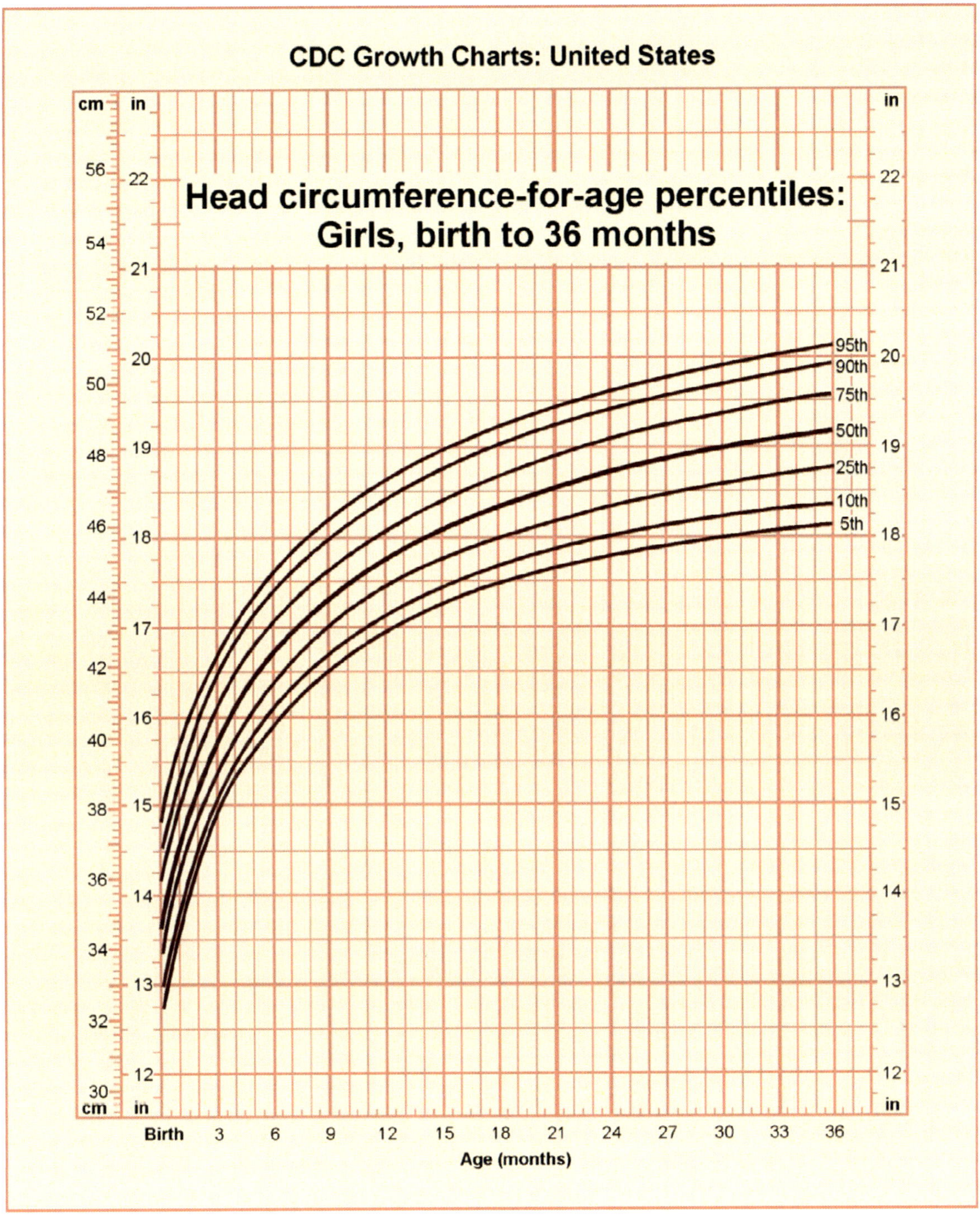

CDC Growth Charts: United States
Head circumference-for-age percentiles:
Girls, birth to 36 months
cm
in
95th
90th
75th
50th
25th
10th
5th
Birth
3
6
9
12
15
18
21
24
27
30
33
36
Age (months)

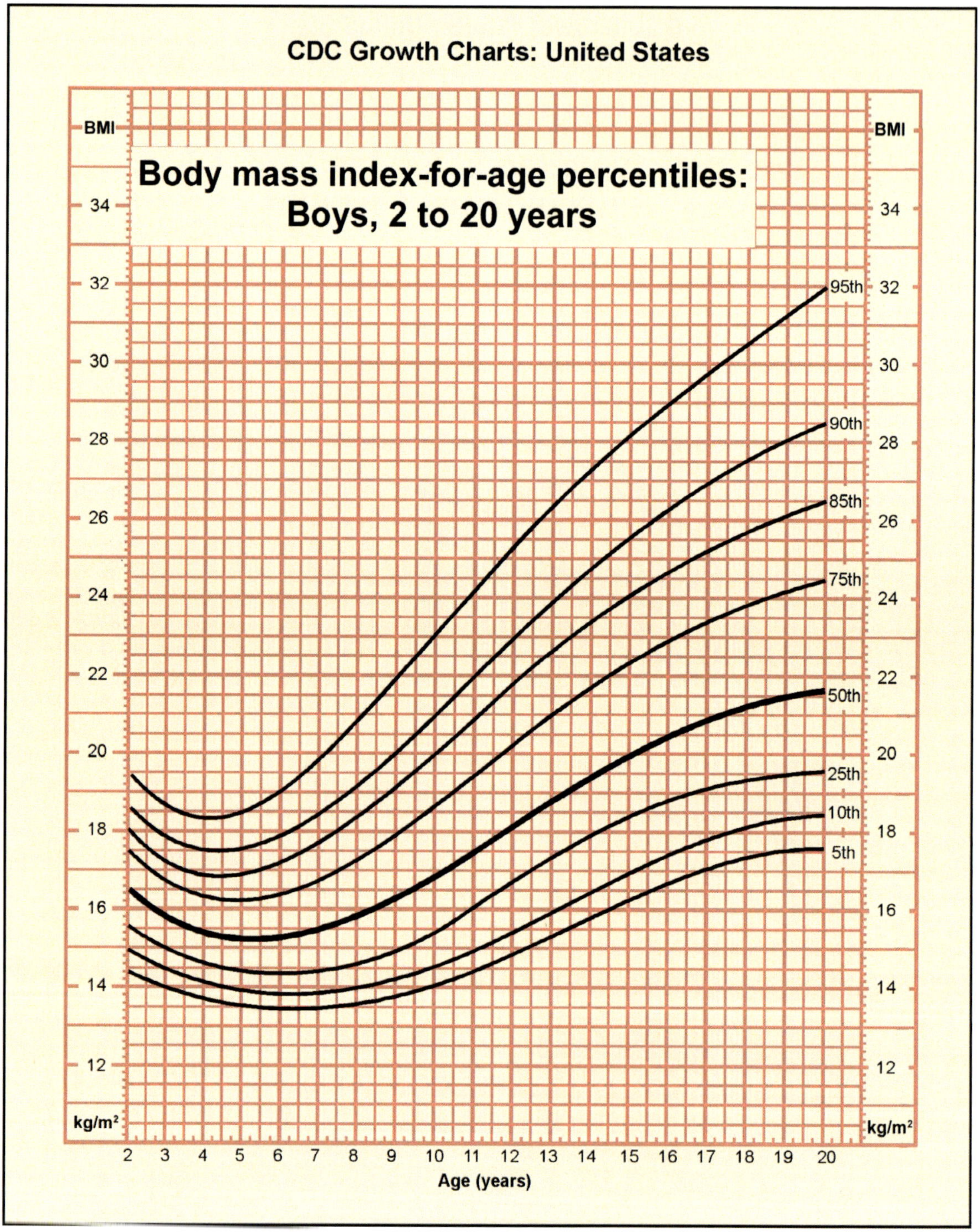
CDC Growth Charts: United States
Body mass index-for-age percentiles:
Boys, 2 to 20 years
BMI
34
32
30
28
26
24
22
20
18
16
14
12
kg/m²
95th
90th
85th
75th
50th
25th
10th
5th
2 3 4 5 6 7 8 9 10 11 12 13 14 15 16 17 18 19 20
Age (years)

CDC Growth Charts: United States

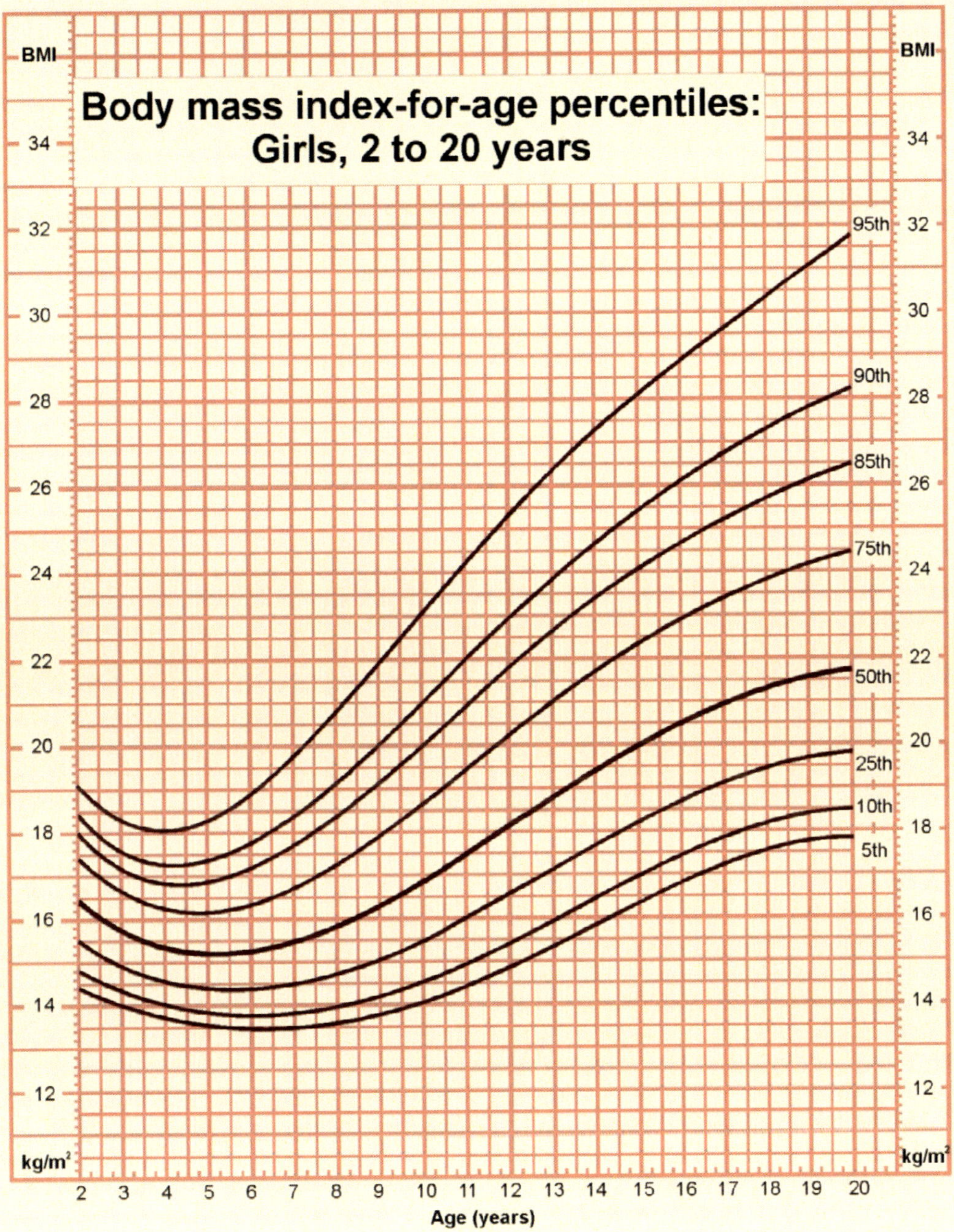

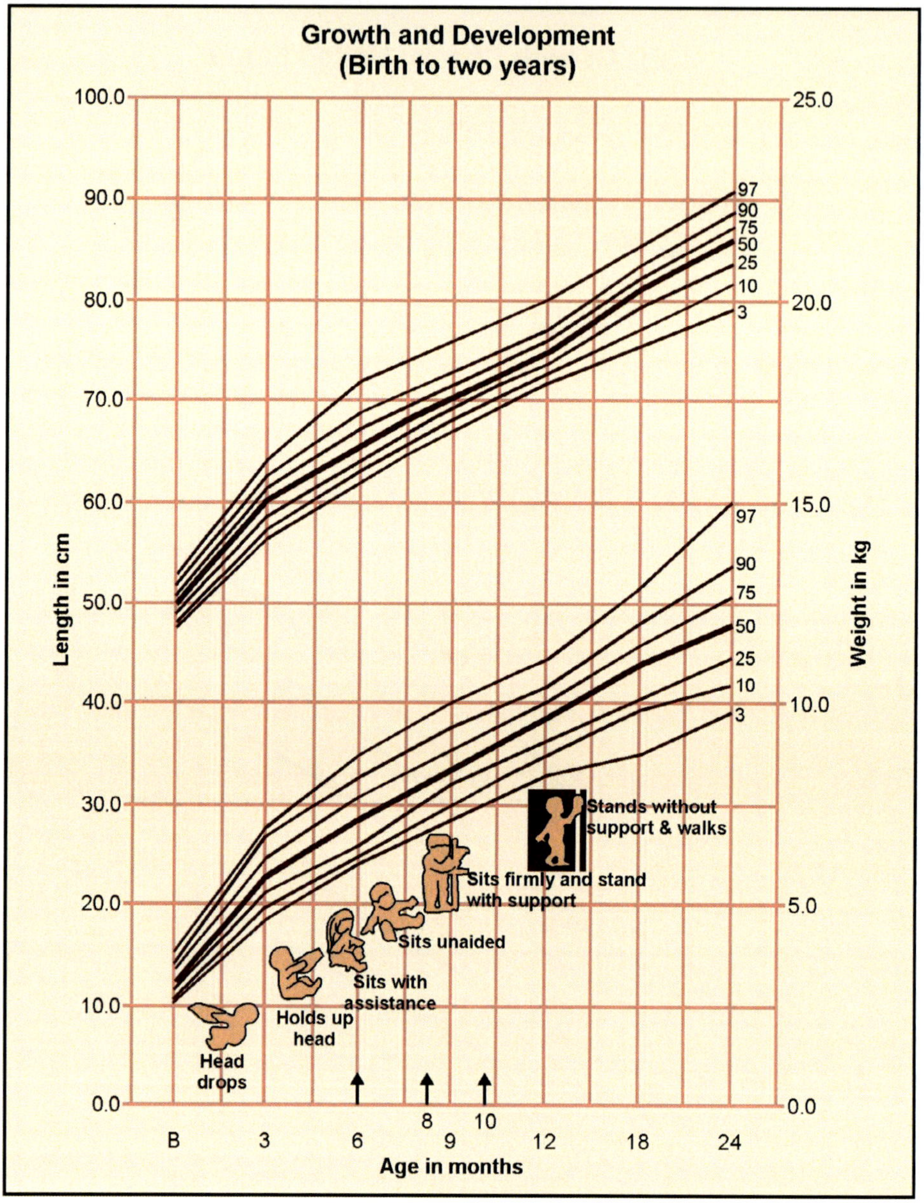
Growth and Development
(Birth to two years)
Length in cm
Weight in kg
Age in months
100.0
90.0
80.0
70.0
60.0
50.0
40.0
30.0
20.0
10.0
0.0
25.0
20.0
15.0
10.0
5.0
0.0
97
90
75
50
25
10
3
B
3
6
8
9
10
12
18
24
Head drops
Holds up head
Sits with assistance
Sits unaided
Sits firmly and stand with support
Stands without support & walks

PERCENTILES FOR HEIGHT AND WEIGHT (BOYS 2-18 YEARS)

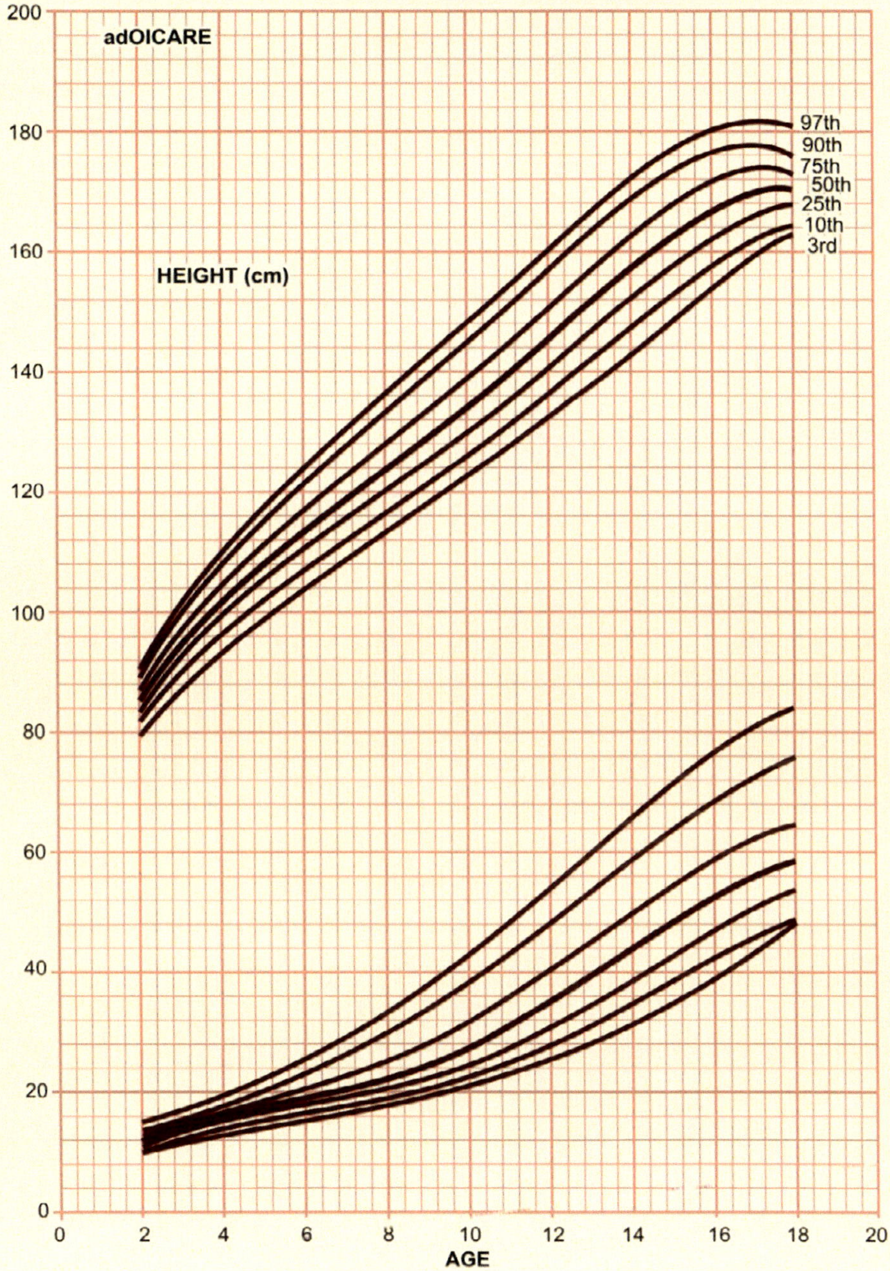

Data Source Agarwal et al. Indian Paediatrics 1992 and 1994 Tables in book The Growth Infancy to adolescence CBS Publ. 2003

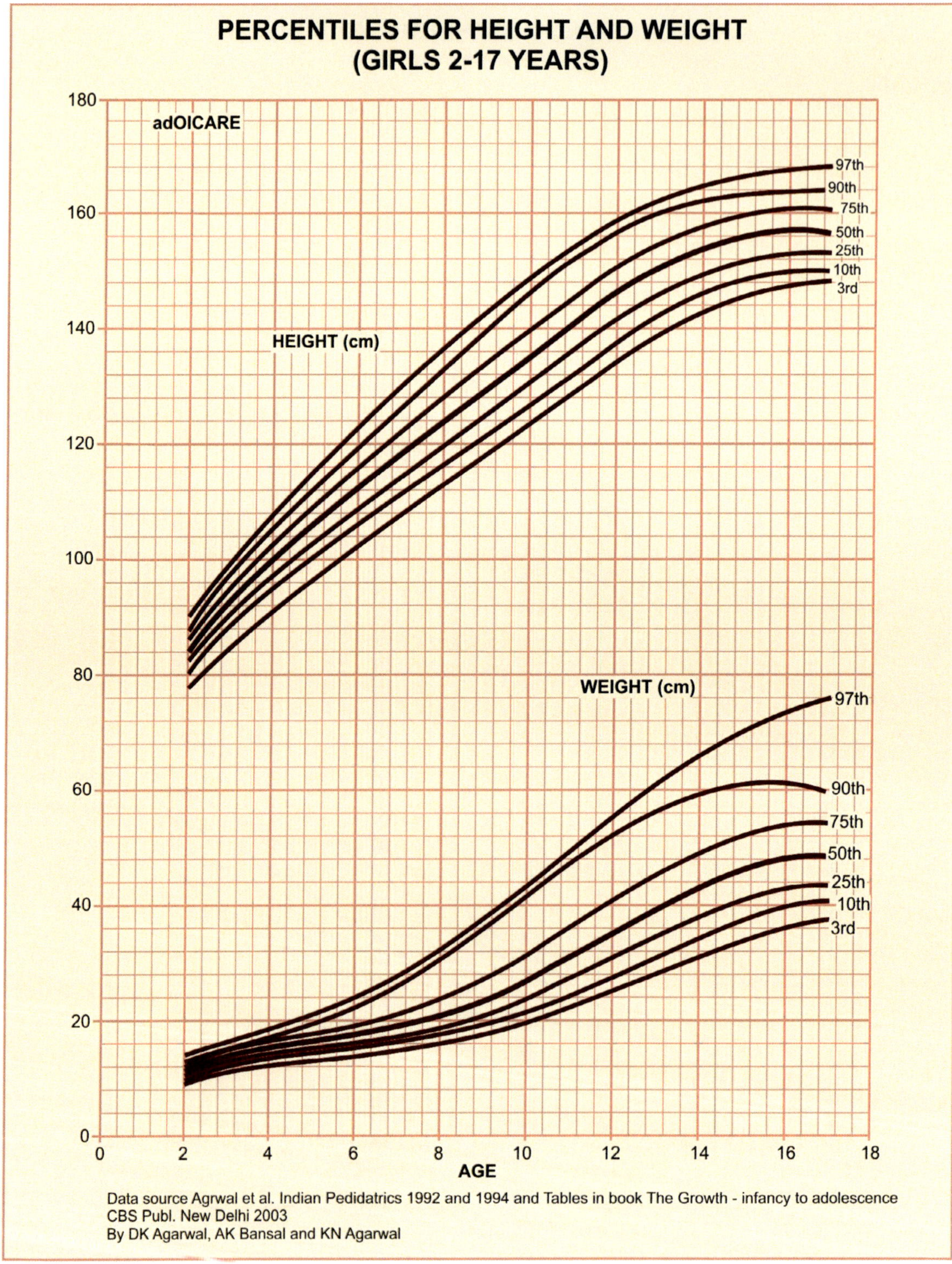
PERCENTILES FOR HEIGHT AND WEIGHT
(GIRLS 2-17 YEARS)
adOICARE
HEIGHT (cm)
WEIGHT (cm)
97th
90th
75th
50th
25th
10th
3rd
0
20
40
60
80
100
120
140
160
180
0
2
4
6
8
10
12
14
16
18
AGE
Data source Agrwal et al. Indian Pedidatrics 1992 and 1994 and Tables in book The Growth - infancy to adolescence
CBS Publ. New Delhi 2003
By DK Agarwal, AK Bansal and KN Agarwal

PERCENTILES FOR BODY MASS INDEX (BMI) (BOYS 2-18 YEARS)

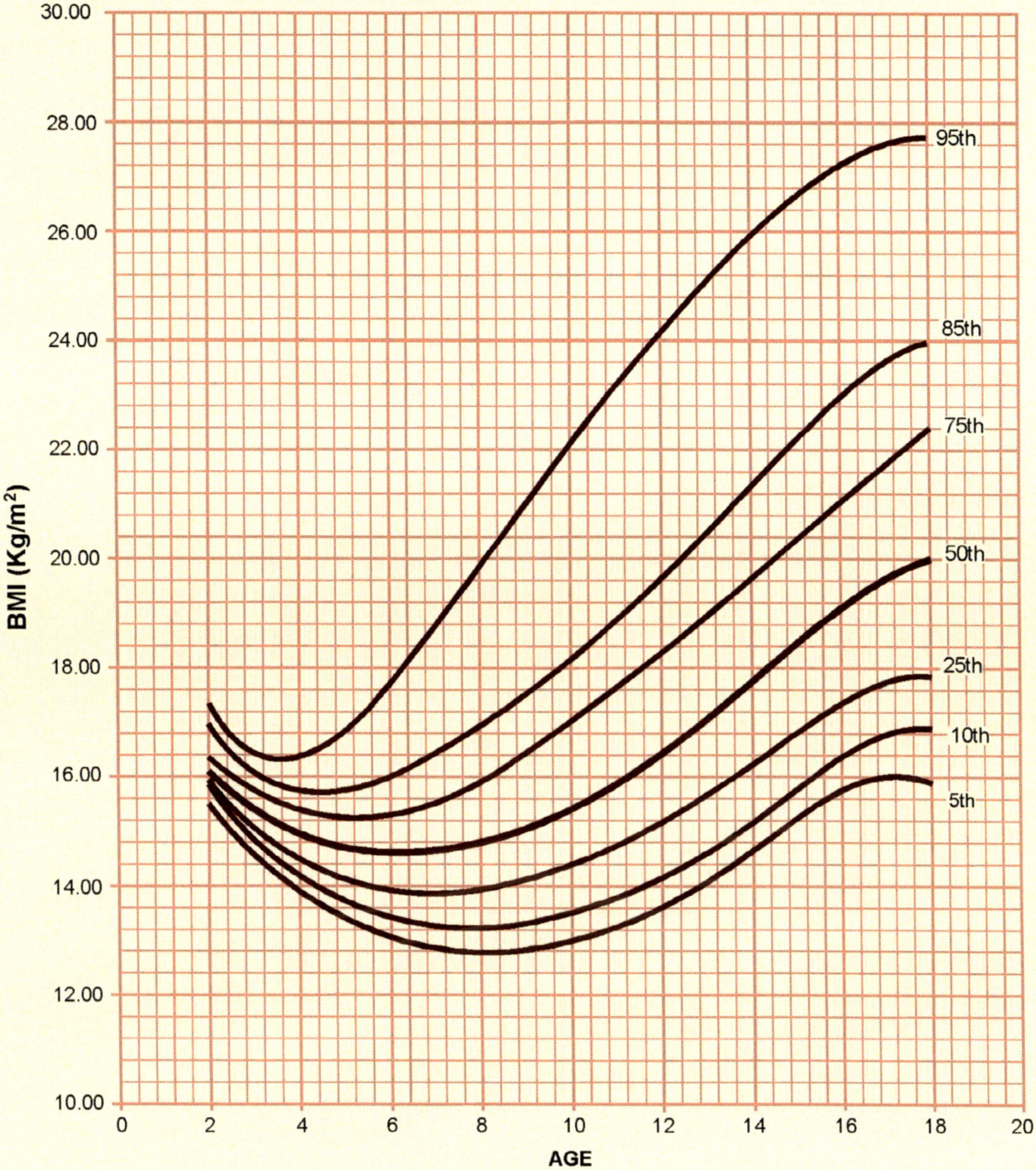

Prepared from Indian Paediatrics 1994; p-377 and 2001; p-1217 (DK Agarwal, AK Bansal and KN Agarwal)

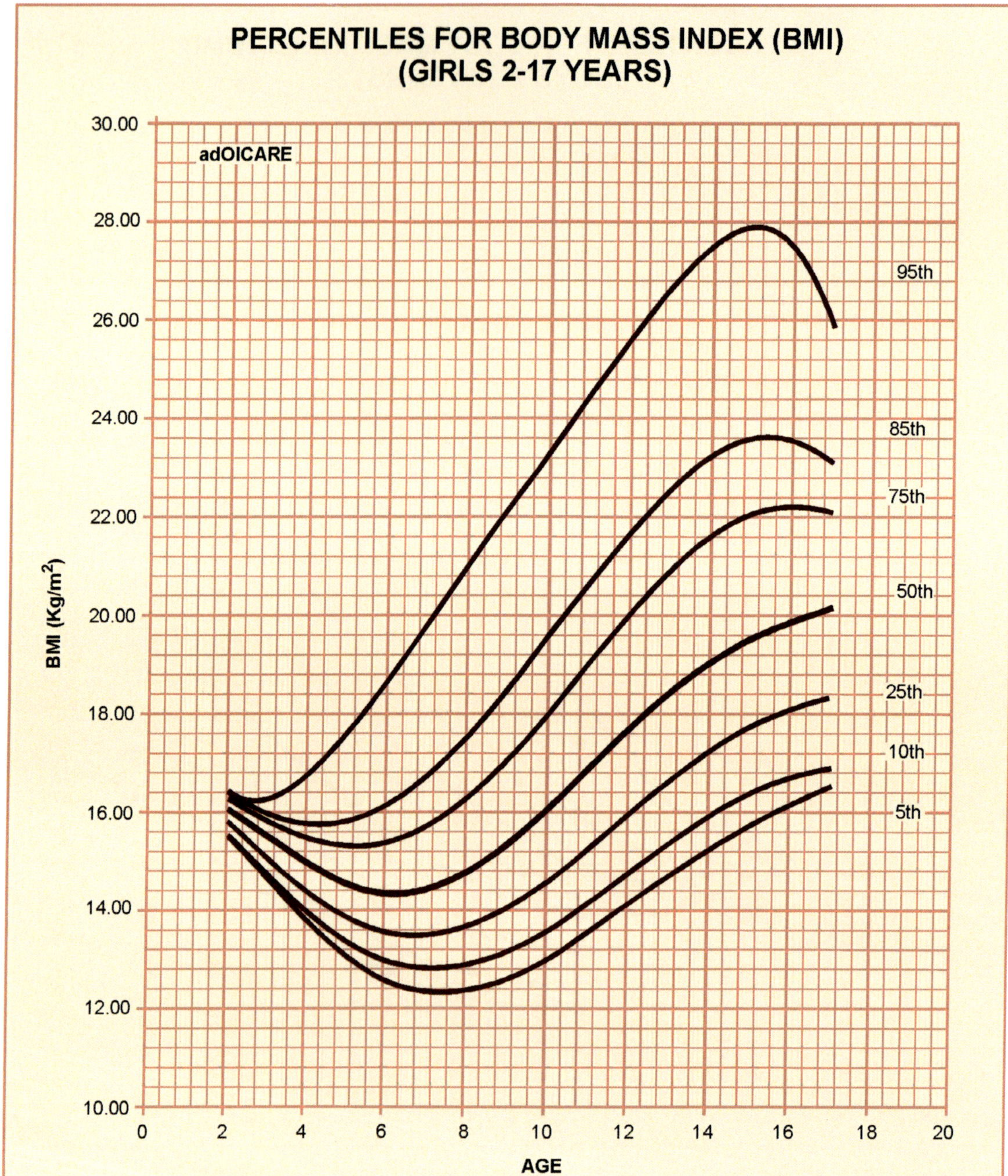

Prepared from Indian Paediatrics 1994; p-377 and 2001; p-1217 (DK Agarwal, AK Bansal and KN Agarwal)

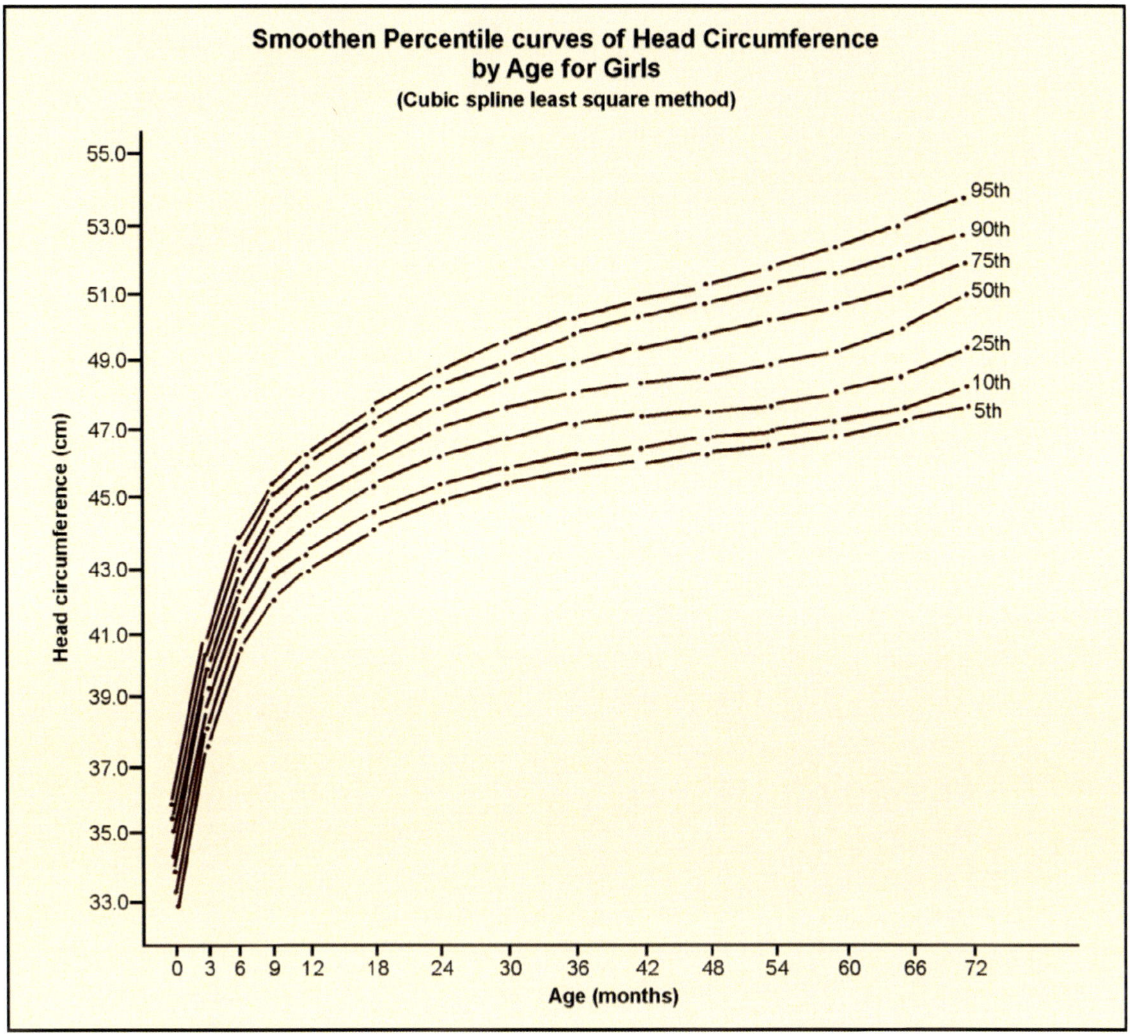
Smoothen Percentile curves of Head Circumference
by Age for Girls
(Cubic spline least square method)
Head circumference (cm)
55.0
53.0
51.0
49.0
47.0
45.0
43.0
41.0
39.0
37.0
35.0
33.0
95th
90th
75th
50th
25th
10th
5th
0
3
6
9
12
18
24
30
36
42
48
54
60
66
72
Age (months)

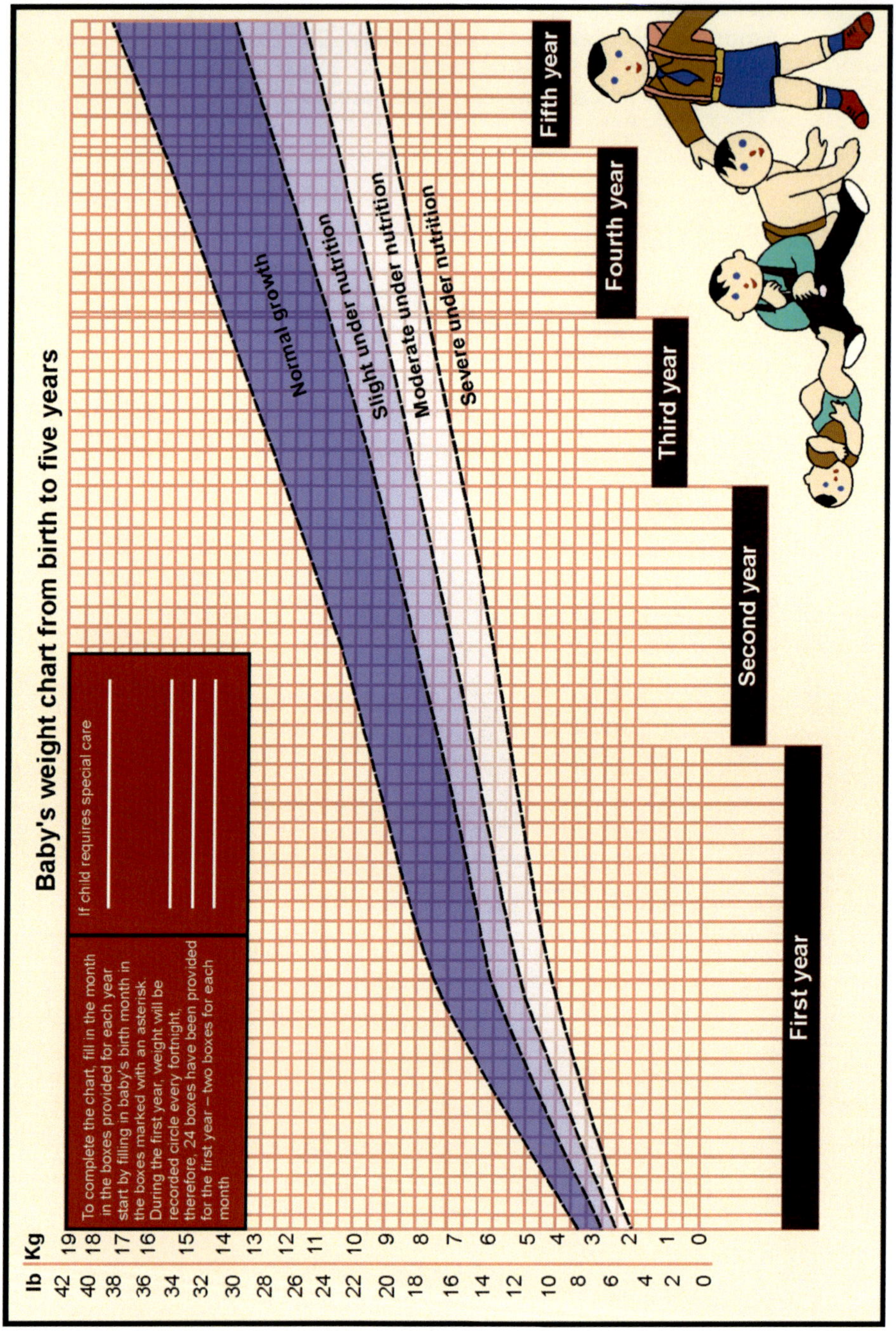

Road to health chart

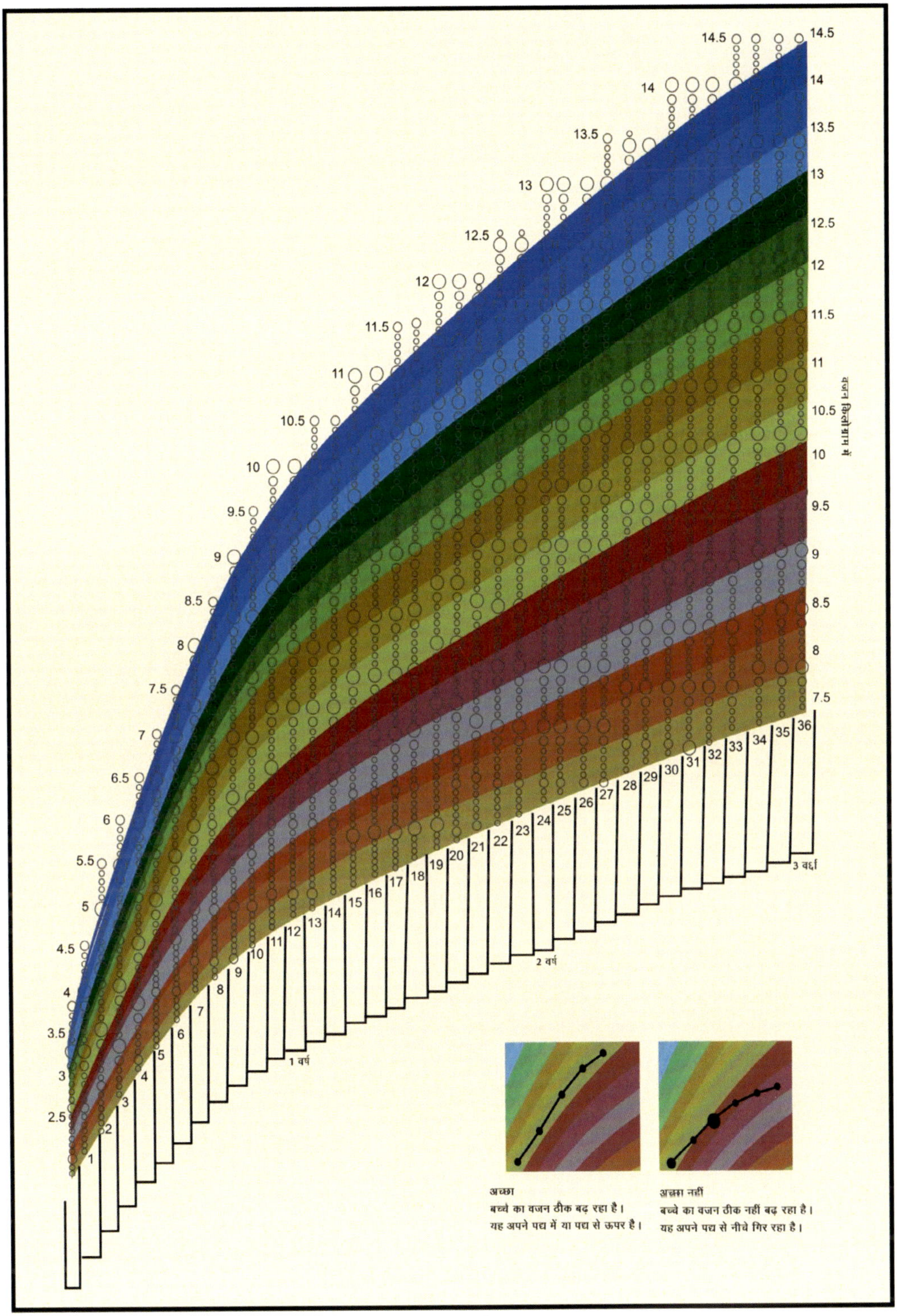

Rainbow chart

NOMOGRAM

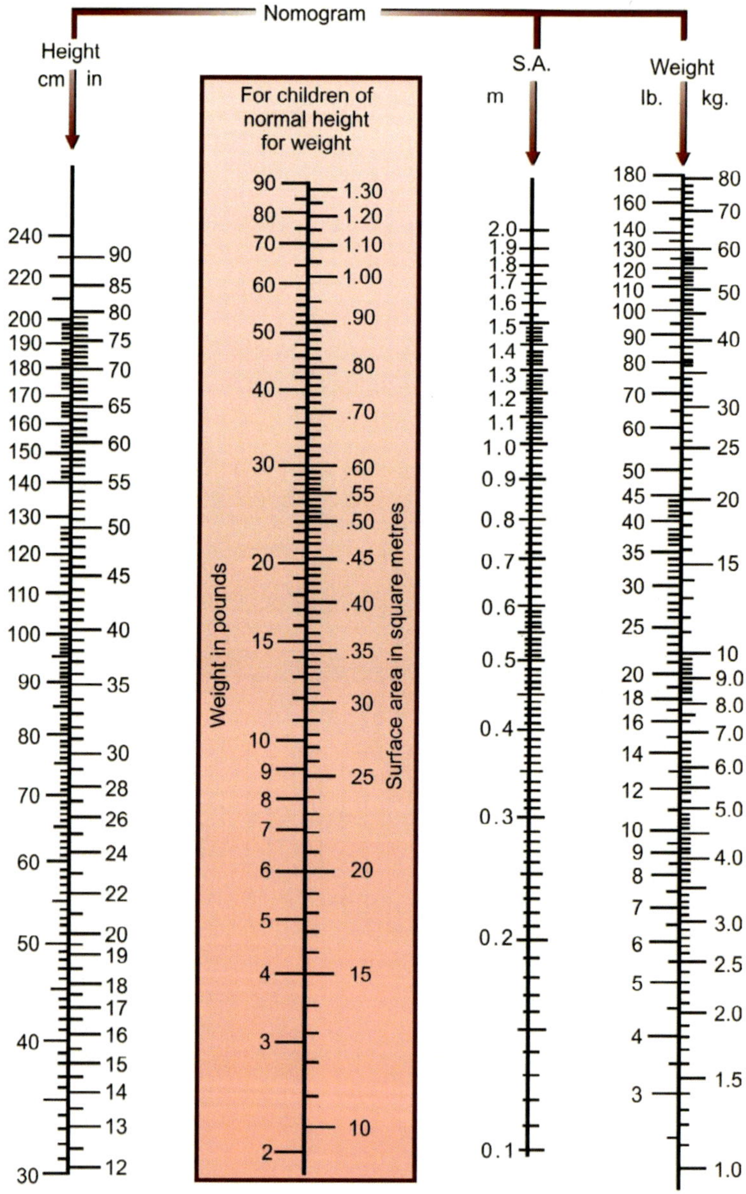

Alternative (mosteller's formula):

$$\text{Surface area } (m^2) = \sqrt{\frac{\text{Height (cm)} \times \text{weight (kg)}}{3600}}$$

SOME CLASSICAL CLINICAL PICTURES

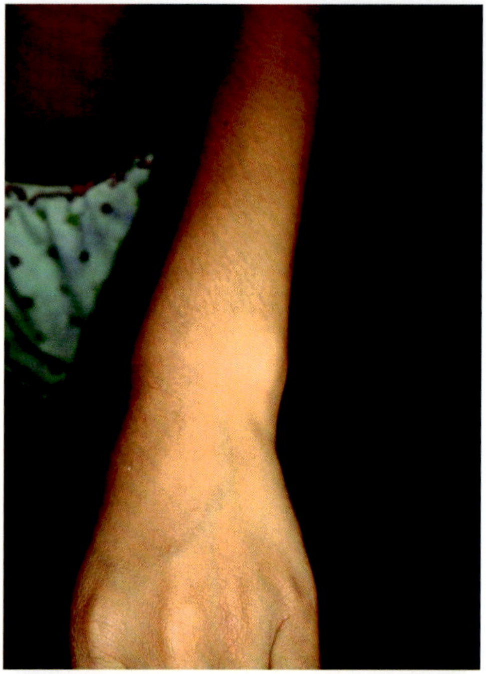

Fig. A.1: Epiphyseal enlargement of wrist in rickets

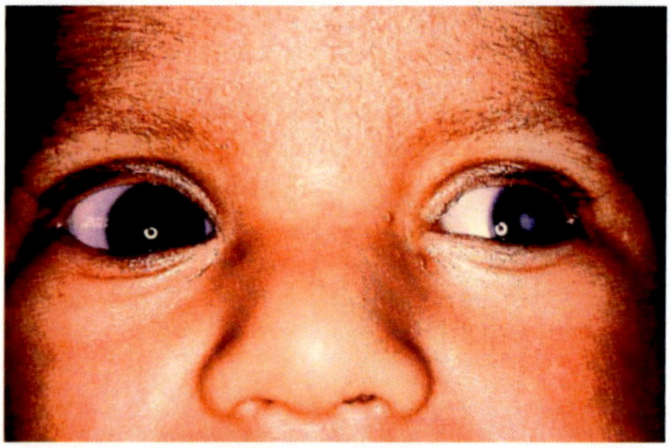

Fig. A.2: Congenital cataract

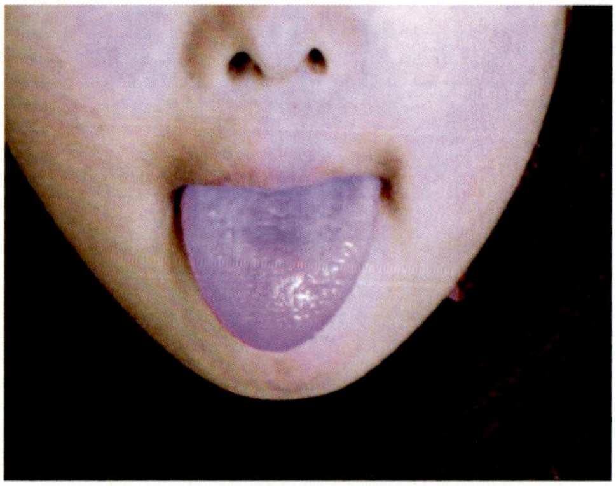

Fig. A.3: Fissured tongue (Down syndrome)

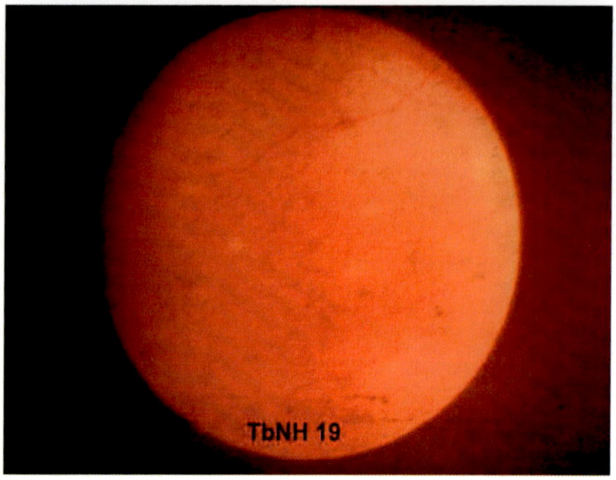

Fig. A.4: Choroid tubercle

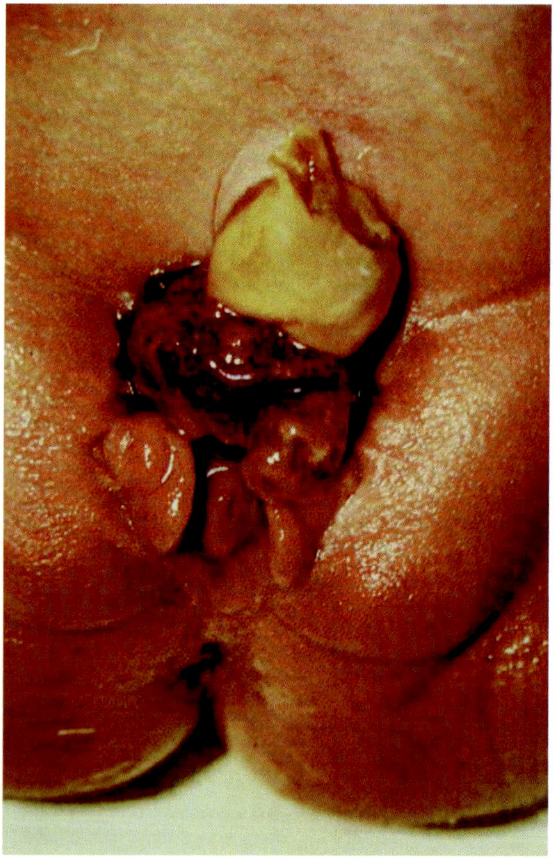

Fig. A.5: Ectopia vesicae

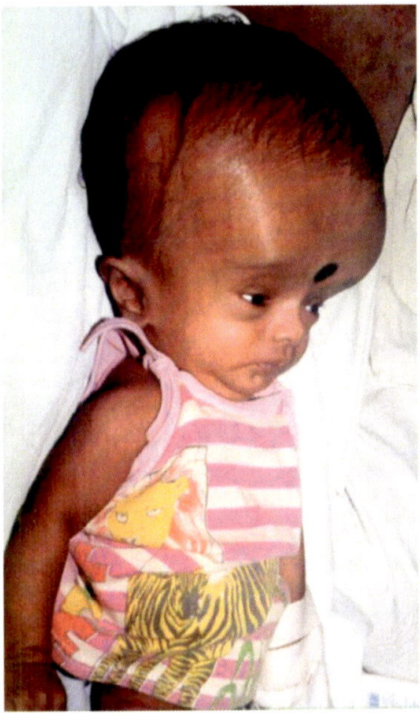

Fig. A.6: Hydrocephalus

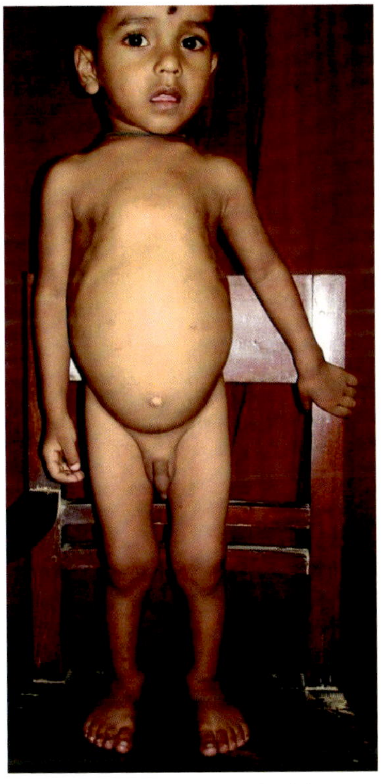

Fig. A.7: Knock knee in ricket

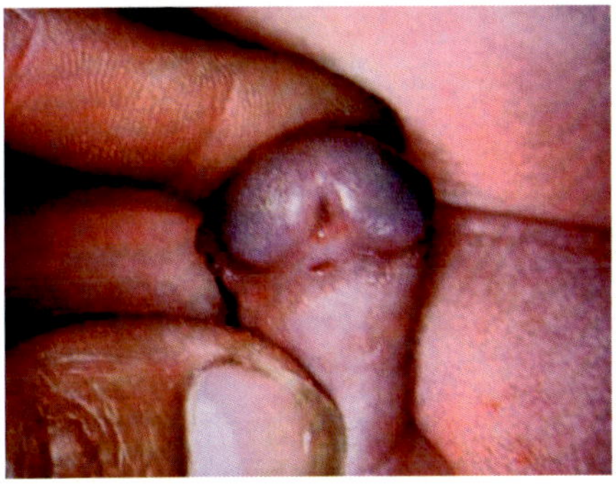

Fig. A.8: Hypospedius

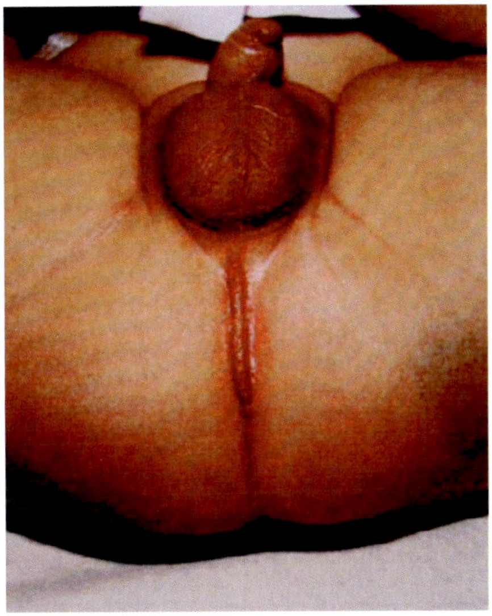

Fig. A.9: Imperforate anus

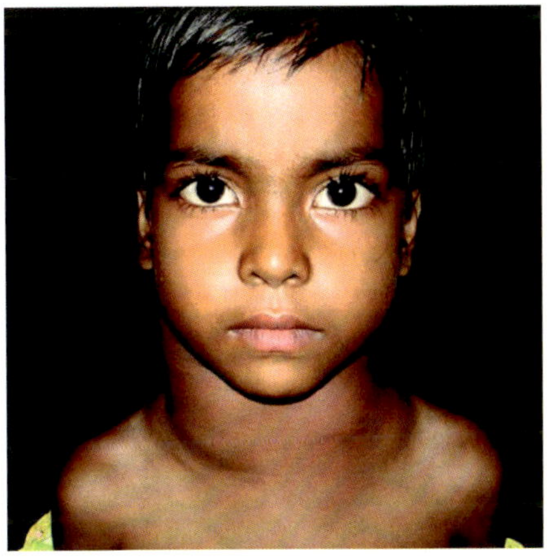

Fig. A.10: Lymphoma

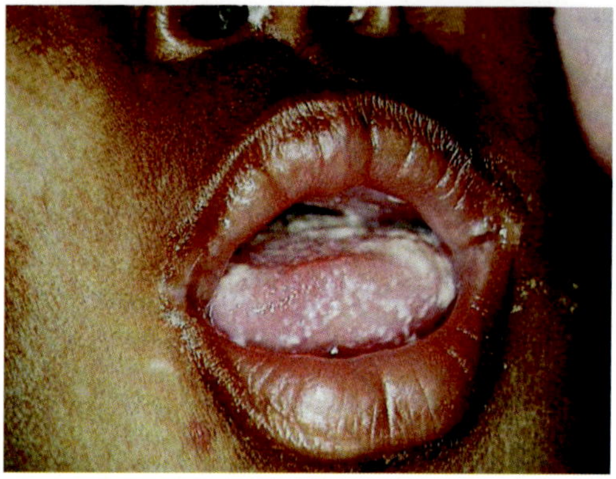

Fig. A.11: Oral thrush

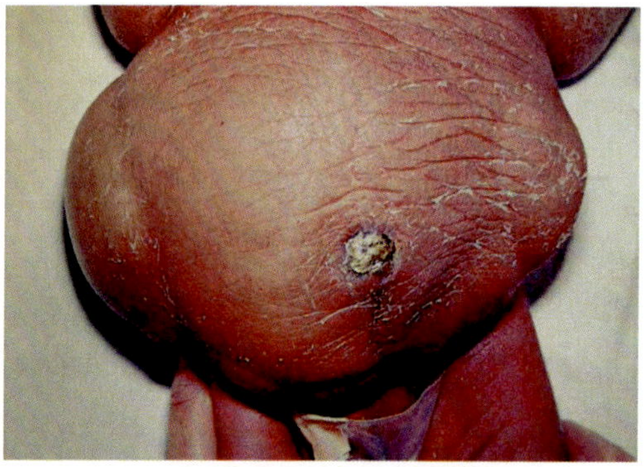

Fig. A.12: Prune belly syndrome

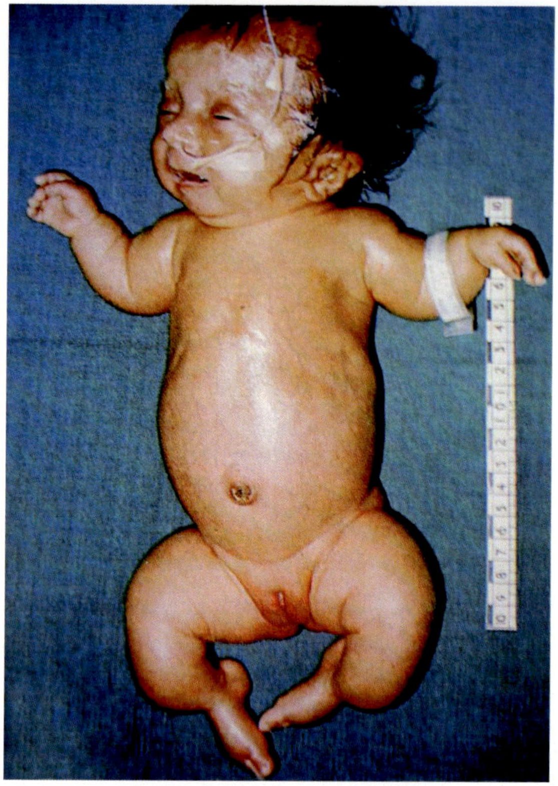

Fig. A.13: Osteogenesis imperfecta

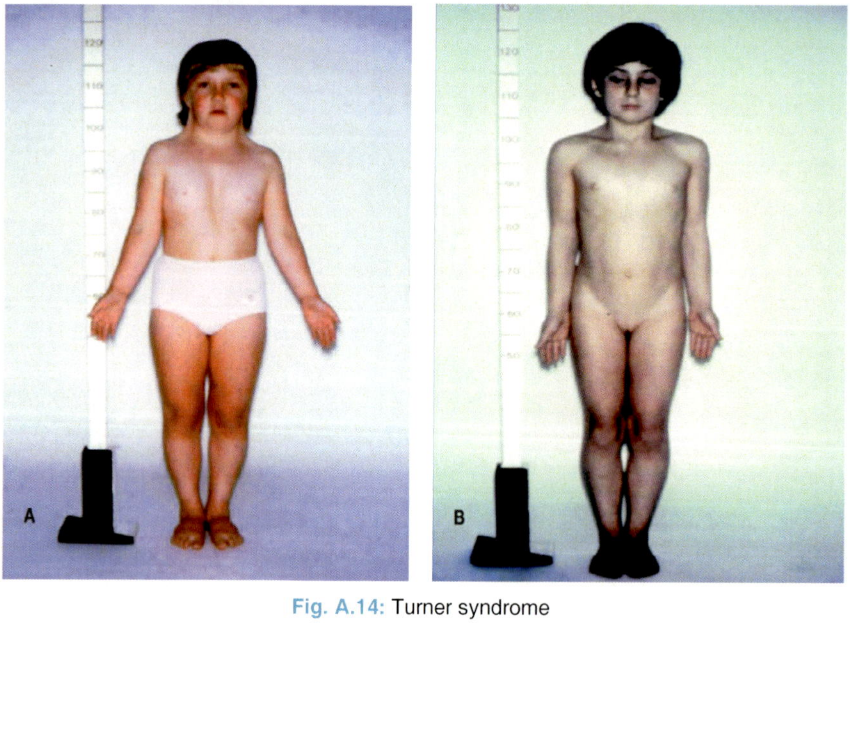

Fig. A.14: Turner syndrome

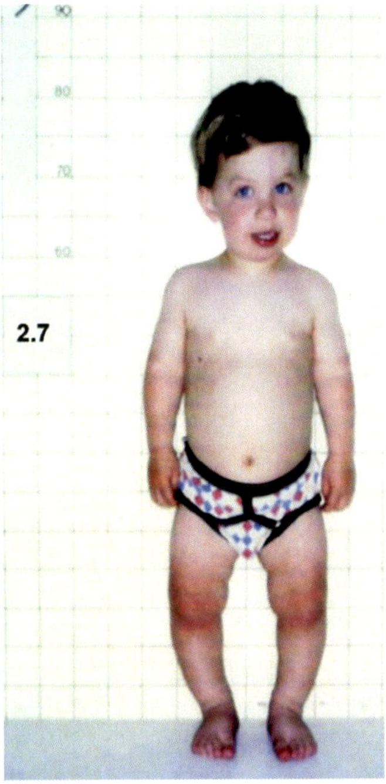

Fig. A.15: Achondroplasia

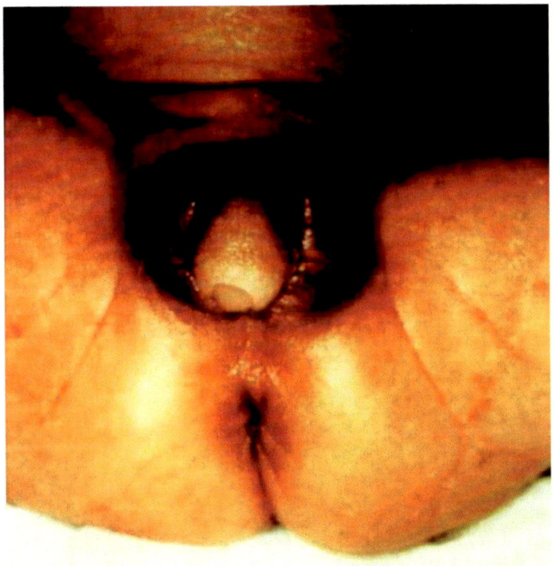

Fig. A.16: Female with congenital adrenal hyperplasia

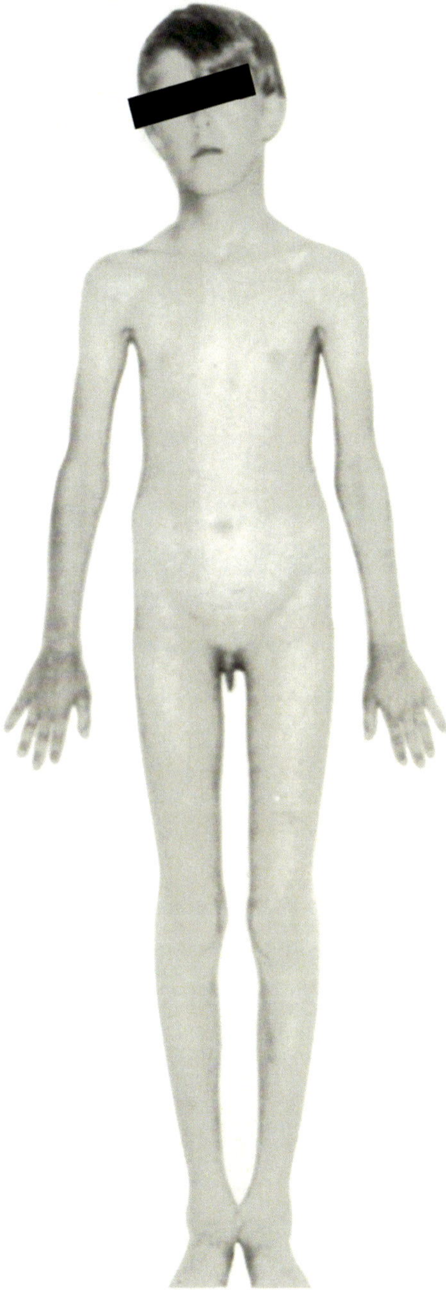

Fig. A.17: Marfan syndrome

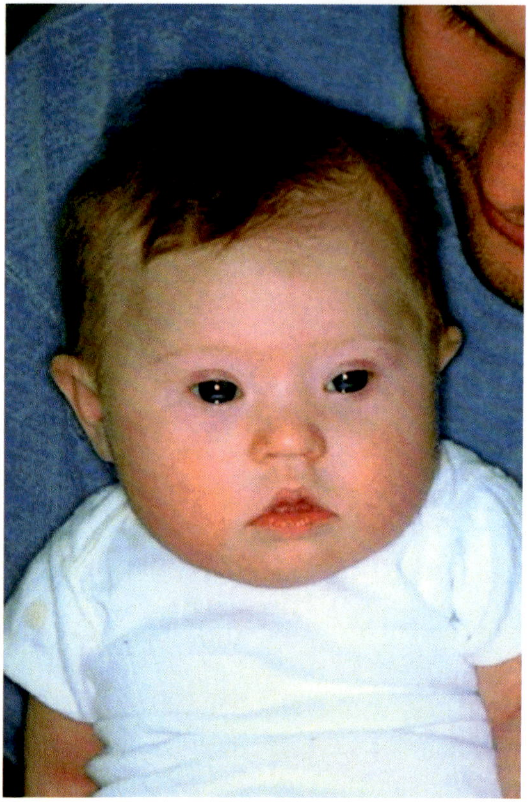

Fig. A.18: Down syndrome

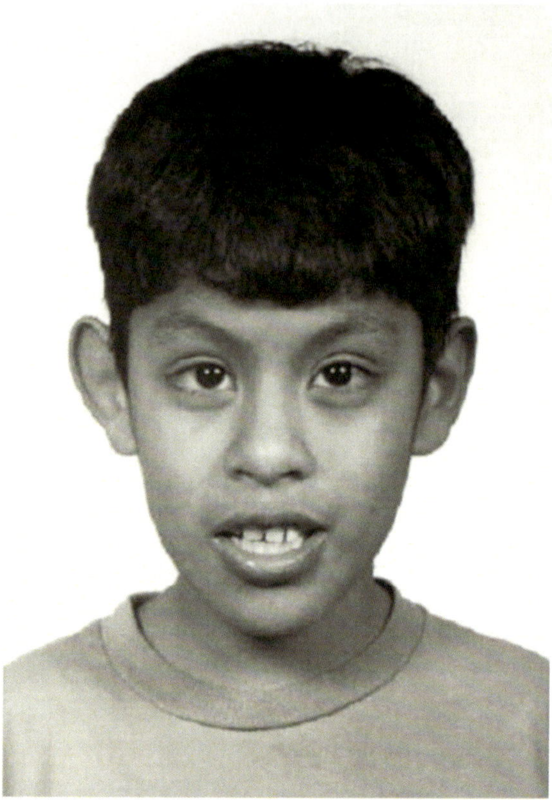

Fig. A.19: Fragile X-syndrome

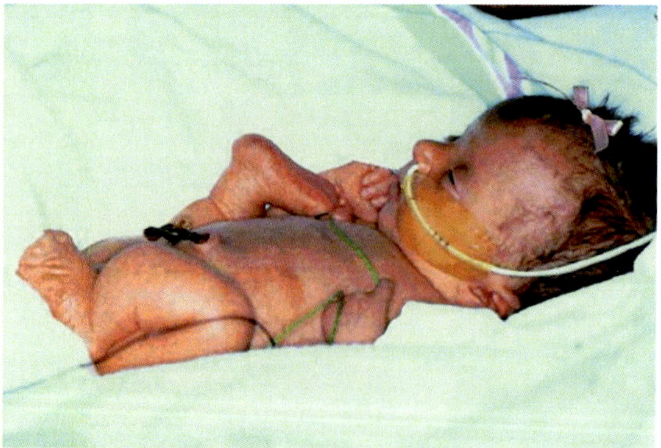

Fig. A.20: Osteogenesis imperfecta

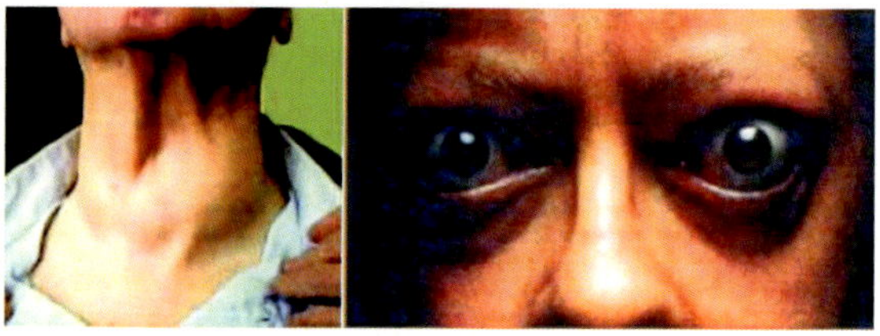

Fig. A.21: Thyrotoxicosis

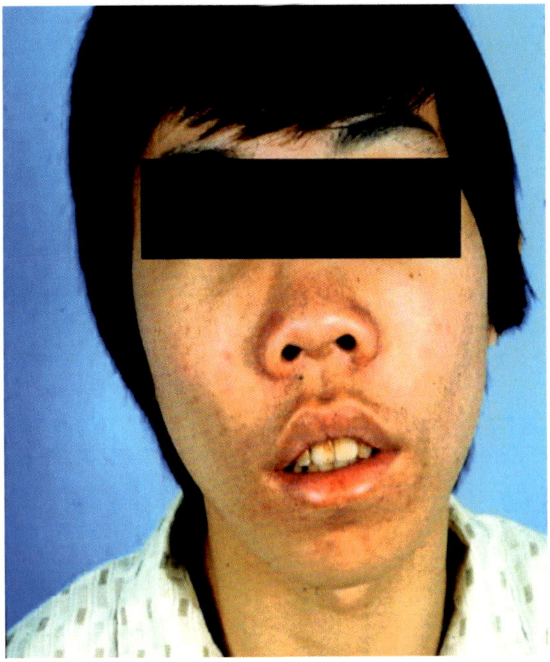

Fig. A.22: Thalassaemic facies

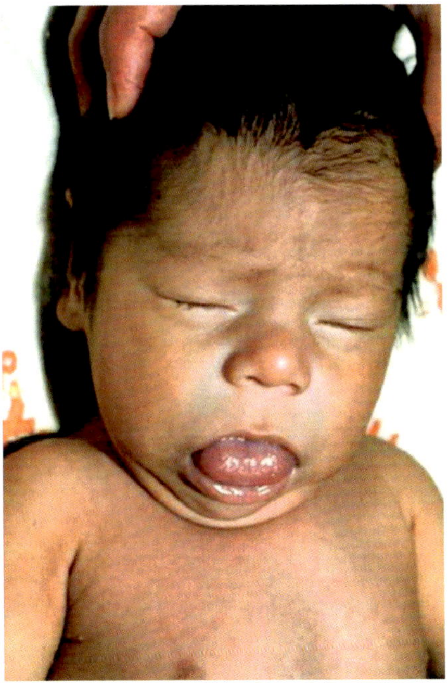

Fig. A.23: Congenital hypothyroidism

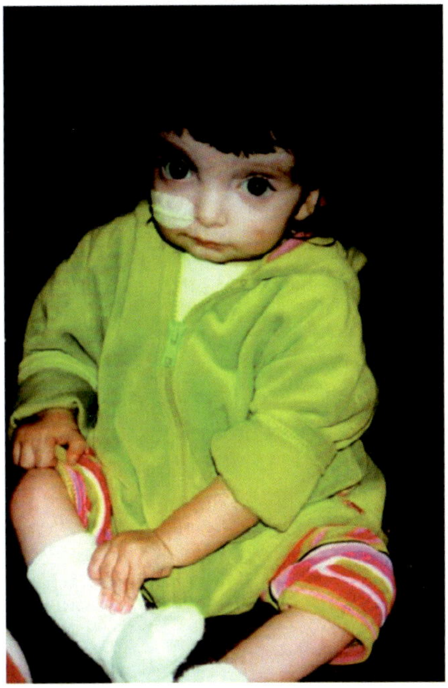

Fig. A.24: Russell-Silver syndrome

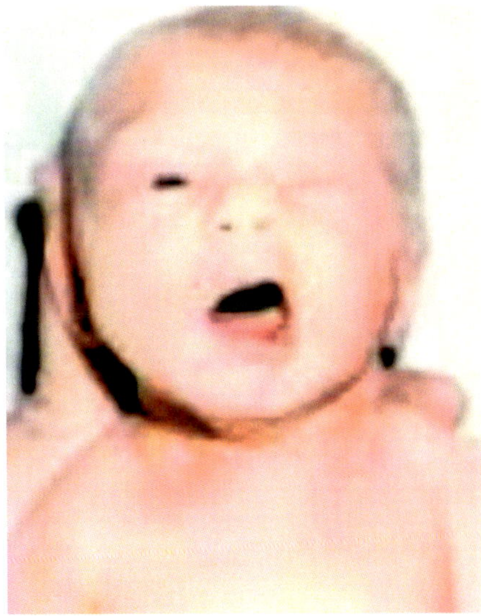

Fig. A.25: Facial palsy

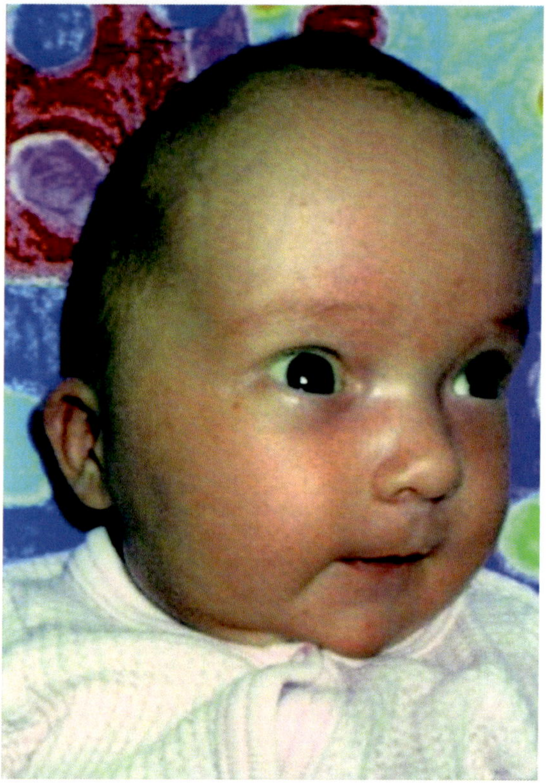

Fig. A.26: Craniosynostosis

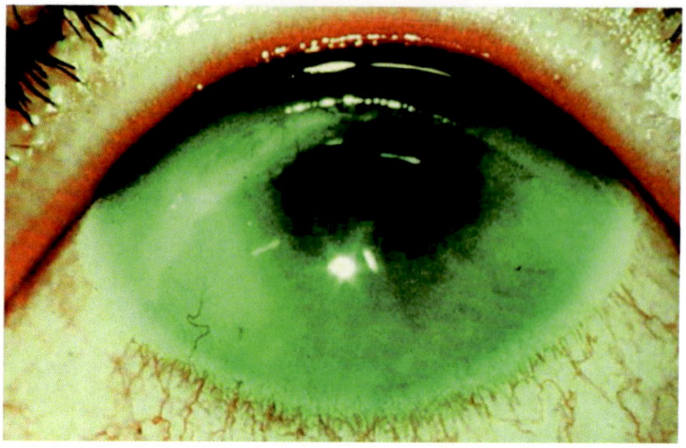

Fig. A.28: Corneal clouding in Hurler syndrome

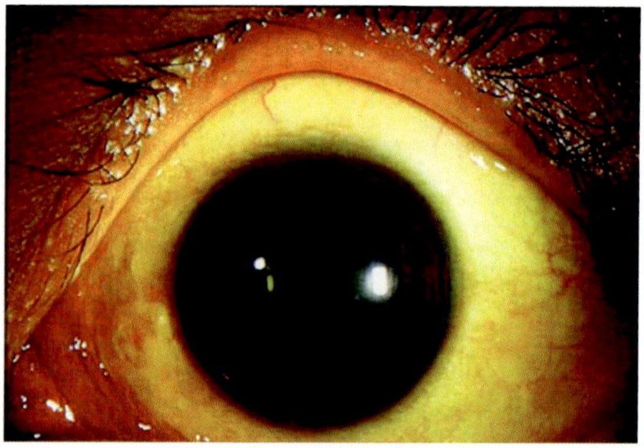

Fig. A.27: KF ring in Wilson disease

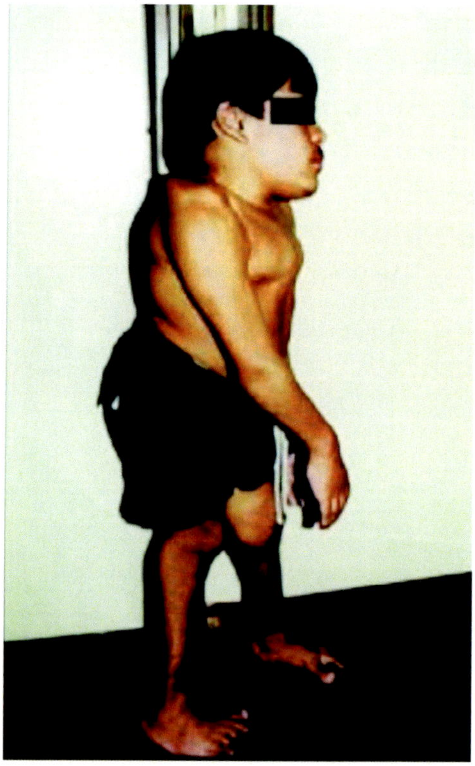

Fig. A.29: Morquio syndrome

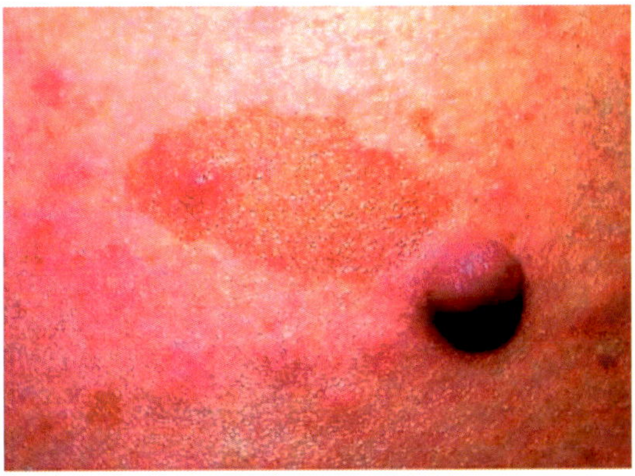

Fig. A.30: Café au lait patch with neurofibroma

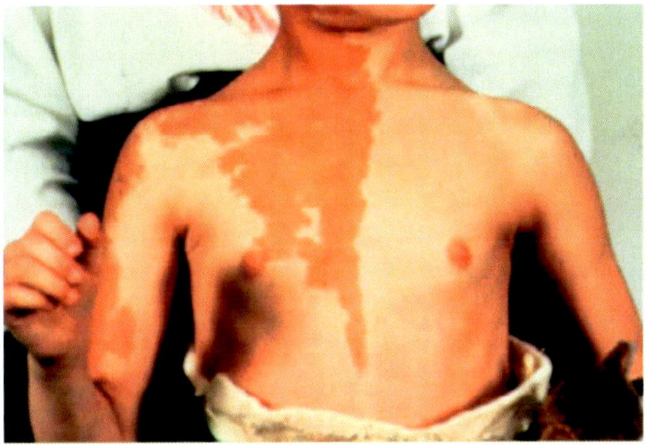

Fig. A.31: Café au lait patch in McCune-Albright syndrome

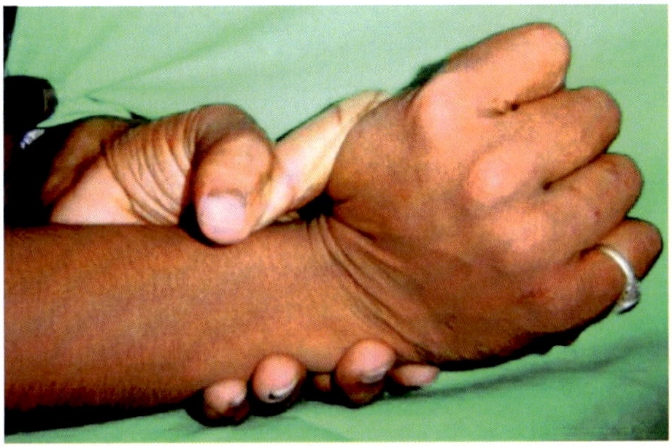

Fig. A.32: Ehlers-Danlos syndrome

X-RAYs

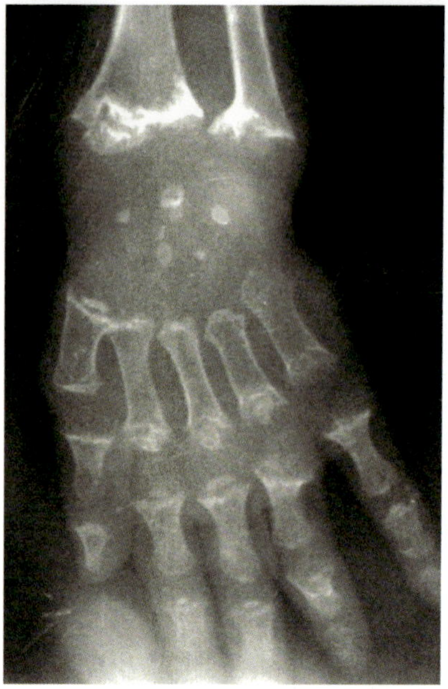

Fig. A.33: Chronic hemolytic anaemia

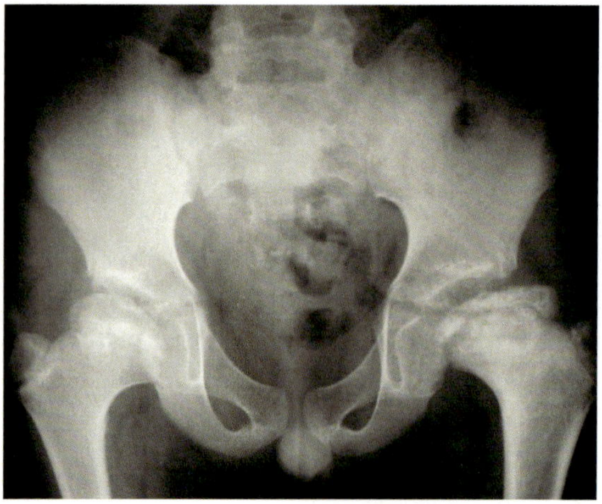

Fig. A.34: Parthe's disease

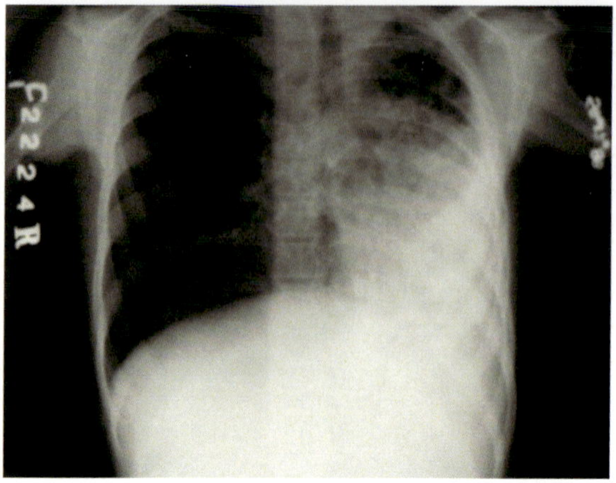

Fig. A.35: Eventration of diaphragm

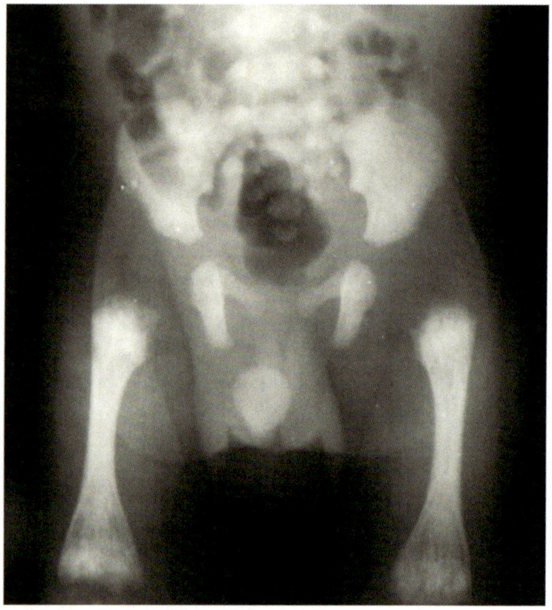

Fig. A.36: Marble bone disease (Osteopetrosis)

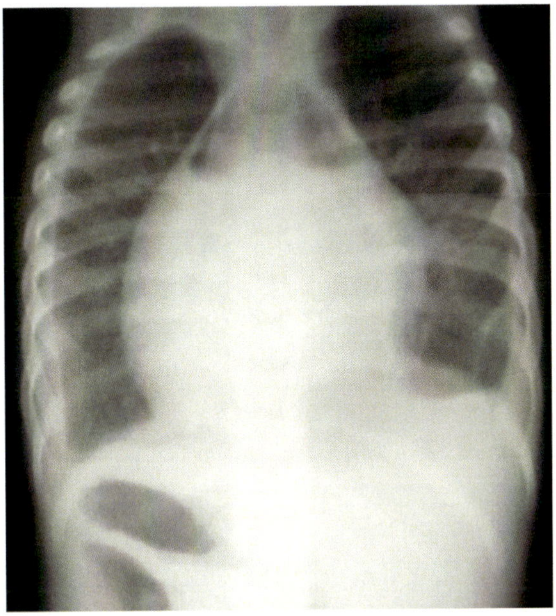

Fig. A.37: Pyopericardium

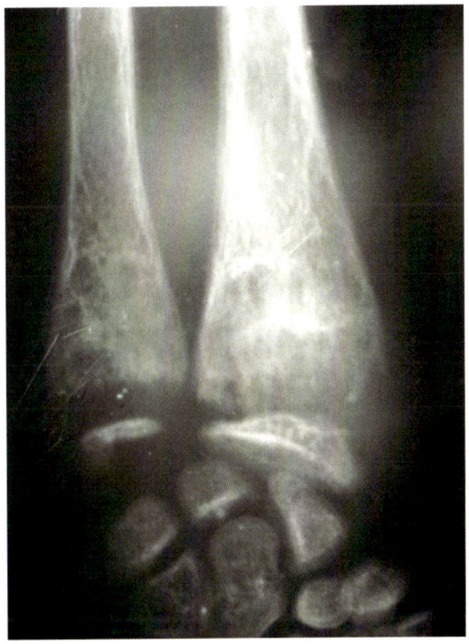

Fig. A.39: Rickets

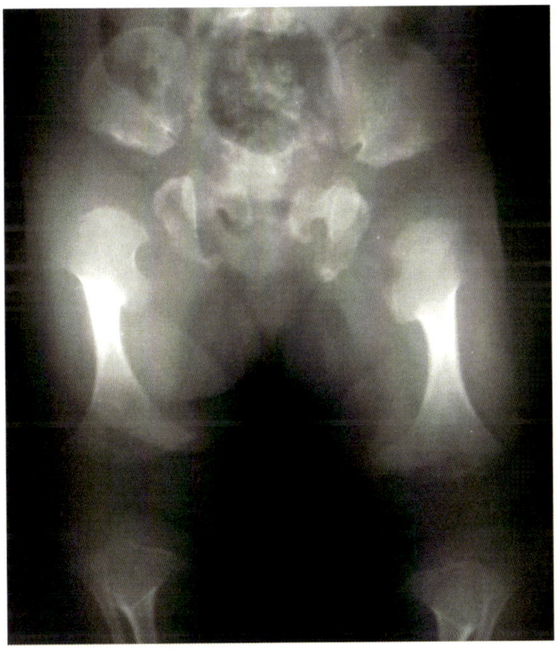

Fig. A.38: Achondroplasia

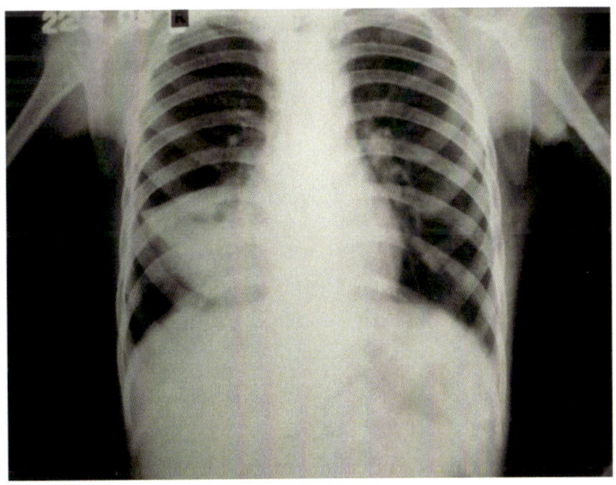

Fig. A.40: Brock's middle lobe syndrome

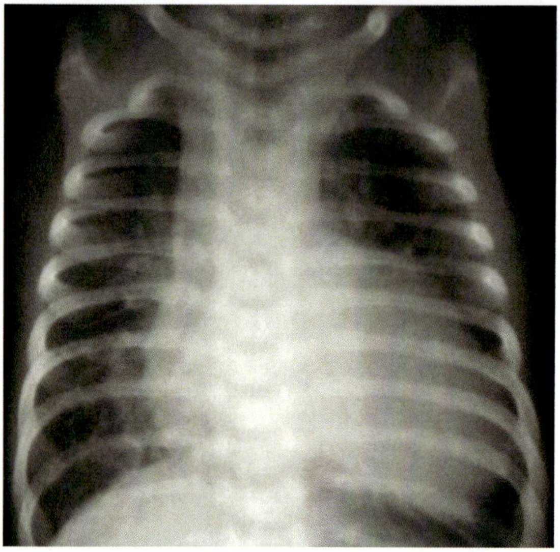

Fig. A.41: Cardiomyopathy

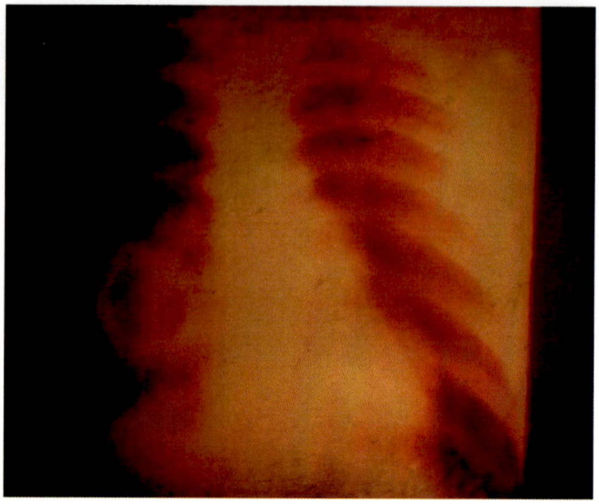

Fig. A.43: Cavity of right lung

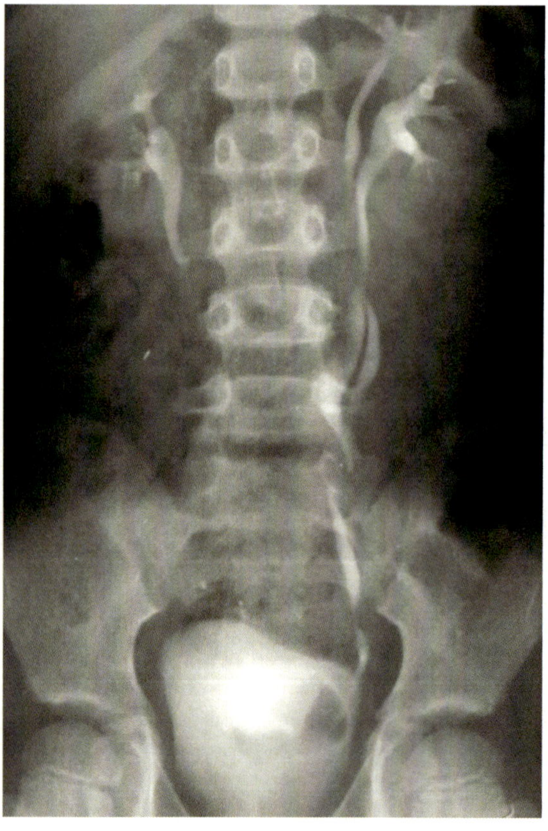

Fig. A.42: Duplication of left ureter

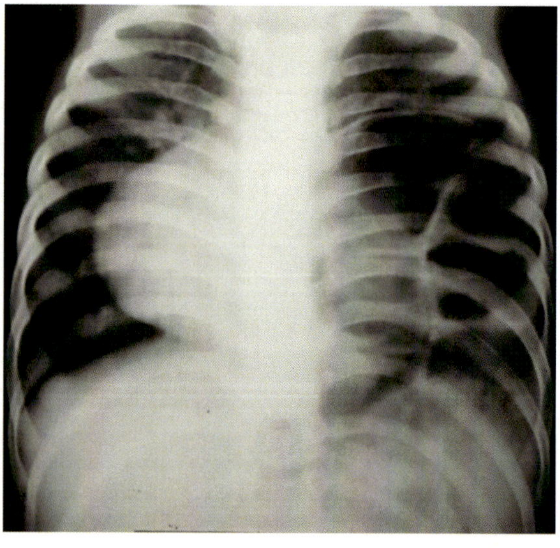

Fig. A.44: Eventration of diaphragm

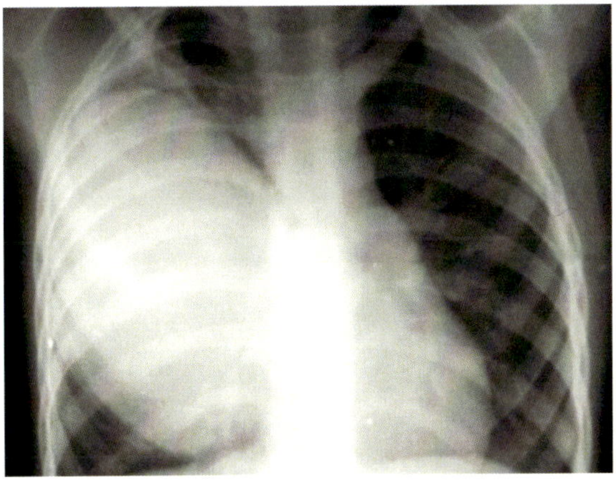

Fig. A.45: Hydatid cyst of left lung

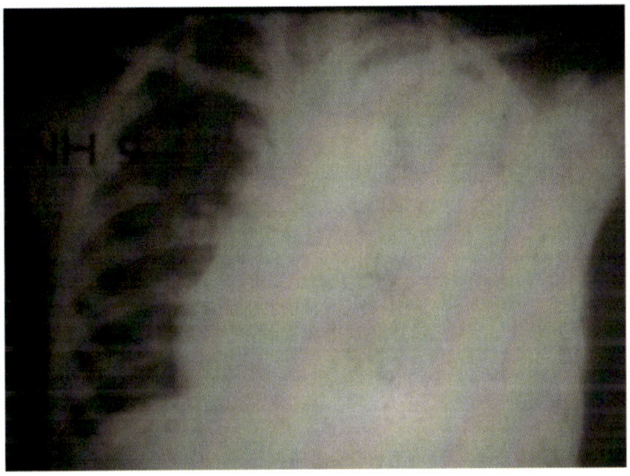

Fig. A.46: Massive pleural effusion (left)

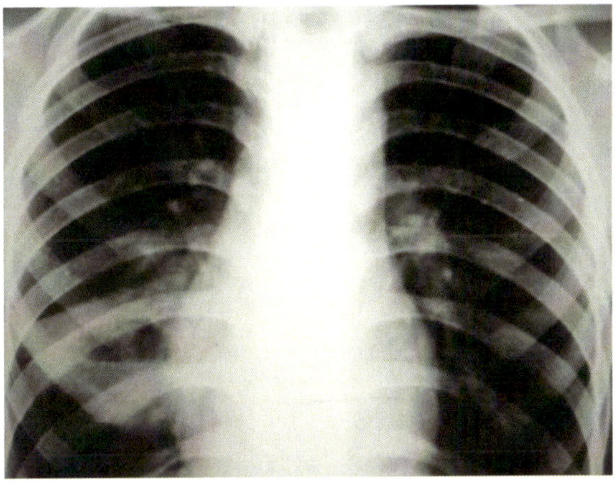

Fig. A.47: Lung abscess

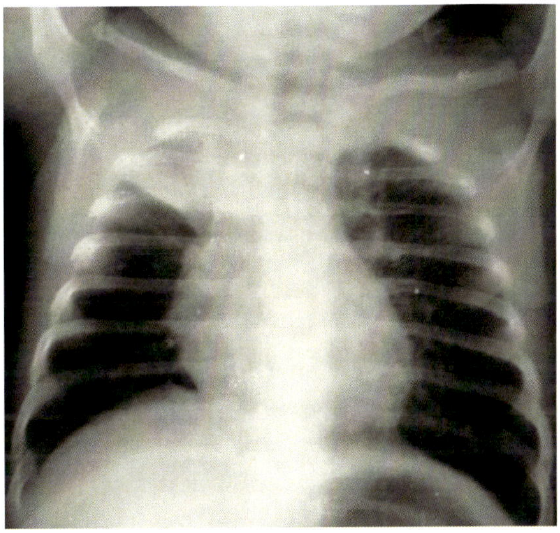

Fig. A.48: Right upper lobe consolidation

ECG

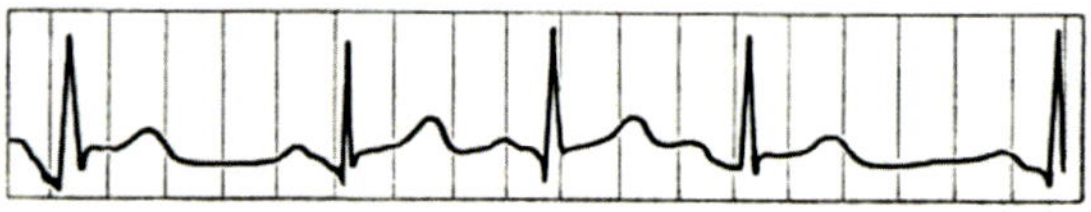

Fig. A.49: Sinus arrhythmia

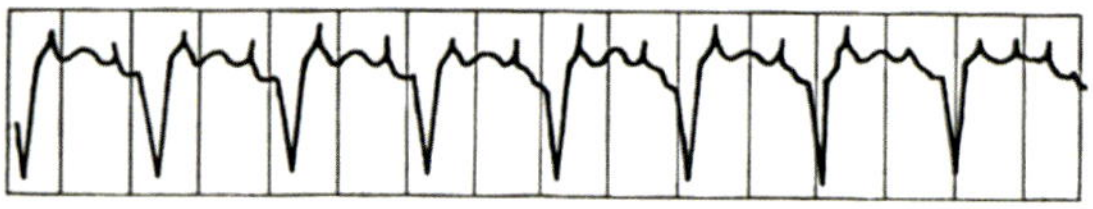

Fig. A.50: Atrial flutter, 2:1 block. Atrial rate about 300. Note the two spiked flutter waves to each ventricular complex

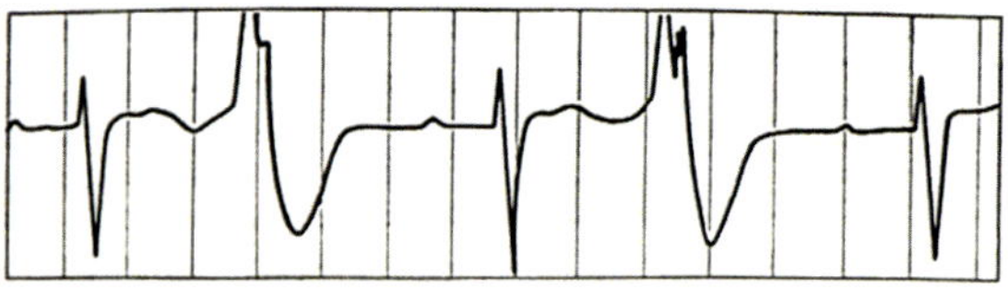

Fig. A.51: Ventricular extrasystoles. Note that there is no P wave before the second extrasystole, and there is an abortive P wave just before the first extrasystole

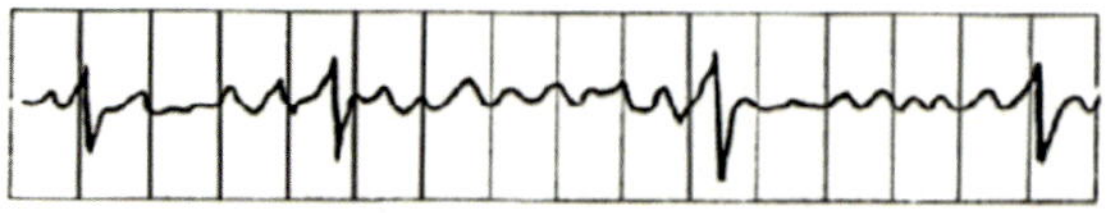

Fig. A.52: Atrial fibrillation. Note the f waves and irregular ventricular rhythm

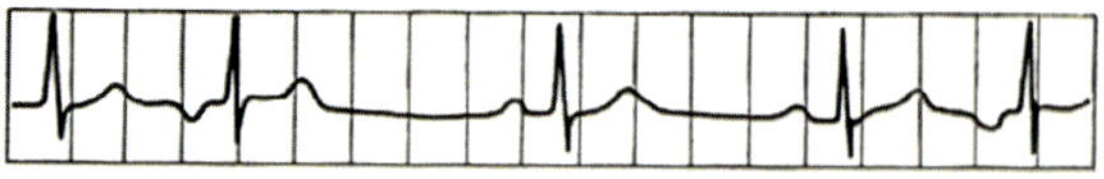

Fig. A.53: Atrial extrasystoles. Note the abnormal (inverted) P wave. The R-R interval is longer after the extrasystole than in the normal cycle

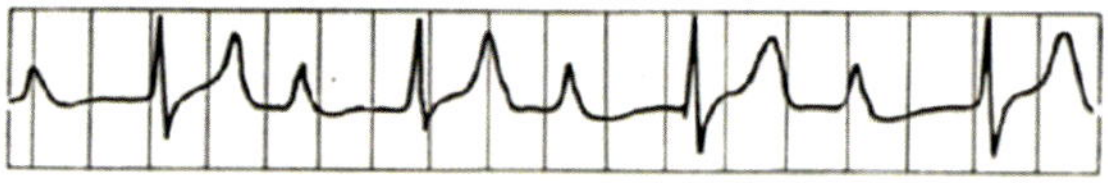

Fig. A.54: First degree heart block. P-R interval = 0.42 second

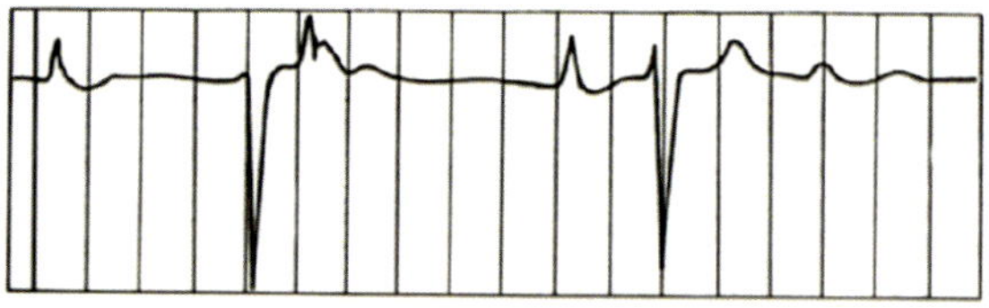

Fig. A.55: Complete heart block. Atrial rate 55; ventricular rate 39

EEG

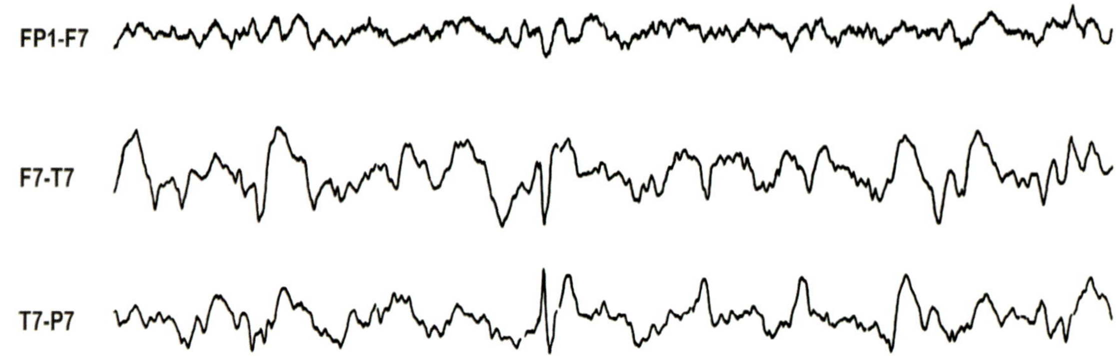

Fig. A.56: Spikes, left temporal

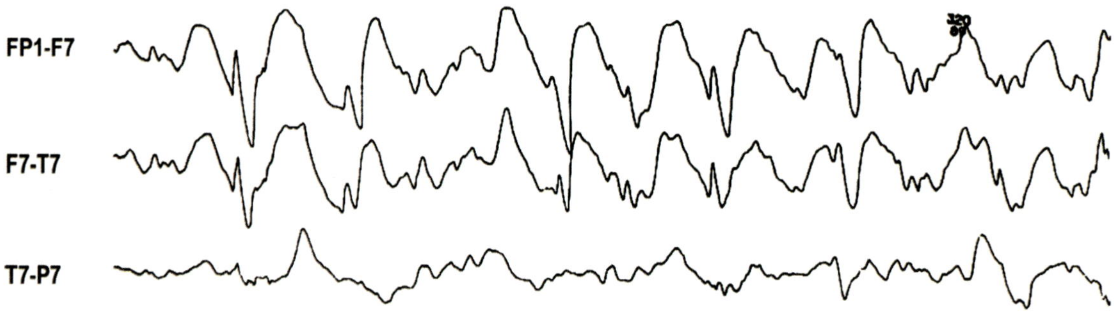

Fig. A.57: Slow spike and wave complexes, generalised

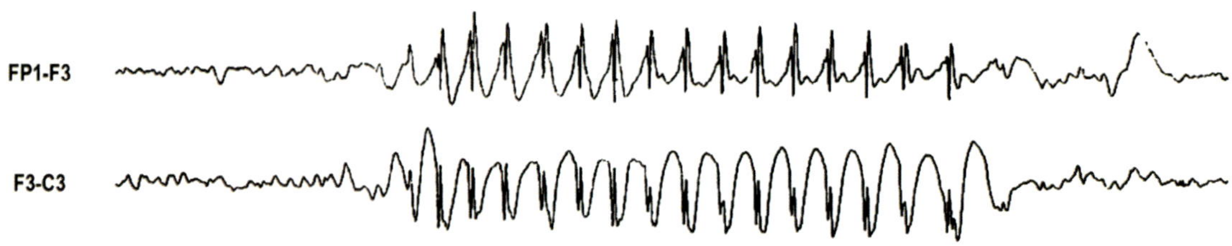

Fig. A.58: 3-Hz spike-and-wave complexes, generalised

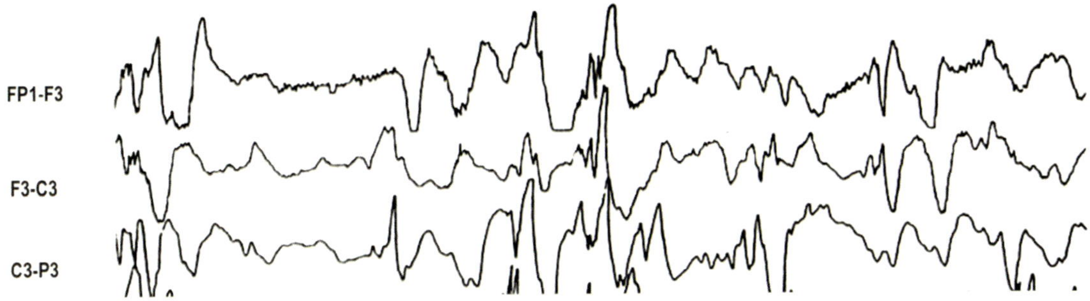

Fig. A.59: Hypsarrhythmia, generalised

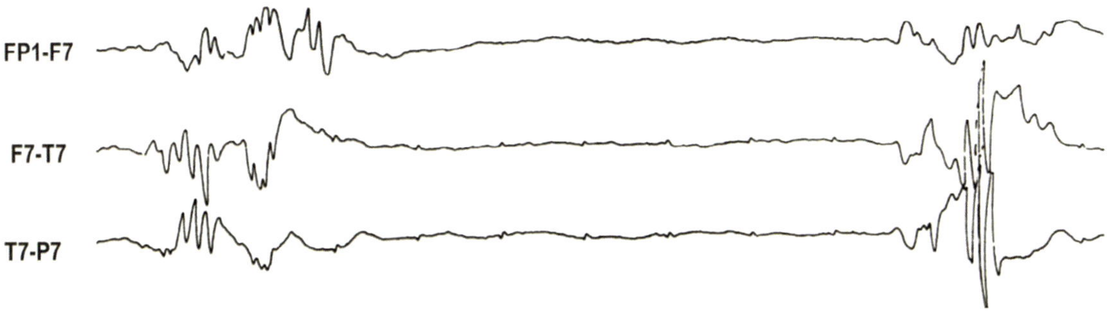

Fig. A.60: Burst suppression, generalised (Coma)

CT SCAN

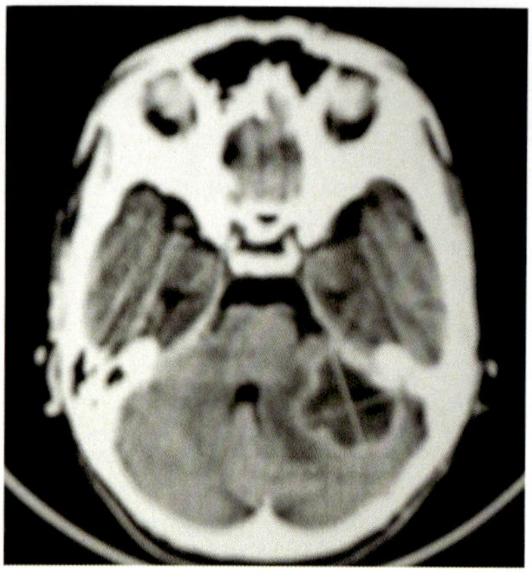

Fig. A.61: Brain abscess

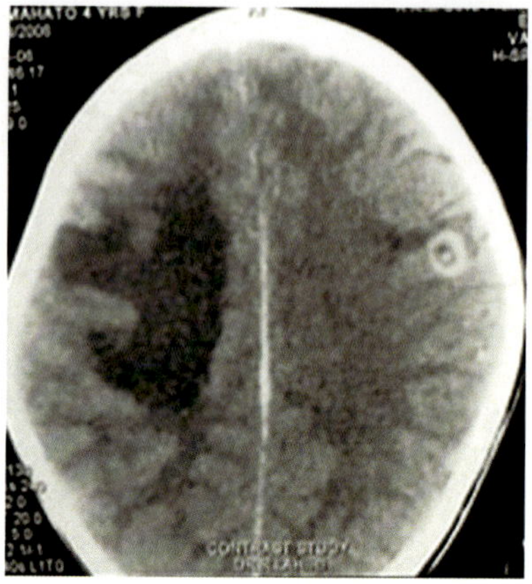

Fig. A.63: Ring enhancing lesion

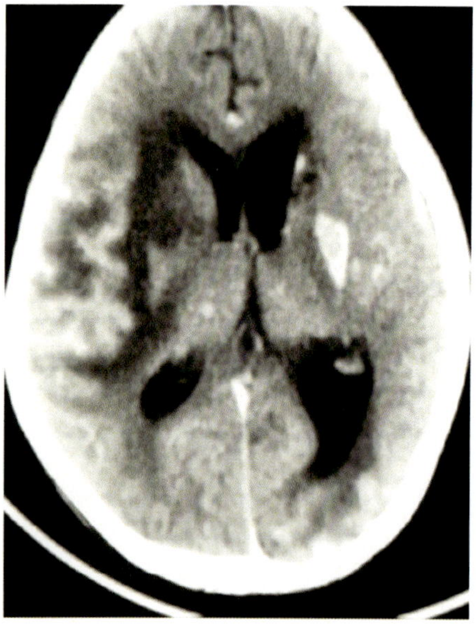

Fig. A.62: Hydrocephalus

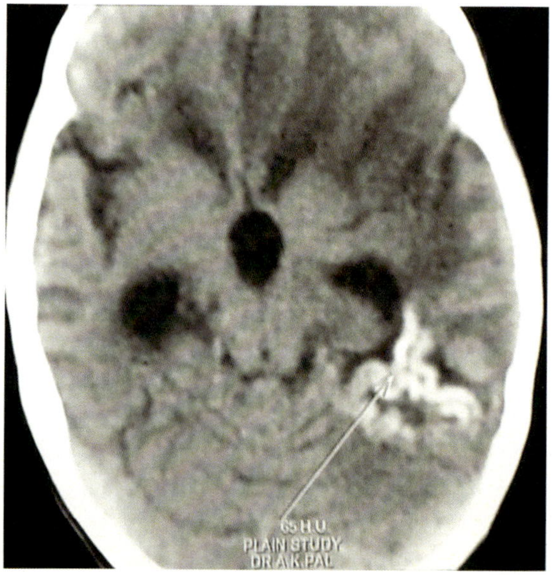

Fig. A.64: Sturge-Weber syndrome

Index